Compendium medicine

Pocket
Obstetrics and Gynaecology

Romée Snijders & Veerle Smit
Maaike van Hoesel, Carlijn Veldman, Gwendolyn Vuurberg

Together for Healthcare

Want to know more about
Compendium Medicine?
Check out our website!

www.compendiummedicine.com

First edition, 2024

ISBN 9789083374017
BISAC MED033000
Thema MKC

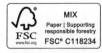

MIX
Paper | Supporting responsible forestry
FSC® C118234

Preface

Welcome to the *Compendium Community!*

'Together for Healthcare' – these three simple words encapsulate the spirit of our collective mission and underscore the essence of our work. In an era where the complexity of healthcare is becoming increasingly interconnected, collaboration is not merely an option but an imperative. Our books symbolise the effectiveness of collaboration, knowledge sharing, and a joint commitment to improve and interconnect healthcare.

We proudly present the first edition of our pocket *Obstetrics and Gynaecology*, with all the information you want to have at your fingertips. This comprehensive guide covers a wide range of clinical topics that will prove invaluable during your internship, traineeship, and night shifts. You can, for instance, explore chapters like gynaelogical examination, diagnostics, conditions, and clinical reasoning.

The innovative *Compendium Method*©, designed for medical students and doctors, employs comprehensible illustrations for every medical condition, straightforward tables, icons, and useful mnemonics. It is visually appealing, to the point, and concise. We only focus on the essentials and make sure all the content is comprehensively presented.

Our strength lies in the diverse expertise of our close-knit medical team, consisting of students, an interdisciplinary team of doctors and medical specialists. This collaborative approach ensures that our content is comprehensive and accurate.

We are committed to inclusivity and aim to make our texts and images a reflection of the diversity of patients our readers provide care to. We aspire for every (future) doctor and patient to find themselves reflected in our books. Our team works continuously to improve and expand the selection of books. We welcome readers to share their feedback and suggestions, contributing to the continual improvement of our pocket series.

We sincerely wish to express immense gratitude to our team of medical students and healthcare professionals. The outstanding result of their contributions is this extraordinary pocket – a pocket for everybody in healthcare.

Enjoy reading and enjoy working, and we hope to hear from you soon!

Amsterdam, August 2024

Veerle Smit, MD & Romée Snijders, MD
Doctors and founders *Compendium Medicine*

Editorial staff

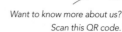

Want to know more about us?
Scan this QR code.

Editorial board

Romée J.A.L.M. Snijders, MD & Veerle L. Smit, MD

Chief editor

Gwendolyn Vuurberg, MD, PhD

Pocket editor

Current edition

Maaike H.T. van Hoesel, MD, University Medical Center Groningen, Groningen

Previous edition

Carlijn Veldman, BSc, University of Groningen
Gwendolyn Vuurberg, BSc, University of Amsterdam

Authors

Current edition

Nathasja van Leeuwen, MD, St. Joseph Hospital, Kagondo
Sherdina E. Romney, MD, St. Antonius Hospital, Nieuwegein

Previous edition

Paul Hendriks, BSc, University of Antwerp
Floortje Opperman, BSc, VU Amsterdam
Guusje Peters, BSc, University of Amsterdam
Kelly Stevens, BSc, Maastricht University
Hagma Workel, BSc, University of Groningen
Lizzy-Sara Zöllner, BSc, University of Groningen

Acknowledgements

Illustrators

Yente S. Beentjes, MD, Utrecht University
Hebe T.A. Boerhout, Utrecht University
Cas van Cruchten, Maastricht University
Susan Deelstra, University of Groningen
Jasmijn M.A. van Es, MD, Utrecht University
Astrid A.H. Feikema, Radboud University Nijmegen
Dite L.C. de Jong, Maastricht University
Didi D.J. Juin, BSc, Hogeschool Utrecht
Jasmin Kaur, BSc, Hogeschool Rotterdam
Koen L.C. Ketelaars, MD, Radboud University Nijmegen
Rosalie C. Krijl, MD, VU Amsterdam
Sybille Lange, Maastricht University
Juliëtte M.E. Linskens, MD, Maastricht University
Kim van den Nobelen, BSc, Radboud Universiteit Nijmegen
Belle van Rosmalen, University of Amsterdam
Laura Sanchez, MSc, KU Leuven
Esther Simons, Radboud University Nijmegen
Flori W. Sintenie, University of Amsterdam
Carlijn Sturm, BSc, Leiden University
Isabel Versmissen, Maastricht University
Linda Xie, MD, Leiden University

Editorial coordinators

Laura M. Barrantes Rodríguez, MD, international relations manager
Pauline Blom, final editor
Vera den Boef, MSc, project manager
Jasmijn M.A. van Es, MD, illustration editor
Melanie Goedegebure, project manager
Qin-ty Janssen-Bouwmeester, MD, manager diversity and inclusivity
Delano Sanches, BSc, illustration manager

Sounding board

Lia C. Bica, BSc, Maastricht University, Maastricht
Eva L. Brunner, MD, Public Health Service Hollands Midden, Hecht
Marijke P. Dorhout Mees, MSc Health Economics Policy and Law, Leiden
Merit E. Maas, MD, MSc, Centre for Youth and Family Rijnmond, Rotterdam
Priscilla A. Maria, MD, Amsterdam University Medical Center, Amsterdam
Daan A. Pijs, Medicine Graduate Entry Program (ZIGMA), University Medical Center Utrecht, Utrecht
Linde Verburgh, MD, Zaans Medical Center, Zaandam

Language support

Translation Agency Perfect
Mark Hannay, translator
Ruth Rose, editor

Graphic designers

Maria van Doorn, BASc
Ivana Kinkel

Content quality assurance

The editorial board extends its sincere appreciation to the many contributions of doctors, specialists, and professors from around the world who played a pivotal role in crafting this pocket. We wish to express our thanks to the entire international team for their dedicated efforts and invaluable expertise. Special appreciation is also extended to the team of specialists who actively participated in shaping the previous edition.

Current edition

Siobhán Corcoran, MD, The National Maternity Hospital, Dublin
Lisa G.H. Cornelissen, MD, Lion Heart Medical Center, Sierra Leone
Charlotte Deltour, MD, Ghent University Hospital, Ghent
Daisy de Groot, MD, Amsterdam University Medical Center, Amsterdam
Prof. Liliana Mereu, MD, PhD, Santa Chiara Hospital, Trento
Assist. prof. Jan Svihra Jr. MD, PhD, Jessenius Faculty of Medicine, Bratislava
Robbert W. Schouten, MD, PhD, Amsterdam University Medical Center, Amsterdam
Bas J.J.W. Schouwenberg, MD, PhD, Radboud UMC, Nijmegen
Vicky Tallentire, MD, PhD, University of Edinburgh, Edinburgh
Koen Traen, MD, OLV Hospital, Aalst
Anna Verhulst, MD, Amsterdam University Medical Center, Amsterdam
Evelien M. Vermeulen, MD, Amsterdam University Medical Center, Amsterdam
Harry Visser, MD, Tergooi Hospital, Hilversum

Previous edition

Nilou Ashtiani, MD, Dijklander Hospital, Hoorn
Juliette O.A.M. van Baal, MD, Amsterdam University Medical Center, Amsterdam
Lisa G.H. Cornelissen, MD, Catharina Hospital, Eindhoven
Sander Dumont, MD, University Hospital Leuven, Leuven
Prof. Sileny Han, MD, PhD, University Hospital Leuven, Leuven
Tom H.M. Hasaart, MD, PhD, Catharina Hospital, Eindhoven
Jason O. van Heesewijk, MD, Amsterdam University Medical Center, Amsterdam
Charlotte H.J.R. Jansen, MD, Amsterdam University Medical Center, Amsterdam
Arnoud W. Kastelein, MD, Amsterdam University Medical Center, Amsterdam
Gunilla Kleiverda, MD, PhD, Flevo Hospital, Almere
Simone M.I. Kuppens, MD, PhD, Catharina Hospital, Eindhoven
Prof. Liesbeth Lewi, MD, PhD, University Hospital Leuven, Leuven
Sharon Lie Fong, MD, PhD, University Hospital Leuven, Leuven
Mette van de Meent, MD, University Medical Center Utrecht, Utrecht
Prof. B.C. (Dick) Schoot, MD, PhD, Catharina Hospital and Ghent University Hospital, Ghent
Kelly Y.R. Stevens, MD, Ghent University Hospital, Ghent
Prof. Jan-Paul Roovers, MD, PhD, Amsterdam University Medical Center, Amsterdam
Philip Voets, MD, Gelre Hospitals, Apeldoorn
Prof. Johanna W. Wilmink, MD, PhD, Amsterdam University Medical Center, Amsterdam

The Compendium Method© Manual

In *Compendium Medicine* we use the same concise, visual and schematic description of the various medical specialties. Everything is geared towards overview and structure, facilitating study and practice. We call this the *Compendium Method©*.

Fixed layout

All our medical specialties are presented in the same, recognisable way and each has its own colour and icon. The pockets have a fixed chapter structure. The table of contents of each pocket tells you exactly which topics are covered. The symbols in the corner of the page show what kind of information is being discussed.

- ATLS
- Anatomy
- Physiology
- Patient history
- Physical examination

- Diagnostics
- Treatment
- Differential diagnosis
- Conditions
- Clinical reasoning

- Appendices
- References
- Abbreviations
- Index

Illustrations

The figures provide at-a-glance insight into topics like anatomy or the typical patient. They are also intended for study and practice, such as checking whether you can identify the letters in a picture without looking at the caption.

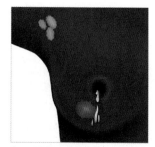

Figure 118 // Breast carcinoma

Conditions

Each condition in this pocket starts with a full-sentence definition followed by a telegram-style explanation. For each condition, the following icons (as applicable) are discussed. These visual cues that convey specific attributes or features of the condition are also useful when studying. You can cover the text and quiz yourself.

Ⓓ Definition
Ⓔ Epidemiology
Ⓐⓔ Aetiology
Ⓡ Risk factors
Ⓗ𝗑 Patient history
Ⓟⓔ Physical examination
Ⓓ𝗑 Diagnostics

Ⓣ𝗑 Treatment
🗨 General
👁 Paramedical care
🖋 Pharmacological treatment
🖊 Invasive, non-pharmacological treatment
Ⓟ Prognosis
❗ Watch out/don´t forget

Tables

We use tables to arrange the information in a clear and structured manner, with columns representing different conditions and rows indicating features or characteristics. Centered formatting for matching features makes it easy to identify similarities and differences.

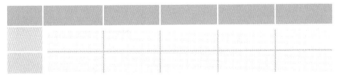

Diagrams

⟶ = positive/yes/+   ⟶ = negative/no/-

Diagrams help you reason clinically, starting from a particular symptom, using the green and red arrows as signposts. Always remember that the full differential diagnosis may consist of additional diagnoses.

Icons & frames

Fun fact: our founders are Dutch, and in the Netherlands, we refer to a mnemonic as a "donkey bridge". That's why the symbol for mnemonics in our books is a donkey.

Throughout this pocket you will find highlighted frames.

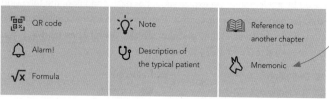

Punctuation marks

The punctuation in our books also focuses on overview and ensures that the subject matters are covered concisely and effectively.

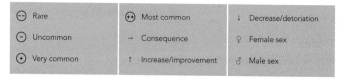

Abbreviations

We make extensive use of abbreviations, medical terms and symbols for scientific units and quantities. Below are some examples of the abbreviations used in this pocket.

sec	second/seconds	d	day/days	min.	minimum
min	minute/minutes	wk	week/weeks	max.	maximum
h	hour/hours	mo	month/months	e.g.	for example
		y/yr	year/years	L	litre/litres

Index

The pockets include a comprehensive and easy-to-use index. It contains all the topics covered in the books so you can quickly navigate and find the information you are looking for.

Appendices

In the pockets, you will find space for your notes, additional information, reminders, or insights. In addition, handy appendices have been added; these contain specific information that you would like to have at hand and are therefore located at the back of the pockets.

They/theirs

We realise that sex and gender identity are not binary and that there is more variation than just 'woman' or 'man'. For readability's sake (as well as for grammatical reasons) we have therefore chosen to use the pronouns 'they/theirs', regardless of sex or gender identity.

Warning

When studying this pocket, be mindful of the protocols within your own facility and adhere to the established guidelines. It is also essential to understand the circumstances under which you may or may not provide assistance in a given country, as this can potentially have legal consequences.

Want to know more about the Compendium Method©? Scan the QR code.

Table of contents
Obstetrics and Gynaecology

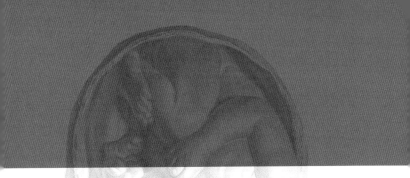

Table of contents
Obstetrics and Gynaecology

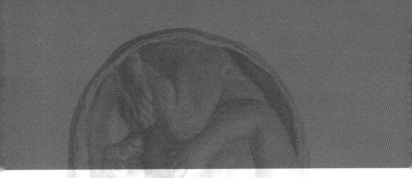

Table of contents
Obstetrics and Gynaecology

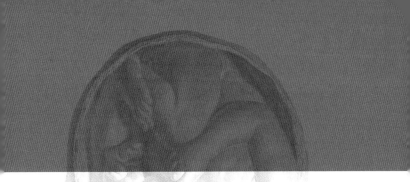

ATLS

ABCDE approach

Advanced Trauma Life Support (ATLS) consists of performing a primary survey using the ABCDE approach (see Diagram 1). The ABCDE approach is a systematic, step-by-step approach to assess and treat trauma patients. Do not continue to the next step until the current step has been found to be stable, or treatment has been started whose effect cannot be evaluated immediately. If the patient deteriorates, restart from the top. If the patient is stable according to the primary survey, the secondary survey is performed (see Diagram 2).

Several function scales can be used to quickly map a patient's neurological condition, such as the Glasgow Coma Scale (GCS, see Table 1) and the AVPU score (see Table 2). The amount of blood loss can be estimated based on vital parameters (see Table 3).

 Keep evaluating the patient throughout the ATLS trauma care. When treatment is started and the primary survey is finished, start from the top to evaluate the effect of the treatment.

EYE OPENING	MOTOR RESPONSE	VERBAL RESPONSE
1 No response	1 No response	1 No response
2 To pain	2 Extension response to pain	2 Sounds
3 To speech	3 Abnormal flexion response to pain	3 Words
4 Spontaneously open	4 Normal flexion response to pain	4 Confused
	5 Moves to localised pain	5 Orientated
	6 Obeys commands	

Table 1 // Glasgow Coma Scale

 A patient with a GCS ≤E1M5V2 is considered to be in a coma.

 Primary survey: care and support based on the ABCDE approach
Secondary survey: complete examination if appropriate response during the primary survey
Tertiary survey: repeat the ABCDE approach and secondary survey one day after admission, incl. evaluation of any interventions

AVPU SCORE

A	Patient is awake and alert
V	Patient responds only to verbal stimulus
P	Patient responds only to pain stimulus
U	Patient is unresponsive

Table 2 // AVPU score (Alert, Verbal, Pain, Unresponsive)

CLASSIFICATION OF HAEMORRHAGIC SHOCK

	I	II	III	IV
Blood loss (ml)	<750	750-1500	1500-2000	>2000
Blood loss (% blood volume)	<15	15-30	30-40	>40
Pulse (per minute)	<100	>100	>120	>140
Blood pressure (mmHg)	=	=	↓	↓
Pulse pressure	=/↑	↓	↓	↓
Respiratory rate (per minute)	14-20	20-30	30-40	>35
Urine production (ml/h)	>30	20-30	5-15	Negligible
Central nervous system/mental status	Slightly anxious	Mildly anxious	Anxious, confused	Confused, lethargic

Table 3 // Classification of haemorrhagic shock

ABC**DE(FG)**: **D**on't **E**ver **F**orget **G**lucose.

ABCDE approach

A Airway (+ C-spine)

PE · In case of no breathing → start CPR
· Airway clear
  - Does the patient talk?
  - Is the breathing audible (stridor, snoring)?
· Inspect mouth (foreign body/blood/vomit)

Dx Maxillofacial CT, C-spine CT, C-spine X-ray (in children)

Tx · Head tilt/chin lift (consider cervical injury → jaw thrust, no head tilt)
· 15L/100% oxygen mask → oropharyngeal airway → orotracheal intubation → cricothyrotomy
· Monitor CO_2 after intubation

! Suspected cervical injury after trauma → immobilise the neck (manual immobilisation or head blocks). If diagnostic imaging is indicated, this is performed in the 5th step (E) when the patient is found stable.

 Possible causes of instability:
· Aspiration of blood/vomit
· Atonia of the tongue due to unconsciousness
· C-spine injury
· Maxillofacial fractures

B Breathing and ventilation

PE · Respiratory rate
· Cyanosis
· Use of auxiliary breathing muscles
· Jugular vein distention
· Tracheal deviation
· Symmetrical chest excursions
· Auscultation of lungs (presence/absence of respiratory sounds, crepitations, rhonchi, wheezing)
· Chest palpation (rib fractures, subcutaneous emphysema)
· Chest percussion

Dx · Oxygen saturation
· Chest X-ray
· Blood gas
· Administration of oxygen therapy/ventilation: 15L/100% non-rebreathing mask, intubation as needed
· Tension pneumothorax → needle decompression at 5th intercostal space, midaxillary line (children: 2nd intercostal space, midclavicular line) and thoracic drain at 5th intercostal space, midaxillary line
· Open pneumothorax → close with valve → final closure in OR
· Massive haemothorax → intravenous (IV) and chest drain at 5th intercostal space, midaxillary line
· Pneumothorax → chest drain at 5th intercostal space, midaxillary line

Possible causes of instability:
· Flail chest with lung contusion
· Haemothorax
· Open pneumothorax
· Tension pneumothorax
· Pulmonary oedema
· Bronchospasm

Diagram 1 // ATLS

C Circulation

PE · Skin (colour, haematomas, clammy)
· Blood pressure, CVP
· Pulse
· Urine production
· Capillary refill
· Auscultation of the heart (heart sounds, murmurs)
· Abdominal palpation (abdominal rigidity with large haematoma)
· Long bone stability
· Rectal examination if indicated

Dx · ECG
· (e)FAST ultrasound (free fluid in peritoneal, pericardial and pleural space, ventral pneumothorax)
· Lab, crossmatch testing
· Pelvic X-ray to diagnose/rule out pelvic fracture as cause of haemorrhagic shock

 Possible causes of instability:
· All forms of shock

Tx · IV access (low-threshold 2nd access route)
· Administer blood/fluids as needed
· Fixate fractures
· External bleeding: compression or tourniquet
· Internal haemorrhage: surgery or angioembolisation as needed, stabilise unstable pelvis with pelvic belt (over greater trochanter)
· Tranexamic acid (1 g in 10 min within 3h of accident, followed by 1 g in 8h at hospital)

! In the event of massive blood loss, atypical symptoms may occur in elderly people, children, athletes, and the chronically ill

D Disability

 Possible causes of instability:
· Cerebral trauma
· Intoxication
· Hypoxaemia
· Hypercapnia   } (back to B and C)
· Hypovolaemia
· Hypoglycaemia
· Meningitis
· Status epilepticus

PE · Consciousness: GCS (see Table 1) and AVPU (see Table 2)
· Lateralisation
· Pupil reflexes
· Neck stiffness

Dx · Blood glucose level
· Brain CT

Tx · Loss of consciousness → return to A; intubate as needed and keep looking for treatable causes (intracerebral haemorrhage, epilepsy, hypoglycaemia, etc.)
· Bedside glucose → treat hypoglycaemia: administer glucose 10 g IV at a slow bolus rate (10 g = 100 ml gluc 10% = 20 ml gluc 50%, expected rise 2 mmol/L per 10 g) and check glucose <10 min, repeat as needed
· Cerebral oedema → hypertonic salt IV (NaCl 10%)

E Exposure

Possible causes of instability:
· Hypothermia

PE · Body temperature
· Check fully undressed patient for wounds and lesions, but try to prevent iatrogenic hypothermia from undressing patient, so cover the patient again as soon as possible
· Assess back and complete spine (log roll)
· Rectal examination (if indicated)

Tx · Hypothermia → warm up patient

In trauma, always consider major bleeding: external, legs, abdomen, chest, and pelvis.

 During the ATLS trauma care, the area to be assessed should be undressed, e.g. to assess symmetrical chest excursions.

 Intact circulation can be measured by e.g. capillary refill (<3 sec) and urine output (catheter urine: >0.5 ml/kg/h).

 GCS ≤8 (in a trauma situation) is an indication for intubation.

 Triad of death: hypothermia, acidosis, and coagulopathy. This triad results in a significant rise in mortality and is often seen in patients who suffered severe trauma.

 Nowadays, single-/multitrauma patients often undergo what is known as a total-body CT. This CT is done as quickly as possible after the primary survey, but not before the patient is stabilised.

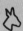 In traumatic resuscitation, consider **HOTT** (**h**ypovolaemia, **o**xygenation, **t**ension pneumothorax and **t**amponade).

 During trauma care the CT is also known as the **Donut of Death**. The indication for a CT scan may be seen during trauma care according to the ABCDE approach, but a patient is not scanned until they are stabilised. An unstable patient may die during a CT scan.

 In pregnant women follow ABCDE and stabilise the mother first. The fetus has no chance of living if the mother is dying.

Secondary survey

1. AMPLE

The AMPLE method can be used to gain a better understanding of the patient's condition.

 AMPLE
A: Allergies
M: Medications currently used
P: Past illness/pregnancy
L: Last meal
E: Events/environment related to injury

2. Head-to-toe examination

- Reassess vital parameters
- Comprehensive head/neck/back examination with log roll
- Comprehensive abdominal examination
- Comprehensive neurological examination with reassessment of GCS
- Comprehensive limb examination

3. Additional tests

- X-rays: chest X-ray (possibly primary), pelvic X-ray (possibly primary), spine X-ray, extremity X-ray.
- CTs: chest CT, abdominal CT, pelvic CT, spine CT. Additional CT scan if necessary.
- (Repeated) (e)FAST
- Lab (type and screen, haemoglobin, kidney and liver function, CRP, lactate)
- Urinalysis

4. Treatment

- Wounds → clean as needed, suture, and/or administer tetanus shot as needed
- Treat fractures and other injuries

Diagram 2 // Secondary survey

In pregnant women fetal monitoring through CTG if fetal heartbeat is present.

Anatomy

Female genitalia

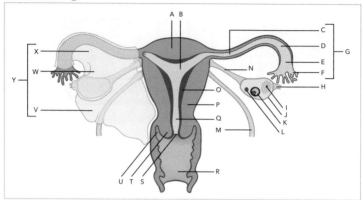

Figure 1 // Transverse section of the internal genitalia

A: Uterine fundus **B:** Uterine cavity **C:** Isthmus **D:** Ampulla **E:** Infundibulum **F:** Fimbriae **G:** Fallopian tube (salpinx) **H:** Infundibulopelvic ligament (suspensory ligament of the ovary) **I:** Corpus luteum **J:** Ovary **K:** Graafian follicle **L:** Primordial follicle **M:** Round ligament of the uterus **N:** Ovarian ligament **O:** Endometrium **P:** Myometrium **Q:** Endocervical canal **R:** Vagina **S:** Vaginal portion of the cervix **T:** Cervix **U:** Lateral fornix **V:** Mesometrium **W:** Mesovarium **X:** Mesosalpinx **Y:** Broad ligament of the uterus (parametrium)

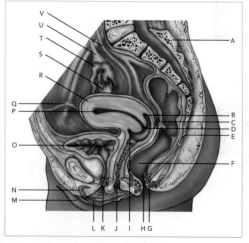

Figure 2 // Anatomy of female internal genitalia

A: Sacrum **B:** Vaginal fornix, posterior recess **C:** Pouch of Douglas **D:** External os **E:** Coccyx **F:** Rectum **G:** External anal sphincter **H:** Anus **I:** Vaginal fornix, anterior recess **J:** Vagina **K:** External urethral orifice **L:** Labium minus **M:** Labium majus **N:** Clitoris **O:** Bladder **P:** Uterine cavity **Q:** Round ligament of the uterus **R:** Uterus **S:** Ovary **T:** Fallopian tube **U:** Infundibulopelvic ligament (suspensory ligament of the ovary) **V:** Ureter

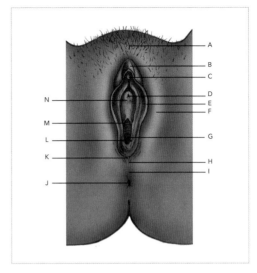

Figure 3 // Anatomy of the female external genitalia

A: Pubic mound **B:** Clitoral hood **C:** Clitoral glans **D:** External urethral orifice **E:** Labium minus **F:** Labium majus **G:** Vagina **H:** Posterior commissure **I:** Perineum **J:** Anus **K:** Frenulum **L:** Greater vestibular gland (Bartholin's gland) **M:** Hymenal ring **N:** Skene's glands

Male genitalia

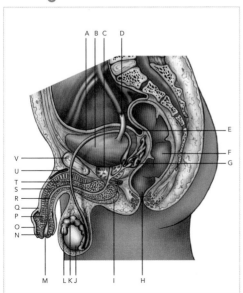

Figure 4 // Anatomy of male internal genitalia

A: Peritoneum **B:** Bladder **C:** Prostate **D:** Ureter **E:** Rectovesical pouch **F:** Rectum **G:** Seminal vesicle **H:** Anus **I:** Bulbospongiosus muscle **J:** Testis **K:** Scrotum **L:** Epididymis **M:** External urethral orifice **N:** Glans penis **O:** Foreskin **P:** Corpus cavernosum **Q:** Penis **R:** Urethra **S:** Corpus spongiosum **T:** Ductus deferens **U:** Dorsal vein of the penis **V:** Pubic symphysis

Pelvic floor musculature

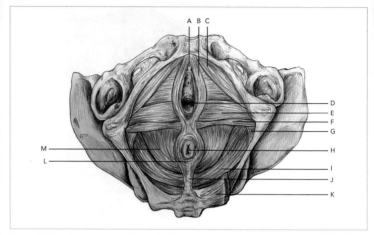

Figure 5 // Superficial vulvar view of the pelvic floor
A: Clitoris **B:** Bulbospongiosus muscle **C:** Ischocavernosus muscle **D:** Vagina **E:** Deep transverse perineal muscle **F:** Superficial transverse perineal muscle **G:** Internal obturator muscle **H:** Anus **I:** Iliococcygeus muscle (part of the levator ani) **J:** Anococcygeal ligament **K:** Gluteus maximus **L:** Superficial part of the external anal sphincter **M:** Puborectalis muscle (part of the levator ani)

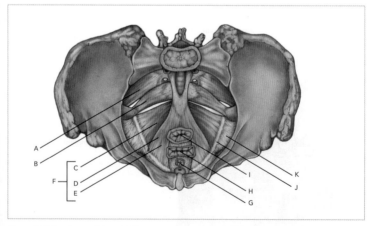

Figure 6 // Musculature of the pelvic floor
A: Piriformis muscle **B:** Coccygeus muscle **C:** Iliococcygeus muscle **D:** Pubococcygeus muscle **E:** Puborectalis muscle **F:** Levator ani **G:** Urethra **H:** Vagina **I:** Rectum **J:** Tendinous arch **K:** Obturator fascia (internal obturator muscle)

Female breast

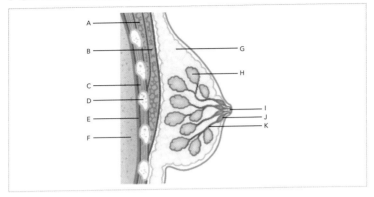

Figure 7 // Cross-section of the female breast
A: Pectoralis minor muscle **B:** Pectoralis major muscle **C:** Intercostal muscles **D:** Rib **E:** Parietal pleura **F:** Lung **G:** Fatty tissue **H:** Mammary gland **I:** Nipple **J:** Lactiferous sinus **K:** Lactiferous duct

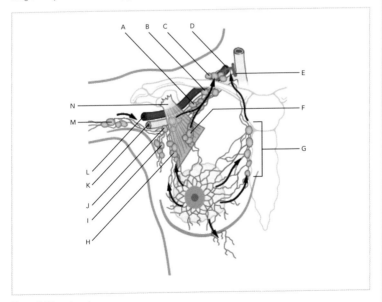

Figure 8 // Lymph nodes
A: Apical **B:** Infraclavicular **C:** Supraclavicular **D:** Subclavian trunk **E:** Right lymphatic duct **F:** Interpectoral **G:** Parasternal **H:** Pectoral (anterior) **I:** Subscapular (posterior) **J:** Central **K:** Right subclavian vein **L:** Right subclavian artery **M:** Humeral (lateral) **N:** Pectoralis minor muscle

Vasculature

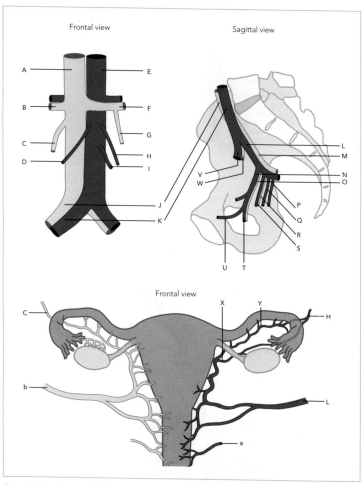

Figure 9 // Vasculature of the lesser pelvis

A: Inferior vena cava **B:** Right renal vein **C:** Right ovarian vein **D:** Right ovarian artery **E:** Abdominal aorta **F:** Left renal vein **G:** Left ovarian vein **H:** Left ovarian artery **I:** Inferior mesenteric artery **J:** Common iliac vein **K:** Common iliac artery **L:** Internal iliac artery **M:** Internal iliac vein **N:** Umbilical artery, patent part **O:** Vesical vein **P:** Inferior vesical artery **Q:** Uterine artery **R:** Obturator vein **S:** Obturator artery **T:** Superior vesical artery **U:** Umbilical artery, closed part **V:** External iliac artery **W:** External iliac vein **X:** Ovarian branch of the uterine artery **Y:** Tubal branch of the uterine artery **Z:** Uterine artery **a:** Vaginal artery **b:** Uterine vein

Innervation

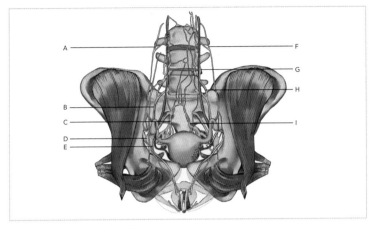

Figure 10 // Innervation female pelvis
A: Right genitofemoral nerve **B:** Right ischiatic nerve **C:** Right inferior hypogastric plexus **D:** N. obturatorius
E: N. pudendus **F:** Left genitofemoral nerve **G:** Left lumbar plexus **H:** Left ischiatic nerve **I:** Left inferior
hypogastric plexus

Lymphatic drainage

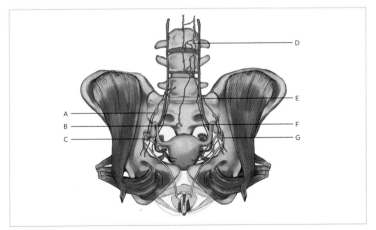

Figure 11 // Lymphatic drainage female pelvis
A: Right external iliac nodes **B:** Right hypogastric lymphnodes **C:** Right obturator lymphnodes **D:** Paraaortic
lymphnodes **E:** Left external iliac lymphnodes **F:** Left hypogastric lymphnodes **G:** Left obturator lymphnodes

Physiology

Gynaecology

Follicular maturation

Primordial follicles develop in the fetal gonads. A primordial follicle consists of an oocyte surrounded by a layer of cuboidal granulosa cells. During puberty, the oocyte grows into a primary follicle. The zona pellucida develops between the oocyte and the granulosa cells. The development into a secondary follicle is characterised by the formation of fluid-filled vesicles. The secondary follicle then proceeds to the ovarian medulla, where three processes take place:

- Formation of adequate blood supply
- Formation of layers of theca cells from surrounding stroma. These theca cells produce androgens that end up in the follicular fluid.
- Formation of insulin-like growth factor (IGF) and androgen receptors. The vesicles also fuse into the antrum, which is formed by oestrogen-producing granulosa cells.

In more than three months, the follicle develops into a tertiary follicle. By this point, the follicle has reached the prophase of meiosis I and will not resume development until puberty.

Granulosa and theca cells play an important role in female hormone regulation, as they produce oestrogens and androgens. Oestrogens and androgens, in turn, exert their effect on the follicles.

Menstrual cycle
Follicular phase

The menstrual cycle begins on the first day of menstruation. The hypothalamus secretes pulsatile gonadotropin releasing hormone (GnRH), causing the pituitary gland to produce luteinising hormone (LH) and follicle stimulating hormone (FSH) (see Diagram 3). Follicles mature in the ovaries, stimulated by FSH (early follicle development is gonadotropin-independent). As the follicles grow, the internal granulosa cells gradually increase inhibin and oestrogen levels, inhibiting the pituitary gland and hypothalamus. This reduces the availability of FSH for all growing follicles. Only the largest follicle, depending less on FSH, will continue to grow autonomously into a dominant Graafian follicle. The other follicles regress (see Figure 12). When inhibin and oestrogen levels reached their threshold values, the negative feedback function immediately transforms into a positive feedback function. This results in an LH surge, which increases intrafollicular pressure along with cyclic adenosine monophosphate (cAMP). An area on the follicle's outer wall (stigma) then begins to soften and vascularise in preparation for ovulation under the influence of prostaglandins and proteolytic enzymes. The remnant of the follicle is converted into the corpus luteum. By that point, oestrogens have also sparked endometrial proliferation and made the cervical mucus clear and stretchy.

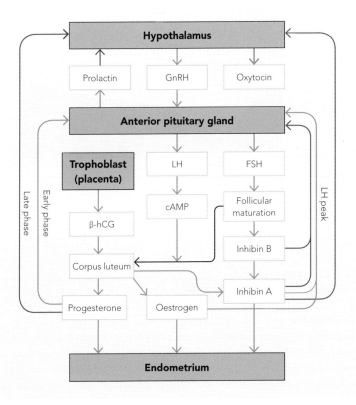

Diagram 3 // Hormonal cycle

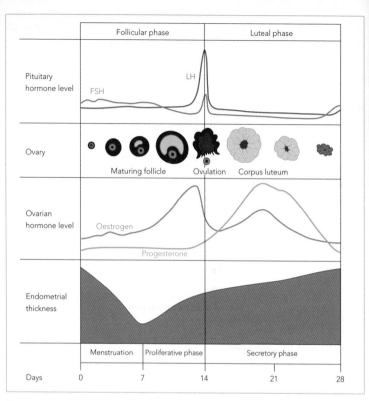

Figure 12 // Menstrual cycle

- **LH** stimulates theca cells. In theca cells, aromatase converts cholesterol into androgens.
- **FSH** stimulates granulosa cells. In granulosa cells, androgens are converted into oestrogens.

Luteal phase

The corpus luteum produces oestrogen, prompting endometrial growth (hyperplasia followed by hypertrophy). The corpus luteum produces progesterone, which is essential for endometrial maintenance. Through negative feedback, progesterone also inhibits the hypothalamus and pituitary gland. In the absence of fertilisation, the corpus luteum can be sustained for only 12-14 days. It then begins to regress and turn into fibrous tissue. The remaining scar is known as corpus albicans. The endometrium is no longer maintained by progesterone and is shed, resulting in menstruation. The negative feedback loop is discontinued and GnRH production in the hypothalamus resumes.

After fertilisation and nidation, the trophoblast produces beta human chorionic gonadotropin (β-hCG) to sustain the corpus luteum. The corpus luteum then begins to regress after 12 weeks, by which point the placenta is capable of completely taking over progesterone and oestrogen production.

Development of secondary sexual characteristics

Female secondary sexual characteristics develop as a result of irregular pulsatile secretion of GnRH and FSH, and later oestrogen production. Menarche is usually an anovulatory breakthrough bleed. Ovulation does not occur until full maturity has been reached and pulsatile secretion of GnRH has stabilised (between ages 10-16, avg. age 13). This is followed by the onset of menstruation. Menarche and a woman's first ovulation can be years apart.

> The first years of menstruation can be anovulatory, resulting in an irregular cycle and heavier bleeds.

Obstetrics

PHYSIOLOGICAL CHANGES	
Hormones	
Corticotropin releasing hormone (CRH)	· Production of ACTH ↑, cortisol levels ↑, and hypertrophy of adrenal cortex · High cortisol levels → Cushing-like symptoms, stretch marks, hyperpigmentation
hCG	· Maintains functional corpus luteum, which produces progesterone · Binds to TSH receptor in thyroid → increased T4 release. Elevated hCG (e.g. in molar pregnancies) can cause goiter.
Oestrogen	· Growth of endometrium (e.g. to enable nidation) and breast tissue, stimulates uterine perfusion, stimulates prolactin secretion · Activates renin-angiotensin-aldosterone system (RAAS) → fluid retention, maturation of fetal adrenal gland, initiates labour · Affects connective tissue composition → laxity ↑

Table 4A // Physiological changes in pregnant women

PHYSIOLOGICAL CHANGES	
Hormones	
Progesterone	Maintains pregnancy: relaxes vascular and uterine smooth muscle → contributes to circulation
Prolactin	· Lactation · Hypothalamus inhibition
Female organs	
Breasts	Number and size of milk ducts ↑ → volume ↑, alveolar hypertrophy, and slight increase in adipose tissue and vascularity → necessary for lactation after delivery
Ovaries	Contain corpus luteum → produce progesterone → maintain pregnancy until ± week 12, after which placenta takes over
Uterus	· Capable of growing from 60 g to ±1200 g and from 10 cm to 30 cm · The capacity of the uterine cavity grows from virtually none at conception to about 5L at term → ample space for child, placenta, and amniotic fluid · Uterine hyperplasia drives growth until week 10, hypertrophy is the main growth mechanism until week 20, followed by uterine stretch
Vagina	· One of the first symptoms of pregnancy is blue-purple discolouration of the vagina and cervix caused by the sharp increase in perfusion · Perfusion ↑ → fluid loss through vaginal wall → discharge ↑
Internal environment	
Respiration	· Sensitivity to pCO_2 ↑, particularly in the 1st trimester → tidal volume ±40% ↑ without increase in respiratory rate → respiratory minute volume ±40% ↑ · Anatomical changes → diaphragm rises ±4 cm → tidal volume ↑ and functional dead space ↓ → more effective respiration (may be perceived as shortness of breath)
Musculoske-letal system	· Frequent exercise → higher maternal fitness → fewer pregnancy symptoms and relatively shorter expulsion stage · Increased laxity of connective tissue and joints due to oestrogen and relaxin → reinforces effect of weight ↑ and extracellular fluid ↑, laxity can cause pelvic pain · Capsular and ligamentous laxity facilitates labour by creating space for fetal descent as the pregnancy progresses and enabling passage of the fetus through the lesser pelvis.

Table 4B // Physiological changes in pregnant women

	PHYSIOLOGICAL CHANGES
	Internal environment
Blood and clotting	• Plasma volume ↑, Hb ↓ and platelets ↓, erythropoietin (EPO) ↑ → erythrocytes ↑ • Blood clotting ↑ and fibrinolysis ↑ during pregnancy → balanced increase means no change in bleeding and clotting time • Relative increased risk of embolism (absolute risk 0.07%) risk is twice as high during pregnancy, 6 times higher in postpartum period (probably to protect mother against excessive blood loss during and shortly after labour and due to low levels of maternal mobility in postpartum period)
Circulation	• Heart rate and stroke volume increase by ±15% at a relatively early stage • Blood volume and cardiac output increase by ±40% during pregnancy • Perfusion demand ↓, vasodilation, extracellular volume ↑ → drop in blood pressure (moderate) • Vena cava inferior syndrome: compression of vena cava inferior (VCI) by uterus in supine position during 3rd trimester → venous return ↓ → cardiac output ↓ → pale face, hypotension, tachycardia, uterine perfusion ↓, possible cardiotoco-graphy (CTG) abnormalities consistent with fetal hypoxia. Quick recovery after left-lateral tilt or lateral positioning.
Immunology	• Immune system suppression → tolerance of maternal antigens → increased risk of viral infections, e.g. influenza • Immunocompetent cells appear to play a role in placental development as well as in remodelling the uterine vasculature • At the end of pregnancy an inflammatory reaction takes place in the cervix, uterus, and membranes, prompting a second episode of remodelling. This remodelling seems to play an important role in the initiation of labour.
Metabolism	Oxygen uptake increases by about 16% in the 2nd and 3rd trimesters in particular, when metabolism in the fetoplacental unit is at its highest.
Renal function	• GFR and renal perfusion ↑ → renal function ↑, waste products and nutrients (e.g. glucose) are filtered from the blood more quickly → mild glucosuria → urine glucose test unreliable during pregnancy • Ureteral obstruction (right>left) by uterus → obstructed urine output → higher risk of asymptomatic bacteriuria, pyelonephritis, or cystitis • Ureteral expansion mediated by progesterone → stasis in renal pelvis → high risk of pyelonephritis gravidarum and mechanical obstruction
	Digestion
Bile	Drainage of bile and bile salts ↓ → risk of cholestasis/cholelithiasis, itching (watch out for cholestasis → risk of IUFD)

Table 4C // Physiological changes in pregnant women

PHYSIOLOGICAL CHANGES

Digestion

Haemorrhoids	Combination of venous outflow obstruction, constipation, pressure ↑ due to pregnancy and venous relaxation → risk of haemorrhoids ↑
Hepatic function	Function remains stable, while liver enzyme activity ↑ → altered medication metabolism → may necessitate dose adjustment (especially in 3rd trimester)
Constipation	• Slowed intestinal peristalsis → fluid absorption from intestinal contents ↑ • Progesterone also causes intestinal dilation → decreased peristalsis
Pancreas	Beta cells increase in size → 2-3 times more insulin → insulin resistance (starting from 2nd trimester) → fetus always gets enough insulin but maternal glucose intake may decrease → switch to lipid metabolism → maternal glucose levels ↑
Reflux	Delayed gastric emptying and displacement of gastroesophageal sphincter into thorax → reflux
Slow digestion	Parasympathetic activity and progesterone levels ↑ → gastric acid production and intestinal peristalsis ↓ → slow digestion
Vomiting in pregnancy	hCG ↑, gastric motility ↓ → vomiting in pregnancy, slow digestion, reflux, constipation, hepatic function ↓

Skin

Palmar erythema	• Vasodilation → cutaneous perfusion ↑ • Also occurs with cholestasis
Skin pigmentation	Increased pigmentation due to melanocyte stimulating hormone (MSH) and melatonin, particularly in areolas, face (melasma/pregnancy mask), linea nigra, and vulva
Stretch marks	Stretching of the skin caused by e.g. relaxation of elastin and collagen fibres (especially around hips, breasts, abdomen, thighs)
Increased hair growth	Resulting from oestrogen levels ↑. Postpartum oestrogen levels ↓ → possible increase in hair loss.

Table 4D // Physiological changes in pregnant women

Circulatory changes during pregnancy may mimic ischaemia/infarction on ECG (deep Q, ST depression, T-wave flattening/inversion).

Functions of the placenta

The functions of the placenta include:

- Production of a plethora of chemicals needed to promote and maintain pregnancy, e.g. β-hCG, oestrogen, progesterone, oxytocinase, and human placental growth hormone.
- Immunological acceptance (to prevent rejection), barrier and filter against microorganisms. Transplacental maternal immunoglobin G (IgG) protects the fetus for up to six months postpartum.
- Nutrient production. About 60% of the glucose used by the placenta is broken down into lactic acid and excreted mainly to the fetus. Lactic acid is an important nutrient for the fetus. The placenta also produces cholesterol and is an important source of glutamine and glycine.
- Exchange of nutrients, blood gases, and waste products.

After the child and placenta are delivered, the negative feedback mechanism affecting the hypothalamus and pituitary gland disappears and the normal cycle resumes. During breastfeeding, the hypothalamus produces oxytocin that can suppress the cycle due to negative hypothalamic feedback.

Normal labour

Latent stage

The latent stage consists of cervical effacement and dilation to 3 cm. This process can take anywhere from several hours to several days and can be accompanied by cramps, lower abdominal pressure, or even contractions. Contractions shorten the cervix and cause the external os to dilate.

Active stage

The active dilation stage begins at 3 cm dilation and ends with full dilation (FD, 10 cm) and reflective pushing. Dilation usually occurs after spontaneous onset of labour. Multiparas reach FD earlier than primiparas, see Figure 13. In order for labour to proceed properly and to minimise the risk of complications, the cervix should dilate at a rate of at least 1cm/h. If dilation stagnates, interventions will be considered (e.g. stimulation with IV oxytocin).

Expulsion stage

The expulsion stage begins when the cervix is fully dilated and effaced. The descent of the fetal head usually prompts a reflective or unstoppable urge to push.

This stage should ideally take no more than one hour. The duration of this stage depends on strength of the contractions, fetal position and engagement, parity, fetal size, and pushing technique.

Afterbirth stage

The afterbirth stage begins when the child is delivered and lasts until the delivery of the placenta. The placenta can be delivered actively or passively:

- Active: oxytocin is administered immediately after birth. The umbilical cord is clamped and cut after minimum 1 minute, approximately after 3-5 minutes. After signs of placental loosening, the woman can actively push to deliver the placenta (see Physical examination).
- Passive: wait for signs of loosening (results in more blood loss): abdominal pain, 'lengthening' of umbilical cord (Ahlfeld's sign) and rise of uterus.

If the placenta is not delivered within one hour, or in the event of 500-1000 ml blood loss, the placenta has to be removed manually (under general or regional anaesthesia). Lastly, the woman should be checked for tears and bleeding. Sutures will be placed when and as needed.

- After week 22, mothers can usually produce milk.
- In the absence of breastfeeding, prolactin levels normalise approximately within 7 days of delivery.

3Ps that determine the course of labour:
- **P**ower: abdominal/pelvic floor muscles, uterine contractions
- **P**assage: bony and soft tissue of the birth canal
- **P**assenger: posture, position, presentation

Embryology

Fertilisation, implantation, and development of the fetus and placenta

Follicles complete meiosis I just before ovulation. In fertilised follicles, meiosis II takes place on average 12 hours after ovulation. The fertilised oocyte transfers from the fallopian tube to the uterus in three days. Here, the oocyte develops into a 16-cell morula before clustering into a 64-cell blastocyst. By that point a fluid-filled cavity has been formed, surrounded by trophoblasts (which will form the placenta) and embryoblasts (which will develop into the embryo). The pre-embryo then remains in the uterus for three days before nidation. During this time the pre-embryo is nourished by endometrial secretion (uterine milk). This stage is followed by decidualisation, an endometrial change characterised by an increase in stromal vascular permeability and secretory activity of the endometrium. Decidualisation is induced by the embryo, mediated by e.g. prostaglandins, cytokines, and β-hCG. The pre-embryo then sheds the zona pellucida (egg coat), allowing it to communicate with the decidual tissue of the uterus. First, this is followed by a process of unstable adhesion known as apposition. Implantation follows as the pre-embryo secretes cytokines, causing trophoblast flakes to intertwine with the decidua. Next, the endometrium forms a stroma around the blastula. After two days, β-hCG production by trophoblasts increases (see Diagram 3).

Fetal development

In the first half of pregnancy, the rate of fetal development is determined primarily by the genetic profile of the fetus. Environmental and epigenetic factors determine the rate of fetal development in the second half of pregnancy.

Each organ and system develops at its own speed (see Table 5). The organs begin to develop separately from week 5, and it isn't until 36 weeks that most organs are fully formed and functional.

Decidualisation can only occur with sufficient progesterone, which is produced by the corpus luteum. After nidation, β-hCG supports the corpus luteum to promote progesterone production.

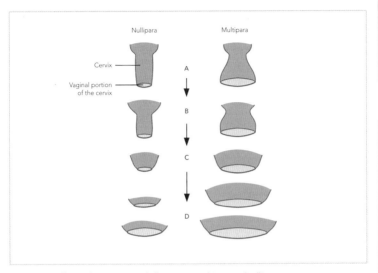

Figure 13 // Difference between cervical effacement in multiparas and nulliparas
A: Upright **B:** Effacement **C:** Full effacement **D:** Dilation

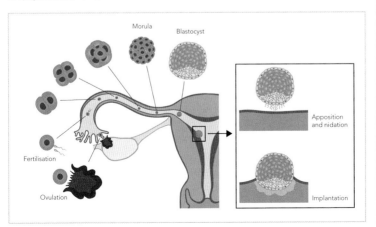

Figure 14 // From ovulation to nidation

CENTRAL NERVOUS SYSTEM	
Gestational age	**Development**
1st half of pregnancy	Neuron generation
2nd half of pregnancy	Glial cell generation and dendrite growth
Week 5	Neural tube formation
Week 6 or 7	First movements
Week 10-12	Fetus can open mouth and swallow
Week 24	Fetus can hear and see
Pregnancy week 26 to 18 months postpartum	Myelination
Week 28	Sense of taste can respond to stimuli

CARDIOVASCULAR	
Gestational age	**Development**
Week 4	Heart begins to beat
Week 5-8	Formation of AV valves
Week 7	Formation of foramen secundum and foramen ovale
Week 9	Aorta and pulmonary artery separation

LUNGS	
Gestational age	**Development**
Week 5	Lungs develop from foregut
Week 6-16	Pseudoglandular stage: bronchi and bronchioles
Week 16-26	Canalicular stage: respiratory bronchioles
Week 26-40	Saccular stage: alveolar duct
Week 31	Alveolar stage: alveoli
From week 34	Surfactant present, lung maturation almost complete

Table 5A // Fetal organ development

IMMUNOLOGY	
Gestational age	**Development**
Week 9	B-lymphocyte production
Week 14	T-lymphocyte production
Week 16	Maternal IgG to fetus
Week 36	Sufficient transfer of maternal IgG to fetus to ensure immunity

KIDNEYS	
Gestational age	**Development**
Week 6-32	Develop from mesonephros
From week 7	• Urine production • Nephron development

DIGESTIVE SYSTEM	
Gestational age	**Development**
Week 5 to toddler age	Digestive system formation
Week 9	Pancreas can produce insulin and glucagon
Week 12	• All structures present, maturation • Adrenal gland and thyroid gland start producing cortisol and thyroxine
Week 16	Starts swallowing amniotic fluid
Week 36	Able to conjugate bilirubin

Table 5B // Fetal organ development

Fetal reproductive system

Development of the fetal reproductive system begins from week 7 of pregnancy. The primitive gonads develop into testes or ovaries based on genetic predisposition (see Diagram 4).

The male Y chromosome is home to the sex-determining region Y (SRY) and the testis-determining factor (TDF). TDF initiates the development of the primitive gonads into testes from week 8 onward, mediated by e.g. Sertoli cells and Leydig cells. Sertoli cells produce anti-Müllerian hormone (AMH), triggering regression of the Müllerian ducts. Leydig cells produce testosterone, allowing the

Wolffian ducts to develop into male internal genitalia. Testosterone is converted to dihydrotestosterone (DHT), prompting the urogenital sinus to develop into the external male genitalia and prostate. Females have no Y chromosome and therefore lack the SRY and the TDF gene. As a result, the primitive gonads develop into ovaries. Without Sertoli cells, no AMH is produced and the Müllerian ducts grow into internal female genitalia. In the absence of testosterone, the Wolffian ducts regress and no DHT is produced. As a result, the urogenital sinus develops into the external female genitalia and the lower $1/3$ portion of the vagina (see Figure 15).

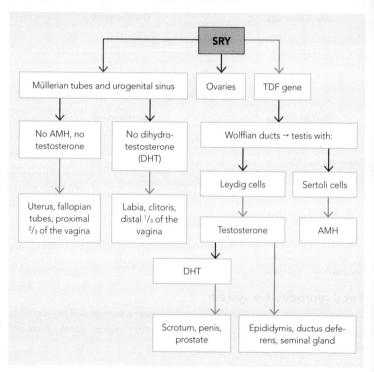

Diagram 4 // Embryology of sex development

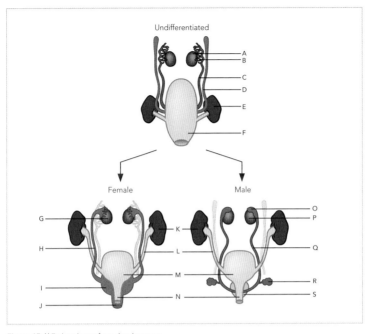

Figure 15 // Embryology of sex development

A: Gonad **B:** Mesonephros **C:** Wolffian duct **D:** Müllerian duct **E:** Metanephros **F:** Urogenital sinus **G:** Ovary **H:** Müllerian duct (fallopian tube) **I:** Uterus **J:** Vagina **K:** Kidney **L:** Ureter **M:** Bladder **N:** Urethra **O:** Epididymis **P:** Testis **Q:** Wolffian duct (ductus deferens) **R:** Seminal vesicle **S:** Prostate

SALT:
Sertoli cells stimulate the production of **A**MH. **L**eydig cells stimulate the production of **t**estosterone.

Patient history

Introduction
- Introduce yourself
- Check personal details
- Assess the patient: acute or non-acute, determine reason for consultation and/or chief complaint, nonverbal communication

Patient history
- General patient history
- History of presenting complaint/current illness
- History of relevant system (full review of systems if necessary)

Concluding
- Summarise your findings
- Patient's remarks and/or questions
- Explain physical examination and/or indicated diagnostics

Consider psychosocial variables such as language barriers, cultural differences between patients and physicians, financial backgrounds, and addiction, which may impact disease progression.

Diagram 5 // Patient history

General patient history

Past medical history (PMHx), medication use (exact dosage, frequency, last dose, administration form), history of substance use (smoking, alcohol, drugs), allergies (latex, plasters, medication, contrast agents), family history (FHx), psychosocial history, travel history, social history (home situation, work, study, social support), vaccinations, ill individuals in immediate vicinity.

In case of male infertility, inquire about cryptorchism, diabetes mellitus (DM), previous ability to conceive, erectile/ejaculation disorders, genital tumours, inguinal hernia, testicular torsion/trauma, neurological disorders, genital surgeries and complications, sexually transmitted infections (STIs), varicocele, cystic fibrosis.

Inquire about medical history:
- Obstetrics: previous pregnancies (e.g. vaginal birth, assisted delivery or caesarean section (CS), episiotomy or perineal tears, haemorrhaging postpartum), gestational diabetes mellitus (GDM), gestational hypertension/pre-eclampsia, congenital malformations (cardiac/vascular malformations, uterine anomalies), autoimmune diseases, clotting disorders, connective tissue disorders, consanguinity, repeated miscarriages, fertility problems, blood transfusions, varicella zoster or herpes, participation in regular vaccination programmes.
- Gynaecology: uterine surgeries (e.g. hysteroscopic surgery, surgical abortion), cervical surgeries, previous screening/diagnostic tests (e.g. most recent PAP smear), prolapse issues, cancers, sexual abuse, female genital mutilation (FGM).
- Fertility: risk of STIs, tubal surgery (tubectomy in ectopic pregnancy), premature menopause, weight fluctuations, excessive exercise, signs of polycystic ovarium syndrome, endometriosis, abdominal surgeries.

Inquire thoroughly about the family history. For example:
- Gynaecology: prevalence of ovarian, breast, uterine, cervical, or colon cancer; hereditary breast and ovarian cancer mutations (*BRCA1/2*, HNPCC); endometriosis, uterine fibroids, or clotting disorders.
- Obstetrics: DM, gestational hypertension and/or congenital malformations, disorders (congenital, carrier, syndromic).
- Fertility: explore family history to rule out a possible genetic cause for fertility problems (e.g. premature ovarian insufficiency (POI)).

Inquire about medication use. For example:
- Gynaecology: use of pain medication (e.g. paracetamol, NSAIDs, opioids), use of hormonal preparations.
- Obstetrics: use of teratogenic medication, DES use (between 1947-1975), thyroid medication.
- Fertility: radiotherapy/chemotherapy treatments.

Review of systems

General system

General well-being, itching, fever, chills, night sweats, appetite, weight change (deliberate/unintended), fatigue, exercise tolerance.

 Watch for red flags/B symptoms (e.g. disabling fatigue, weight loss, unexplained fever, night sweats, itching, icterus). These symptoms may be associated with a serious condition, such as malignancy.

Circulatory system

Dizziness/lightheadedness (orthostatic), chest pain (on exertion or at rest), palpitations (e.g. fluttering, pounding, racing), dyspnoea (e.g. dyspnoea on exertion or at rest, orthopnoea), nycturia, intermittent claudication, cold extremities, peripheral oedema.

 Palpitations can occur in relation to the use of tocolytics or antihypertensive medication. Peripheral, facial, and sacral oedema can arise in pre-eclampsia. The amount of vaginal blood loss is important in case of abnormal menstrual bleeding, a miscarriage, or postpartum haemorrhaging.

Respiratory system

Dyspnoea, coughing (dry, sputum, nocturnal), audible breathing (e.g. wheezing, rhonchi), chest pain (worsens when breathing deeply), sputum (e.g. consistency, colour, blood), haemoptysis. ENT: sore throat, earache, tinnitus, voice (hoarse), recurrent respiratory infections.

 Dyspnoea in pregnant patients can occur in case of severe hypertension or severe pre-eclampsia. The combination of dyspnoea, pain on the chest or between shoulder blades, and/or palpitations could be a sign of pulmonary embolism.

Digestive system

Vomiting (e.g. frequency, blood), nausea, reflux, regurgitations, swallowing problems, abdominal pain, stool pattern (e.g. frequency, consistency, colour, blood or mucus, tenesmus), flatus, jaundice, diet, appetite changes.

Inquire about:
- Abdominal pain or discomfort when pregnant: could indicate HELLP syndrome, severe pre-eclampsia, or acute fatty liver.
- Dysmenorrhoea: could indicate endometriosis/adenomyosis.
- Abnormal stool pattern (frequency, consistency, colour, blood or mucus, tenesmus): could indicate involvement of the rectum in deep infiltrating endometriosis.
- Changes in bowel habits or appetite, constipation, diarrhoea, or weight loss: could be signs of malignancy.

Obstetric and gynaecological history

Some system-specific complaints and questions will be discussed in the following section.

Hypertension

Headache, nausea, vomiting, pulmonary oedema, peripheral oedema, oliguria, pain (upper abdomen/epigastrium or between shoulder blades that does not improve with painkillers), retrosternal pain, visual disturbances (starry vision).

Fever

Pain type (e.g. acute/subacute/slow) and duration (e.g. long/short, continuous/intermittent), malodorous lochia, temperature differences (cold/hot/chills), headache, general malaise, anorexia, fever, palpitations, state of consciousness.

Abdominal pain

Lower abdominal pain (worsens with intercourse), vaginal bleeding (intermenstrual, menorrhagia, postcoital), pain type (e.g. acute/subacute/slow), additional complaints (e.g. nausea, vomiting, malaise, fever), discharge (e.g. odour, colour, consistency), number of sexual partners, unprotected intercourse, previous *Chlamydia* infection, burning sensation/pain on urination, recent intrauterine device insertion, abdominal surgery, abdominal distension (e.g. mass in abdomen, ascites), change in stool pattern (e.g. frequency, consistency, blood, mucus), B symptoms (e.g. weight change/weight loss, lymphadenopathy).

Vaginal blood loss

Intermenstrual, postcoital, postmenopausal, last menstrual period, amount of blood loss (e.g. menorrhagia, leaking, large clots), abdominal pain, history of STIs, ectopic pregnancy, history of cervical issues (e.g. cervicitis, ectropion, abnormal cervical cytology), recent PAP smear (participation in population screening), vaginal/vulva varices, regular menstrual cycle, symptoms of anaemia, use of contraception, medication use (e.g. antiplatelets).

 Consider the possibility of rectal blood loss in patients who complain of vaginal blood loss (e.g. in endometriosis, haemorrhoids in pregnancy).

Dysmenorrhoea

Age of menarche, menstrual cycle (e.g. duration, amount of bleeding), secondary dysmenorrhoea, pain (cyclical/continuous, chronic/acute), nausea, vomiting, diarrhoea, malaise, dyspareunia (superficial/deep), subfertility, menorrhagia, influence on personal life (absenteeism from work), use of contraceptives/analgesics, abnormalities of internal genitalia (endometriosis, fibroids), other chronic pain (e.g. chronic abdominal pain), irritable bowel syndrome, fibromyalgia, premenstrual syndrome.

 The essential components of a pain history can be recalled using the mnemonic SOCRATES.

Pain (SOCRATES)
Site
Onset (sudden/gradual)
Character (dull, sharp, stinging)
Radiation
Associated symptoms
Time course/duration
Exacerbating, relieving factors (urge to move, pain during transport)
Severity

Reproductive system
Premenopausal

Pain, vaginal discharge (odour, colour, amount, consistency); use of irrigation (vaginal showers); frequency of coitus; vaginal bleeding; last menstrual period; menstrual cycle (age at menarche, regularity, duration, intensity, dysmenorrhoea); impact on activities of daily living (ADL); frequency of usage of tampons, pads, or menstrual cup; intermenstrual bleeding; menopausal/perimenopausal symptoms (e.g. menstrual irregularities, hot flashes, vaginal dryness, impaired sleep, mood swings); contraception (e.g. oral contraceptives, intrauterine device, condom).

Postmenopausal

Postmenopausal blood loss, use of medication (e.g. antiplatelets), pain/other symptoms, B symptoms (e.g. weight loss, nocturnal sweating).

Course of pregnancy

Time since last period; due date; prenatal care (planned/unplanned, wanted/unwanted, feelings regarding continuation or termination, if applicable); nutritional status; fatigue and physical activity during pregnancy; use of folic acid; course of pregnancy (gestational age, weight gain, illness during pregnancy (e.g. hyperemesis gravidarum); prenatal testing, OGTT); pregnancy symptoms (e.g. nausea, vomiting), awareness of fetal movement (from 20 weeks gestation), Braxton-Hicks contractions.

 Pregnancy complications are vaginal bleeding, preterm contractions (amount, intensity, urge to push), preterm fluid loss (premature rupture of membranes), other abdominal pain (e.g. persistently hypertonic uterus, round ligament pain), itching and/or pruritis (gestational cholestasis), dyspnoea, fever, symptoms of pre-eclampsia (e.g. headache, dizziness, visual complaints, tingling in hands and/or feet, oedema).

Fertility history

Intention and active attempts to conceive, regularity of attempts, previous pregnancy, secondary sexual characteristics, onset of pubarche and thelarche, regularity of menstrual cycle, weight loss/weight gain, amount of exercise, menopausal symptoms, use of alcohol/drugs, smoking, maternal age, gynaecomastia, profession.

Sexual history

Intercourse (sexual orientation, types of sex, multiple partners, safe/unsafe), satisfaction with sex life (stress during sexual activity, lubrication, relationship with partner, partner's attitude towards complaint, triggering factor), postcoital blood loss, dyspareunia (superficial or deep), negative sexual experiences, previous experiences with gynaecological examination, use of pelvic floor physiotherapy.

Urogenital system

Miction (e.g. dysuria, stranguria, haematuria, pollakisuria, polyuria), bladder function, incontinence, flank pain, changes in bowel habits, sexual history. ♀: vaginal discharge, menstrual cycle, hot flashes. ♂: weak stream, feeling of incomplete emptying, dribbling, discharge, erectile dysfunction, testicular pain or swelling.

 Inquire about dysuria or haematuria to determine the possible involvement of the bladder in endometriosis. Stranguria, incontinence, and/or feeling incomplete emptying could be a sign of prolapse.

Endocrine system

Changes in bowel habits (e.g. diarrhoea/constipation), polydipsia, polyuria, menstrual irregularities, agitation/inertia, cold or heat intolerance, exopthalmos, enlarged thyroid, muscle problems, skin/hair changes, sweating, oedema, weight changes, mood swings, alterations in libido or sexual function.

 In case of primary or secondary amenorrhoea ask about development of secondary sexual characteristics, weight gain or weight loss, acne, abnormal hair growth, and other endocrine disorders. Use the World Health Organisation (WHO) classification to distinguish between the different causes of amenorrhoea (see Table 39).

 Diseases and factors that may affect the cycle include anorexia nervosa, DM, weight fluctuations, adiposity, hypothyroidism and hyperthyroidism, hyperprolactinaemia, frequent exercise, stress, clotting disorders.

Locomotor system

Warmth, redness, swelling, cramps, restless legs, joint pain, joint instability, morning stiffness, loss of function, action radius, muscle atrophy.

Haematological system

Bone pain, epistaxis, haematomas, heavy menstrual bleeding, prolonged bleeding, petechiae, lymph node swelling, night sweats, fever, fatigue.

 Ask about the duration of the menstruation, products used (tampons, pads, or cups), and how often they need to be changed.

Inquiring about prolonged bleeding and haematomas could help predict the risk of postpartum haemorrhaging.

 Risk factors for deep venous thromboembolism should be considered when prescribing oral contraceptives (e.g. history of deep venous thromboembolism (DVT)/pulmonary embolism, oestrogen-dependent tumours, pre-eclampsia, smoking, clotting disorders).

Central nervous system

Concentration difficulties, amnesia, dizziness (spinning rotation), loss of consciousness, seizures, headache, impaired senses (e.g. hearing, smell, taste, vision), language, speech, mastication, swallowing, diplopia, abnormal sensation (e.g. numbness, tingling), loss of strength, gait disorders, balance problems, tremors or involuntary movements, psychiatric symptoms.

 Headaches, impaired vision, and tremors could indicate severe pre-eclampsia. Seizures during pregnancy can be a sign of eclampsia.

 Chronic abdominal pain can persist due to sensitisation of the nervous system.

Skin and mucous membranes system

Skin rash (efflorescence, redness), skin discolouration, nail/finger abnormalities, itching.

Mental health

Cognitive functioning, sleep problems, anxiety, depression, mood swings, delusions, hallucinations, suicidal thoughts or self-harm.

 Anxiety, depression, and/or sleeping problems in pregnancy can be a sign of posttraumatic stress disorder (PTSD) after a previous traumatic labour. Consider postpartum depression or psychosis in case of anxiety, depression, delusions, suicidal thoughts, sleeping problems, or self-harm.

Physical examination

The next chapter provides a systematic guide to performing a general physical examination. Emphasis is placed on the importance of clear communication and patient comfort throughout the examination. The most important aspects of the obstetric and gynaecological examination are presented.

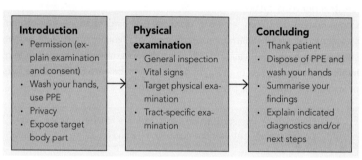

Introduction
- Permission (explain examination and consent)
- Wash your hands, use PPE
- Privacy
- Expose target body part

Physical examination
- General inspection
- Vital signs
- Target physical examination
- Tract-specific examination

Concluding
- Thank patient
- Dispose of PPE and wash your hands
- Summarise your findings
- Explain indicated diagnostics and/or next steps

Diagram 6 // Physical examination
PPE, personal protective equipment

General inspection

Gender, age (biological vs. calendar), state of consciousness (GCS and AVPU score, see Tables 1 and 2), mental state, posture, skin colour (e.g. pale, cyanotic, flushing/blushing, icteric), mobility, grooming, nutritional status (e.g. cachexia, BMI), and any medical equipment attached to the patient or in the bedspace.

- Skin colour (e.g. icteric) could indicate underlying acute fatty liver in pregnancy. Pale skin in postpartum patients could indicate severe blood loss during labour.
- Specific features can be a sign of chromosomal disorders (e.g. Turner, Swyer, Klinefelter).
- Nutritional status and weight loss could indicate malignancy.

During inspection, be mindful that change in colour (e.g. cyanosis, bruises) in patients with dark skin can be more subtle.

Anthropometric data

Abdominal circumference, weight, height, BMI.

Vital signs

REFERENCE RANGES					
RR	15-20/min	**Systolic BP**	100-140 mmHg	**T**	36-38°C/ 96.8-100.4°F
SpO$_2$	>95%	**Diastolic BP**	60-90 mmHg	**CRT**	<2-3 sec
HR/pulse rate	60-100/min	**CVP**	R 4-9 cm H$_2$O (3-8 mmHg)		

Table 6 // Normal vital signs (Vx)

BP, blood pressure; CRT, capillary refill time; CVP, central venous pressure; HR, heart rate; RR, respiratory rate; SpO$_2$, oxygen saturation; T, temperature

 A capillary refill time (CRT) >3 sec suggests poor peripheral perfusion.

 An elongated CRT may be caused by e.g. dehydration, hypovolaemia due to postpartum haemorrhage (degree of shock), sepsis.

Pulse

- Heart rate: 60-100 bpm
- Heart rhythm: regular or irregular rhythm (e.g. atrial fibrillation, atrioventricular blocks)
- Pulse character/pulse force: full, normal, weak, absent/non-palpable
- In emergency situations or when access to the radial artery is challenging, the carotid or femoral pulse can be palpated for assessment

MEWS

The modified early warning score (MEWS) is an objective parameter for early recognition of patients who are at risk of rapid deterioration (see Table 7). Different hospitals have different trigger scores for notifying physicians: verify that your facility uses the same point assignments listed here.

	+3	+2	+1	0	+1	+2	+3
RR (per min)		<9		9-14	15-20	21-29	≥30
Saturation (%)	<92	92-93	94-95	>95			
Supplemental O$_2$		Yes		No			
Temperature		<35°C/<95°F		35.0-38.4°C/95-101.1°F		≥38.5°C/101.3°F	
Systolic BP (mmHg)	≤70	71-80	81-100	101-199		≥200	
HR (per min)		≤40	41-50	51-100	101-110	111-129	≥130
Consciousness (AVPU score)				Alert	Responds to voice	Responds to pain	Unresponsive

Table 7 // Modified early warning score
AVPU, Alert Verbal Pain Unresponsive; BP, blood pressure; HR, heart rate; RR, respiratory rate

General physical examination

 Always perform the physical examination according to the patient's specific complaints and clinical history. Consider indications or any red flags for additional diagnostics. This chapter provides a focused exploration of the most common general and system-specific aspects of physical examination in Obstetrics and Gynaecology rather than attempting to cover all aspects comprehensively.

Thorax
Lungs
🔍 Inspection

Skin abnormalities (e.g. thoracic scars, rash, peripheral and central cyanosis), breathing pattern (e.g. depth, rate, sound, posture, use of accessory breathing muscles, rhythm, asymmetry in the expiratory and inspiratory phases), chest wall deformities (e.g. asymmetry, pectus carinatum, pectus excavatum, hyperexpansion/barrel chest), extremities (e.g. colour, clubbed fingers, nail clubbing), respiratory effort.

PHYSICAL EXAMINATION

➤ Percussion

Air resonance (normal), dullness (increased tissue density, e.g. pneumonia, pleural effusion), stony dullness (e.g. pleural effusion), hyperresonance (increased air, e.g. emphysema, pneumothorax), symmetry, lower lung border, shifting lung borders, lung-liver border, diaphragm.

⚕ Auscultation

Breathing sounds (vesicular/normal, bronchial/harsh-sounding (e.g. consolidation)), quiet/reduced breath sounds (e.g. silent chest in COPD), symmetry, vocal resonance (volume), inhalation/exhalation ratio, abnormal breath sounds (fine end-inspiratory crackles indicating opening of obstructed central bronchi, coarse crackles indicating opening of distal airways, pleural rub, rhonchi, inspiratory/expiratory stridor, wheezing, muffles, absent breath sounds).

 Thoracic examination is performed during a gynaecological consultation as clinically indicated. For example, examine the lungs when suspecting pulmonary embolism, noting potential manifestations such as tachycardia, tachypnoea, pale or cyanotic skin, or abnormal breath sounds, which could include basilar crackles or wheezing.

 Pulmonary oedema is a sign of severe pre-eclampsia. You may hear crackles during auscultation.

Heart
🔍 Inspection

Skin abnormalities (e.g. thoracic scars, rash, petechiae/Osler's node/Janeway lesion/splinter haemorrhages (e.g. endocarditis stigmata)), neck veins (pulsations, CVP ↑), peripheral pitting oedema.

⚕ Auscultation

Heart rate, heart sounds (S1 and S2), S2 splitting, presence of S3 (e.g. in athletes or pathological cause, e.g. post-myocardial infarction, mitral regurgitation, ventricle septum defect, dilated cardiomyopathy) and/or S4 (decreased ventricular compliance, e.g. in hypertrophic cardiomyopathy, aortic stenosis), cardiac rhythm (regular/irregular, breathing-based or unrelated to breathing), murmurs (timing in systole or diastole, high/low frequency, loudness, radiation over carotid arteries, valve locations, see Figure 16 and Table 8), pericardial friction rub.

Percussion and palpation of the heart play no role in obstetrics and gynaecology. Inspection and auscultation play a relatively minor role in clinical examination and are performed on indication. For example, auscultation of pregnant patients with congenital heart disease may show signs of abnormal heart sounds, which can exacerbate during pregnancy and/or postpartum (<48h).

PHYSICAL EXAMINATION

VALVE DEFECTS	PHASE OF HEART CYCLE	SHAPE	PMI	ILLUSTRATION
Aortic valve regurgitation	Diastole	Decrescendo	3 ICS left	
Aortic valve stenosis	Systole	Crescendo-decrescendo	• 2 ICS right • Radiation: carotid artery	
Mitral valve regurgitation	Systole	Holosystolic	• Apex • Radiation: left flank and axilla	
Mitral valve stenosis	Diastole	Opening snap, presystolic murmur	Apex	
Pulmonary valve regurgitation	Diastole	Decrescendo	2 ICS left	
Pulmonary valve stenosis	Systole	Crescendo-decrescendo	2 ICS left	
Tricuspid valve regurgitation	Systole	Holosystolic	4 ICS left	

Table 8 // Characteristics of cardiac murmurs caused by valvular heart disease
ICS, intercostal space; PMI, point of maximum intensity

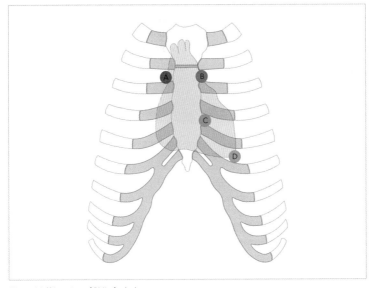

Figure 16 // Location of PMI of valvular murmers
A: Aortic valve **B:** Pulmonary valve **C:** Tricuspid valve **D:** Mitral valve

Abdomen

🔍 Inspection

Shape/symmetry (e.g. flanks, swelling, abdominal distension: fat, fluid, flatus, faeces, fetus, fulminant mass), skin abnormalities (e.g. scars, striae, rash, discolouration, caput medusae), abdominal hernias, navel, visible peristalsis.

🩺 Auscultation

Bowel sounds (normal, absent, tinkling indicative of mechanical bowel obstruction), bruits (e.g. abdominal aorta aneurysm, renal artery stenosis).

👆 Percussion

Quality (e.g. dull sounds, resonant sounds), organs (e.g. bladder contours, liver contours, spleen contours), pain, shifting dullness (when suspect ascites).

👆 Palpation

Superficial palpation: tenderness, voluntary guarding, involuntary guarding/rigidity (e.g. peritonitis).

Deep palpation: rebound tenderness (e.g. peritoneal irritation), organomegaly (liver, spleen), masses (e.g. location, size, shape, consistency, mobility), organs (aorta, bladder, colon, gallbladder, liver, spleen, kidneys).

 During obstetrical abdominal inspection, it is crucial to consistently assess for peripheral oedema at the sacrum, as oedema may gravitate towards this region in severe pre-eclampsia.

 In gynaecological patients with abdominal pain, differentiate between abdominal wall pain and intra-abdominal pain. A positive Carnett sign indicates pain deriving from the abdominal wall. A negative Carnett sign suggests an intra-abdominal issue (visceral). To perform Carnett's test, position the patient on the examination table lying supine. Have the patient elevate one leg with a straight knee. Palpate the lower abdomen on the ipsilateral side. If the pain increases when muscles of the abdominal wall are tensed, it is a sign of abdominal wall pain and a positive Carnett sign.

Inguinal region
🔍 Inspection
Skin abnormalities (e.g. scars, rash), swelling, herniations (with and without Valsalva).

👉 Palpation
Femoral artery, herniations (with and without Valsalva), lymph nodes.

Extremities
🔍 Inspection
Hair growth, skin abnormalities (e.g. scars, rash, bruises), contours of arms and legs (e.g. muscle atrophy), symmetrical spacing between extremities and torso, joints (e.g. redness, position, swelling), oedema, trophic disorders (e.g. shiny skin, lack of hair, brittle nails), varicose veins.

👉 Palpation
Capillary refill, peripheral oedema (e.g. pitting/non-pitting), arterial pulsations (brachial, radial, femoral, popliteal, posterior tibial, dorsalis pedis arteries), reflexes (biceps , brachioradialis, triceps, quadriceps muscles, Achilles tendon),

sensation, temperature, swelling, joint (e.g. range of motion (ROM), stiffness, stability), muscles (e.g. tension, tenderness, eccentric and concentric strength).

 Klinefelter syndrome (47 XXY) can be a cause of infertility in male patients because it affects testicular growth, often with lower testosterone production and low to no sperm count. Inspection of limbs is important, because patients with Klinefelter have a taller-than-average stature, a shorter torso, longer legs, and broader hips.

 Examine reflexes in patients with hypertension and pre-eclampsia. Hyperreflexia could indicate neurological involvement and be a sign of existing or impending eclampsia.

Gynaecological examination

 It is important to ask about previous experiences prior to the gynaecological exam and to communicate clearly with the patient throughout the exam, maintaining eye contact and announcing physical contact. Ask permission for each step of the exam and keep reassuring the patient. Explain what you will be doing and ask if the patient wants a mirror to follow along. In some countries you are required to offer a chaperone for gynaecological exams.

General impression

When the patient enters the room, when taking her history, and when conducting the physical examination, pay attention to the following:

- Physique: anorexia nervosa, adiposity, posture (e.g. in case of abdominal pain)
- Dysmorphic facial features, webbed neck (Turner syndrome), or other dysmorphic features
- Hygiene
- Hair: hair in the usual places (e.g. around external genitalia, under armpits), hirsutism (e.g. facial hair, abdominal hair, excessive hair growth elsewhere, like the extremities)
- Skin pathology: non-facial acne, skin pathology around external genitalia
- Tanner stages and puberty development

Signs of hormonal imbalance include abnormal hair distribution, abnormal physique, absence of secondary sexual characteristics, skin pathology.

External genitalia
🔍 Inspection

Perineum, vulva, labia majora, labia minora, clitoris, vagina, introitus, hymenal remnants, Bartholin's and Skene's glands, urethra, prolapse prompted by Valsalva manoeuvre, discharge (odour, colour, blood, volume), skin pathology, scratch marks, scarring, perineum, mucosal pathology, ulcers, warts, masses, lichenification (figure of eight (vulvar/perineal/anal), burying of the clitoris under preputium, hyperkeratosis, hypopigmentation, vaginal introitus narrowing), signs of virilisation (e.g. clitoral megaly).

 Visible scratch marks, abnormal discharge (e.g. odour, colour, volume), and red discolouration of the vulva/labia may be consistent with candidiasis. Vesicles, ulcers, and warts may be signs of an STI.

🖢 Palpation

Vulva, labia majora, labia minora, femoral artery, inguinal canal (suspected inguinal/femoral hernia, with/without Valsalva manoeuvre), inguinal lymph nodes.

Internal genitalia
🔍 Inspection (speculum exam):

- Vagina: vaginal wall (e.g. atrophy, colour, abnormalities), macroscopic abnormalities, blood/contact bleeding, discharge (e.g. odour, colour, amount, consistency), prolapse (e.g. cystocele, rectocele, uterine – can be evaluated by rotating speculum to a vertical position and partially opening it (this will cause a cystocele or rectocele to bulge)).
- Cervix: appearance of transitional zone epithelium, Nabothian cysts, intrauterine device (wires in situ), ectropion (position, shape, size), colour, external os (size, position, discharge, shape (pinpoint/slit)), vaginal portion, uterine prolapse, suspected cervical tumour.
- Fornices: atrophy, epithelial defects, fistulas, discolouration, location (superficial/deep), signs of inflammation, trauma, anterior and posterior wall, masses, dark spots in posterior fornix (e.g. in endometriosis).
- If indicated, a PAP smear can be performed during the speculum exam as well

as a PCR (e.g. for *Chlamydia* and/or *gonorrhoea*). Figure 18 shows a normal cervix during a speculum exam.

 To properly assess a vaginal prolapse, use a single-blade Sims' speculum if available or with the patient in a lateral position.

 Practitioners are warned against using lubricant when performing a PCR test, although there is no evidence supporting this. Use a small amount of lubricant when performing a smear test. Cytology results may be unreliable/uninterpretable if too much lubricant is used. If possible, avoid performing a smear test during menstruation or pregnancy as this may also lead to inconclusive results.

 Speculum and vaginal examinations in virgins are typically reserved for situations with hard indications when alternative diagnostics are insufficient, and the patient may undergo anaesthesia for the examination if deemed necessary.

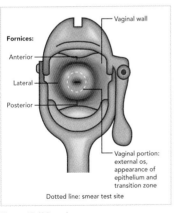

Fornices:
Anterior
Lateral
Posterior

Vaginal wall

Vaginal portion: external os, appearance of epithelium and transition zone

Dotted line: smear test site

Figure 17 // Speculum exam

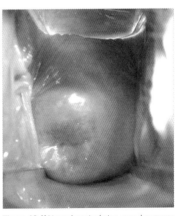

Figure 18 // Normal cervix during speculum exam

➤ Palpation

Vaginal exam

- Vaginal portion: motility, consistency (firm, firm-elastic, weak), tenderness, size, surface, shape, uterine prolapse.

- External os: size, position, shape, is the os open (e.g. in retained placenta, incomplete miscarriage) or closed.
- Adnexal motion tenderness: tenderness when the cervix and uterus are pushed up towards the abdominal wall. To check this, the examiner places their fingers in the posterior fornix.
- Cervical motion tenderness: tenderness when the cervix is gently moved back and forth between two fingers. Uterine mobility should also be checked.
- Pelvic floor: muscle tone (e.g. strength, ability to relax, contraction endurance) and prolapse (e.g. urethral mobility, bladder, uterine or rectal prolapse prompted by coughing/straining/Valsalva manoeuvre).
- Pouch of Douglas: pain on palpation, palpable thickening consistent with endometriosis or other tumours.
- Uterosacral ligaments: palpable thickening (e.g. in endometriosis).

 Discreetly inspect the glove for blood, mucus, smelly/inodorous discharge, or pus after vaginal and rectal exams (in pregnant women, also check for signs of amniotic fluid and meconium).

 Pouch of Douglas pain can indicate various pathologies, e.g. endometriosis, tubal rupture in ectopic pregnancy, colitis, tumours.

Bimanual exam
- Uterus: uterine position (anteversion-flexion (AVF)/retroversion-flexion (RVF)/anteversion-retroflection (AVRF)), motility, consistency, tenderness, size, surface, shape.
- Adnexa: location, size, consistency, pain (e.g. adnexitis, cysts).

Rectovaginal exam
- Assess sphincter tone, rectovaginal septum, posterior side of the vaginal portion and uterus, bulging pouch of Douglas, and uterosacral ligament (e.g. involvement of surrounding structures in endometriosis, suspected pelvic tumour).

Performing the Valsalva manoeuvre during inspection or during a speculum exam, vaginal exam, or rectovaginal exam may reveal a prolapse (depending on location and severity). The POP-Q quantification system is used for prolapse staging (see the section on General Gynaecology, Prolapse).

Touch test

The touch test, or Q-tip test, involves touching the vulva with a cotton swab. The test is positive if the patient reports severe pain when the vulva is gently touched between 4 and 8 o'clock (posterior commissure) relative to the introitus (see Figure 20). Indications for this test include suspected provoked vulvodynia (PVD) and vaginismus. The touch test should be performed prior to the speculum exam and vaginal exam if the differential diagnosis includes one of the above-mentioned diagnoses. It may not be possible to perform a speculum exam or vaginal exam if this test is positive.

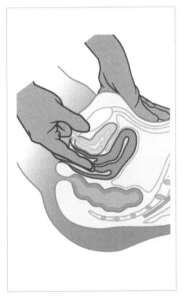

Figure 19 // Bimanual exam

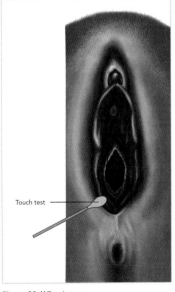

Touch test

Figure 20 // Touch test

Breast examination
🔍 Inspection

Symmetry, size, contour variations, retraction phenomenon (dimpling), skin discolouration, shape, masses, peau d'orange, nipple (eczema, discolouration, retraction, discharge), ulceration.

 Breast exam should be performed from the front, left and right, with both arms raised and abducted, with pectoralis major contraction and bending forward.

👉 Palpation

Nipple fixation, axillary, supraclavicular and infraclavicular lymph nodes, nipple discharge, masses.

 The breast can be examined with the patient lying down, sitting, or standing. When examining the breast lying down, ask the patient to prop up her head with her ipsilateral hand. The breast is divided into four quadrants: start palpation in the medial upper quadrant and palpate around the nipple, the breast, and the axillary tail (see Figure 21). Abnormalities should be described in the same order.

 There are two methods for palpating the breast: the concentric circle method (moving around the nipple and breast in two circles) and the wagon wheel or spoke method. It is particularly important that all breast tissue be examined.

 When performing a breast exam, adhesions must be ruled out, as they may be suggestive of malignancies or other pathology. When evaluating masses, note their size, shape, consistency, margins, motility, and pain.

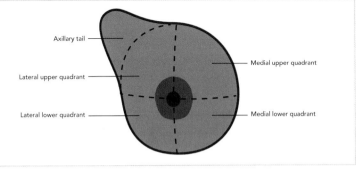

Figure 21 // Breast exam quadrants (right breast)

Obstetrical examination

1st trimester

🔍 Inspection

Anorexia/adiposity, congenital abnormalities/pathology, pelvic shape/position, skin pathology, scarring (e.g. previous caesarean section).

Speculum exam

Cervical assessment if indicated: position, cervical dilation, possible blue discoloration due to venous stasis, macroscopic abnormalities, bleeding, vaginal discharge (odour, colour, amount, consistency), amniotic fluid prompted by Valsalva manoeuvre.

🖐 Palpation

Tingling/tenderness, masses, fundal height (fetal growth).

2nd/3rd trimester

🔍 Inspection

Weight gain, peripheral oedema, abdominal circumference, striae, navel and umbilical hernia, scarring, wounds, signs of infection, pigmentation, petechiae (possible risk of bleeding), jaundice, scratch marks, spider naevi.

🖐 Palpation

- Fundal height: measured to chart uterine growth (see Figure 22).
- Leopold manoeuvres (see Figure 23): estimate fetal weight and position

(cephalic, breech or transverse), amniotic fluid (oligohydramnios, polyhydramnios), fetal engagement.

- Vaginal exam: presentation (cephalic/breech), cervical effacement, dilation, ruptured membranes, engagement (Hodge plane 1-4), anterior part: head (e.g. left occipitooccipital-anterior, right occipitooccipital-posterior), breech (complete, incomplete, complete footling).

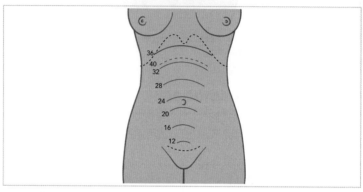

Figure 22 // Fundal height in relation to gestational age

 Fundal height is generally calculated in centimetres, e.g. gestational age ±2 cm. At a gestational age of 20 weeks, fundal height should be approximately 18 cm.

Leopold manoeuvres
Leopold 1: measurement of fundal height and cephalic or breech presentation
Place both hands on either side of the fundus and gently apply pressure to identify which fetal part is present. The first manoeuvre aims to determine fundal height and fetal position. The podalic pole is softer than the cephalic pole (see Figure 23).

Leopold 2: evaluation of back position
Place both hands flat on either side of the uterus. The position of the back can be determined by palpating for varying levels of resistance, with the back of the fetus providing the most uniform resistance. The back of the fetus cannot be palpated in transverse position.

Leopold 3: evaluation of descent and mobility of presenting part

The presenting part is determined by grasping the lowest part of the fetus. To assess the engagement of the head, move the presenting part from left to right. The head can be distinguished from the rest of the fetus because it moves separately from the trunk (ballottement).

Leopold 4: evaluation of descent

For this manoeuvre, the examiner faces away from the patient and looks at their feet. The examiner asks the patient to exhale and partially raise her legs. The nature and degree of descent are determined by palpating the area between the pubic symphysis and the presenting part with the fingertips of both hands.

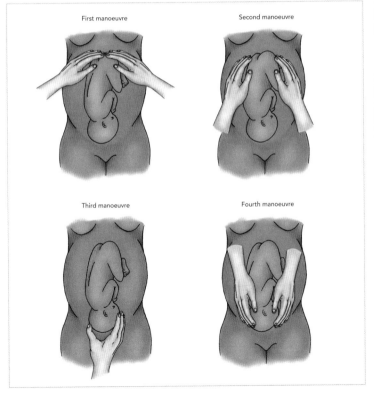

First manoeuvre

Second manoeuvre

Third manoeuvre

Fourth manoeuvre

Figure 23 // Leopold manoeuvres

Modified early obstetric warning score (MEOWS)

MEOWS is a scale used to score vital signs in ill pregnant patients. These scores may indicate the need for further diagnostics or active intervention (see Table 9). Indications for further diagnostics or treatment based on MEOWS score:

- One yellow flag: increase monitoring frequency
- Two yellow flags or one red flag: monitor <15 minutes and initiate diagnostics and treatment.

PARAMETER	YELLOW FLAG	RED FLAG
Systolic BP	150-160 mmHg	≥160 mmHg
Diastolic BP	100-110 mmHg	≥110 mmHg
Mean arterial pressure (MAP)	110-125 mmHg	≥125 mmHg
Pulse	100-120 bpm 40-50 bpm	≥120 bpm ≤40 bpm
Respiratory rate (RR)	20-30/min	≥30/min ≤8/min
Oxygen saturation	N/A	≤94%
Decreased consciousness	V = verbal: response to voice	P = pain: response to pain
Temperature	N/A	≥38°C, ≥100.4°F
Urine production		≤30 ml/h

Table 9 // Modified early obstetric warning score (MEOWS)

Fertility examination

Fertility evaluation aims to detect possible signs of anatomical or endocrine abnormalities that may explain subfertility or infertility.

 Abnormalities regarding the general impression of the patient may be indicative of an endocrine disorder (e.g. hormonal hirsutism due to overproduction of DHT in women, or gynaecomastia due to hypogonadism or medication in men).

Female fertility testing

🔍 Inspection

Acne, hair distribution, clitoromegaly, genitalia, weight, BMI, hirsutism, Tanner stage (see Table 10 and Figure 24).

Speculum exam

Scarring (surgery), vaginal portion (anatomic variation), blind vagina/absent vagina (in Mayer-Rokitansky-Küster-Hauser (MRKH) syndrome), vaginal septum.

Male fertility testing

🔍 Inspection

External genitalia (perineum, scrotum, foreskin and foreskin retraction, glans penis), testis (descended/undescended), hair distribution, inguinal hernia (with/without Valsalva manoeuvre), urethral meatus, Tanner stage (see Figure 24).

👉 Palpation

Corpora cavernosa and spongiosum, dribbling (before and after emptying urethra), epididymis (spermatocele), funiculus, rectal exam incl. prostate palpation (consistency, tenderness, size, irregularities, surface, sulcus, symmetry), testes (size, location, hydrocele, seminoma, varicocele, masses), ductus deferens, femoral artery, inguinal hernia (with/without Valsalva manoeuvre).

Stage 1	No glandular breast tissue palpable, no hair
Stage 2	Breast bud palpable under areola, downy hair
Stage 3	Breast tissue palpable outside areola, scant terminal hair
Stage 4	Elevated areola above the breast contour, terminal hair at the entire triangle overlying the pubic region
Stage 5	Visible breast contour with papillae development, areolar hyperpigmentation and nipple protrusion, terminal hair extending beyond the inguinal creases and thighs

Table 10 // Tanner stages women

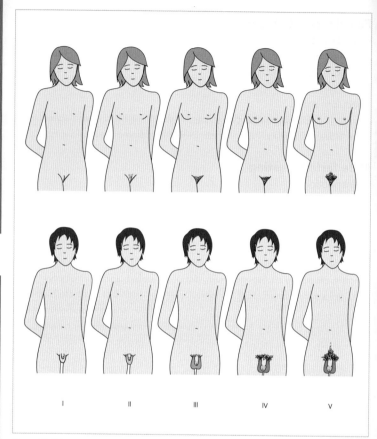

Figure 24 // Tanner stages

Determine Tanner stages in case of primary amenorrhoea, e.g.:
- Delay in breast development or discrepancy with pubic hair development could indicate a disturbance in the hypothalamic-pituitary-ovarian axis.
- When menarche does not start within five years of breast development (thelarche), it may be a sign of abnormalities of the internal genitalia.
- Absence or minimal pubic hair development can be a sign of androgen insensitivity syndrome.

Diagnostics

Lab values

 Reference values may vary between laboratories. Test results should preferably be compared to previous values. Request them from the patient's GP or another hospital if necessary.

While the following section provides examples of conditions associated with altered lab values, it is essential to acknowledge that the scope of medical diagnoses is vast and varied.

 When interpreting laboratory results, it is crucial to consider them in the context of all findings. For example, an isolated thrombocytopaenia has a completely different differential diagnosis than thrombocytopaenia with anaemia and leukopaenia (pancytopaenia).

General blood count

LAB VALUE	EXPLANATION	INTERPRETATION

Haemoglobin (Hb)	Protein in erythrocytes that can bind and carry oxygen	↑ Polycythaemia:
		• Primary polycythaemia:
		  - Congenital
		  - Acquired: malignant bone marrow disease
		• Secondary polycythaemia:
		  - Secondary to hypoxia: e.g. COPD or smoking, sleep apnoea, high altitudes, right-to-left shunts, congestive heart failure
		  - Secondary to kidney disease
		  - Secondary to EPO-producing tumour
		  - Secondary to alcohol use disorder
		↓ Anaemia, see Table 12

Haematocrit (Ht)	Measure of red blood cell volume in relation to total blood volume	↑ • Dehydration • Primary or secondary polycythaemia ↓ • Anaemia

Table 11A // General blood count

LAB VALUE	EXPLANATION	INTERPRETATION
Mean corpuscular volume (MCV)	Measure of the average volume of erythrocytes, see Table 12	↑ Macrocytic = Normocytic ↓ Microcytic
Platelet count (PLT)	• Platelets/thrombocytes • Are primary haemostasis by aggregation	↑ Thrombocytosis: • During/after infection/inflammation • Splenectomy/hyposplenism • Iron deficiency • Myeloproliferative disease • Paraneoplastic ↓ Thrombocytopaenia: • Synthesis ↓: bone marrow insufficiency, e.g. tumour invasion/medication-induced, deficiencies (vitamin B12, folic acid), liver disease (e.g. liver cirrhosis), hyperthyroidism/hypothyroidism • Utilisation/degradation ↑: disseminated intravascular coagulation (DIC), immune thrombocytopaenia (ITP), medication-induced immune thrombocytopaenia, post-transfusion, pre-eclampsia/HELLP, viral infection (e.g. CMV, EBV, hepatitis B/C, HIV), parasitic infection (malaria), idiopathic, heparin-induced thrombocytopaenia (HIT) • Loss ↑: blood loss, splenomegaly (e.g. in portal hypertension) • Other causes: gestational thrombocytopaenia, hereditary thrombocytopaenia (e.g. Bernard-Soulier syndrome) • Watch out for pseudothrombocytopenia: false lower result due to agglutination in EDTA tube

Table 11B // General blood count

DIAGNOSTICS

Anaemia - interpretation

HB	MCV	DIFFERENTIAL DIAGNOSIS
↓	↓	• Iron-deficiency anaemia (chronic blood loss) • Haemoglobinopathy • Other causes: lead poisoning ⊖, sideroblastic anaemia ⊖, hookworm infection ⊖
	↓/=	Anaemia of chronic disease (e.g. infections, malignancy, autoimmune diseases)
	=	• Acute blood loss • Long-term chronic kidney disease (EPO deficiency) • Malnutrition • Mixed-aetiology anaemias • Multiple myeloma

	=/↑	• Haemolysis
		• Medication-induced
		• Thyroid dysfunction (specifically hypothyroidism)
		• Haematological malignancy
		• Bone marrow disease:
		  - Aplastic anaemia
		  - Bone marrow filtration
		  - Myelodysplastic syndrome

↓	↑	• Vitamin B12 deficiency (e.g. malabsorption, HIV) • Folic acid deficiency • Pregnancy • Toxic: alcohol use disorder, medication-induced (e.g. cytostatics)

Table 12 // Anaemia - interpretation

 For the differential diagnosis of anaemia, the iron panel is essential, see Iron panel.

Arterial blood gas (ABG)

LAB VALUE	EXPLANATION	INTERPRETATION
1. pH 7.35-7.45	Hydrogen ion concentration in the blood	↑ Alkalosis ↓ Acidosis

2. $PaCO_2$
35-45 mmHg
(4.7-6.0 kPa)
	Partial pressure of carbon dioxide	↑ • Respiratory acidosis: hypoventilation, type II respiratory insufficiency (e.g. COPD)
		  • Respiratory compensation in metabolic alkalosis
		↓ • Respiratory alkalosis: hyperventilation
		  • Respiratory compensation in metabolic acidosis

Table 13A // Arterial blood gas (ABG)

LAB VALUE	EXPLANATION	INTERPRETATION

3. HCO_3^- 22-26 mEQ/L	Buffer for H^+	↑ Metabolic alkalosis:
		• Loss of H^+:
		  - Gastrointestinal loss (e.g. vomiting, diarrhoea (with Cl^-))
		  - Renal loss (e.g. activation of RAAS due to primary hyperaldosteronism, heart failure, cirrhosis)
		  - Intracellular H^+ shift (as in hypokalaemia)
		• Increase in HCO_3^-:
		  - Renal retention (e.g. loop and thiazide diuretics)
		  - Cystic fibrosis
		↓ Metabolic acidosis:
		• Increase in H^+:
		  - Excessive production (e.g. ketoacidosis, lactate acidosis, rhabdomyolysis)
		  - Renal insufficiency (impaired H^+ excretion)
		  - Intoxications with exogenous acids (e.g. toxic alcohols, salicylates)
		  - Hyperchloraemia
		• Loss of HCO_3^-:
		  - Gastrointestinal (e.g. severe diarrhoea, laxative use, gastrointestinal fistulas)
		  - Renal loss
		  - Medication (e.g. spironolactone)

4. HCO_3^- 22-26 mEQ/L	Base excess or deficit needed to get pH to 7.40	↑ • Metabolic alkalosis • Metabolic compensation in respiratory acidosis ↓ • Metabolic acidosis • Metabolic compensation in respiratory alkalosis
5. Anion gap (only in metabolic acidosis) 4-12 mmol/L	• Number of unmeasured anions (negatively charged particles, including albumin, SO_4^{2-} and HPO_4^{2-}) • Formula: $[Na^+]$ - $([Cl^-] + [HCO_3^-])$	↑ Due to increase in H^+: • Endogenous: lactic acidosis, ketoacidosis, renal insufficiency • Exogenous: intoxications, e.g. ethylene glycol, methanol, salicylate = Due to loss of HCO_3^- (compensated by higher levels of chloride): • Gastrointestinal loss of HCO_3^- (urine anion gap -) (accompanied by Cl^- retention in the kidneys), e.g. diarrhoea • Renal loss (urine anion gap +), e.g. hyperchloraemia • Addison's disease
6. PaO_2 75-100 mmHg 10.0-13.3 kPa	Partial pressure of oxygen	↑ Hyperventilation ↓ Type I respiratory insufficiency: • Hypoventilation • Ventilation perfusion mismatch • Diffusion disorder • Right-to-left shunt

Table 13B // Arterial blood gas (ABG)

LAB VALUE	EXPLANATION	INTERPRETATION
7. SaO$_2$ ≥95%	Oxygen saturation of haemoglobin	↓ Oxygen deficiency, e.g. carbon monoxide poisoning
8. Lactate 0.5-1.7 mmol/L	End product of anaerobic glycolysis	↑ Diminished tissue oxygenation (lactate acidosis), e.g. sepsis, hypoxaemia

Table 13C // Arterial blood gas (ABG)

- Decreased albumin can result in a false low anion gap (AG) AG = $Na^+ - (Cl^- + HCO_3^-)$.
- Oxygen saturation (sO$_2$) measures the saturation of functional Hb = $O_2Hb/(O_2Hb + deoxyHb)$. As a result, the saturation of haemoglobinopathies such as carboxyHb, MetHb, and SulfHb is not measured. In the presence of dyshaemoglobins, oxygen saturation is an unreliable metric (overestimation) and measuring the oxygen fraction is preferred.
- An air bubble in the sample will produce anomalous pCO$_2$ (decreased) and pO$_2$ (increased) values due to gas diffusion.

In practice, a venous or capillary blood gas test usually provides the necessary information and is more comfortable for the patient. Arterial blood gas tests are only needed for measuring the Aa gradient (difference between pO$_2$ in alveoli vs. in arterial blood).

The common causes of anion gap acidosis can be recalled using the mnemonic MUDPILES: **m**ethanol, **u**raemia, **d**iabetic ketoacidosis, **p**ropylene glycol, **i**soniazid, **i**ron, **l**actic acidosis, **e**thylene glycol, **s**alicylates.

Blood gas - interpretation

	PH	pCO$_2$	HCO$_3^-$	ANION GAP	COMPENSATION MECHANISM
Respiratory alkalosis	↑/=	↓	↓/=		↓ Renal [HCO$_3$] reabsorption (slow)
Metabolic alkalosis	↑/=	↑/=	↑		Hypoventilation (fast)

Table 14A // Blood gas - interpretation

DIAGNOSTICS

	PH	pCO$_2$	HCO$_3^-$	ANION GAP	COMPENSATION MECHANISM
Respiratory acidosis	↓/=	↑	↑/=		↑ Renal [HCO$_3$] reabsorption (slow)
High anion gap metabolic acidosis	↓/=	↓/=	↓	↑	Hyperventilation
Normal anion gap metabolic acidosis	↓/=	↓/=	↓	=	Hyperventilation

Table 14B // Blood gas - interpretation

Electrolytes

LAB VALUE	EXPLANATION	INTERPRETATION

Sodium (Na⁺)	• Main extracellular cation
	• Very important in water management
		↑ Hypernatraemia:
		  • Increased water loss:
		    - Osmotic diarrhoea or diuresis (e.g. hyperglycaemia, mannitol)
		    - Arginine vasopressin deficiency (e.g. cranial trauma, infections, autoimmune)
		    - Arginine vasopressin resistance (e.g. drugs, amyloidosis, hereditary)
		  • Increased sodium retention (iatrogenic with unchecked IV drip)
		  • Insufficient fluid intake (with or without intact thirst stimulus)
		↓ Hyponatraemia: often multiple causes
		  • Water retention:
		    - Syndrome of inappropriate antidiuretic hormone secretion (SIADH)
		    - Renal insufficiency stage 5
		    - Congestive heart failure
		    - Liver cirrhosis
		    - Blood loss (resulting in ADH ↑ to preserve volume)
		    - Nephrotic syndrome
		  • Increased sodium loss:
		    - Gastrointestinal, e.g. diarrhoea, small bowel obstruction
		    - Renal, e.g. diuretics, renal failure, osmotic diuresis (severe hyperglycaemia), Addison's disease
		    - Transdermal, e.g. burns, excessive sweating
		  • Other:
		    - Tea & toast (malnutrition)
		    - Polydipsia

Table 15A // Electrolytes

LAB VALUE	EXPLANATION	INTERPRETATION

Potassium (K^+)	• Main intracellular cation
	• Regulates e.g. nerve impulse transmission, glycogen and protein synthesis
		↑ Hyperkalaemia:
		• Extracellular redistribution (shift):
		  - Metabolic or respiratory acidosis
		  - Hyperosmolality
		  - Insulin deficiency
		  - Medication-induced, e.g. beta blockers, digoxin
		• Tissue breakdown (often in combination with LDH, AST, bilirubin):
		  - Haemolysis
		  - Tumorlysis
		  - Rhabdomyolysis
		  - Distal arterial occlusion
		• Impaired renal excretion:
		  - Mineralocorticoid deficiency
		  - Renal insufficiency
		  - Medication-induced, e.g. ACE inhibitors, NSAIDs, potassium-sparing diuretics
		  - Type IV renal tubular acidosis
		• Pseudohyperkalaemia (e.g. following blood collection)
		↓ Hypokalaemia:
		• Intracellular redistribution:
		  - Metabolic or respiratory alkalosis
		  - Insulin use
		• Renal loss:
		  - Renal conditions, e.g. type I and II renal tubular acidosis
		  - Hyperaldosteronism
		  - Medication-induced, e.g. diuretics, glucocorticoids
		  - Hypomagnesaemia
		  - Chronic metabolic acidosis
		• Extrarenal loss, e.g. gastrointestinal (diarrhoea)
		• Insufficient intake, e.g. chronic alcohol use disorder

Table 15B // Electrolytes

Liver tests and pancreatic tests

LAB VALUE	EXPLANATION	INTERPRETATION

Alanine transaminase (ALT)	Enzyme found primarily in hepatocytes	↑ • Liver conditions:
		   - Hepatitis, e.g. viral, toxic, alcoholic (ALT<AST), autoimmune, ischaemic
		   - Non-alcoholic steatohepatitis
		   - Liver cirrhosis
		   - Hepatocellular carcinoma/liver metastases
		   - Medication-induced liver injury
		   - Liver abscess
		   - Acute liver failure
		   - Haemochromatosis
		   - Wilson's disease
		   - Primary biliary cholangitis/primary sclerosing cholangitis
		 • Bile duct obstruction, see ALP
		 • Chronic/acute pancreatitis
		 • Budd-Chiari syndrome
		 • Pre-eclampsia/HELLP
		 • Hypotension, i.e. septic shock

Aspartate aminotransferase (AST)	Enzyme found mainly in liver and striated (i.e. cardiac, skeletal) muscle tissue	↑ • In all diagnoses mentioned in ALT
		 • May also be elevated in:
		   - Myocardial infarction/heart failure
		   - Muscle conditions, e.g. rhabdomyolysis, dermatomyositis

Alkaline phosphatase (ALP)	Enzyme found primarily in liver parenchyma, bile epithelium, and osteoblasts	↑ • Bile duct obstruction:
		   - Cholelithiasis
		   - Cholangitis
		   - Hepatocellular carcinoma, cholangiocarcinoma, liver metastases
		   - Pancreatic malignancy
		   - Medication-induced
		   - Pregnancy
		 • Liver conditions:
		   - Hepatitis, e.g. alcoholic
		   - Primary biliary cholangitis
		   - Primary sclerosing cholangitis
		 • Bone disease (isolated elevation of ALP):
		   - Hyperparathyroidism
		   - Bone metastases
		   - Paget's disease
		   - Osteomyelitis or fractures

Table 16A // Liver tests and pancreatic tests

LAB VALUE	EXPLANATION	INTERPRETATION

Gamma-glu-tamyltrans-ferase (GGT)	· Enzyme present in virtually all cells
	· Serum GGT generally comes from the hepato-biliary system
		↑ · Bile duct obstruction, see ALP
		· Liver conditions:
		  - Primary biliary cholangitis
		  - Primary sclerosing cholangitis
		  - Hepatitis, e.g. alcoholic
		· Alcohol use
		· Obesity

Bilirubin	· Degradation product of haemoglobin · Mainly formed in the spleen → conjugated in the liver → excreted with bile	↑ Hyperbilirubinaemia: · Prehepatic (unconjugated): excessive formation of bilirubin (direct bilirubin <20%), e.g. haemolysis, haematoma resorption · Hepatic (unconjugated and conjugated): liver disease, Gilbert's disease · Posthepatic (conjugated): bile duct obstruction (direct bilirubin >50%, ALP ↑, GGT ↑)

Lactate de-hydrogenase (LDH)	Enzyme involved in glycolysis in various tissues	↑ · Increased cellular death in:
		  - Liver conditions
		  - Myocardial infarction
		  - Muscle conditions
		  - Haemolysis
		· Malignancies (specifically lymphoma, haema-tological malignancy)

Lipase	· Enzyme that hydroly-ses triglycerides to fatty acids and glycerides
	· Serum lipase is largely pancreas-specific
	· Released into circulation during autolysis of pan-creatic tissue
	· Lipase has a higher sen-sitivity for pancreatitis and is released more of-ten than amylase
		↑ · Acute pancreatitis (with acute or chronic pan-creatitis there might be no elevation)
		· May also be elevated in:
		  - Renal insufficiency
		  - Diabetic ketoacidosis
		  - Bile duct disease
		↓ Exocrine pancreatic insufficiency

Table 16B // Liver tests and pancreatic tests

A combination of elevated AST and ALT (liver enzymes) indicates hepatocellular damage. The AST/ALT ratio can provide information about the underlying condition. ALT>AST could indicate viral or au-toimmune hepatitis and AST>ALT could indicate alcoholic hepatitis. A combination of bilirubin ↑, ALP ↑, and GGT ↑ indicates cholestasis.

DIAGNOSTICS

A decrease in the synthetic function of the liver indicates severe liver disease. The common assessing liver synthetic function are albumin, PT/INR, and glucose.

Proteins

LAB VALUE	EXPLANATION	INTERPRETATION

Albumin	· Half of all blood proteins
	· Produced by the liver
	· Main protein for osmotic pressure, also a transport protein
	· Negative acute-phase protein
	· Non-specific marker of liver synthetic function
	· Necessary for interpretation of calcium level
		↑ Hyperalbuminaemia:
		  · Dehydration
		↓ Hypoalbuminaemia:
		  · Reduced synthesis:
		    - Liver disease (e.g. liver cirrhosis, hepatitis, malignancy)
		    - Inflammatory processes
		    - Malnutrition/malabsorption
		    - Hypothyroidism
		  · Increased degradation:
		    - Cushing's syndrome
		    - Malignancies
		    - Hyperthyroidism
		  · Increased loss:
		    - Renal, e.g. nephrotic syndrome
		    - Gastrointestinal, e.g. IBD
		    - Ascites (exudate)
		    - Burns
		  · Haemodilution

Haptoglobin	· Protein that binds free haemoglobin · Positive acute-phase protein	↑ Inflammation ↓ · Utilisation in haemolysis (thus the haptoglobin is often suppressed or lowered due to haemolysis) or high cell turnover, e.g. sickle cell disease · Also reduced in impaired synthesis, e.g. severe liver disease, severe malnutrition

Table 17 // Proteins

DIAGNOSTICS

Inflammatory markers

LAB VALUE	EXPLANATION	INTERPRETATION
C-reactive protein (CRP)	• Positive acute-phase protein • Produced in the liver	↑ • Infections • Inflammation • Rheumatic conditions • Malignancies • Trauma • Thrombosis
White blood cell (WBC) count	• Leukocytes: white blood cells • Part of the immune system	↑ Leukocytosis: • Infections • Inflammatory processes • Autoimmune diseases • Myeloproliferative disease, e.g. leukaemia • Medication-induced, e.g. steroids • Smoking ↓ Leukopaenia: • Infections (due to utilisation) • Medication-induced/iatrogenic, e.g. chemotherapy, immunosupressants, antibiotics • Bone marrow deficiency • Splenomegaly (e.g. in portal hypertension) • Benign leukopaenia, seen in individuals of African, Middle Eastern, and West Indian descent • Other causes: B12 and folate deficiency

Table 18A // Inflammatory markers

 In various inflammations, e.g. in acute pancreatitis an elevated WBC precedes an increase in CRP (approx. 24 hours).

LAB VALUE	EXPLANATION	INTERPRETATION

Leukocyte differential	Breakdown of total leukocytes by subtype	↑ Neutrophilia:
		  • Bacterial infection, sepsis, myeloproliferative diseases
		↓ Neutropenia:
		  • Decreased production: severe infections, medication-induced/iatrogenic
		  • Increased utilisation/destruction: medication-induced antibody formation
		↑ Lymphocytosis:
		  • Infection, smoking, hyposplenism, lymphoproliferative disease
		↓ Lymphopenia:
		  • Infection, HIV, renal failure
		↑ Monocytosis:
		  • Bacterial/parasitic infection, myeloproliferative diseases, Hodgkin's disease, neutropenia, steroids
		↓ Monopenia:
		  • In neutropenia, hairy cell leukaemia, cytotoxic agents (e.g. chemotherapy)
		↑ Eosinophilia:
		  • Parasitic infection, allergic reactions, skin diseases, myeloproliferative diseases, hypereosinophilic syndrome
		↑ Basophilia:
		  • Allergic reactions, iron deficiency, chronic myeloid leukaemia, systemic mastocytosis, allergic reaction

Table 18B // Inflammatory markers

Renal function tests

LAB VALUE	EXPLANATION	INTERPRETATION

Creatinine	Degradation product of creatinine phosphate from muscle tissue, mainly excreted by glomerular filtration	↑ • Acute kidney injury, chronic kidney disease
		  • Medication-induced, e.g. trimethoprim, supplements
		  • Dehydration
		  • Muscle breakdown (e.g. rhabdomyolysis, myocardial infarction)
		  • Excessive meat consumption
		↓ • Significant fluid overload
		  • Low protein intake, e.g. malnutrition
		  • Reduced muscle mass, e.g. increasing age, females
		  • Hyperthyroidism

Table 19A // Renal function tests

LAB VALUE	EXPLANATION	INTERPRETATION
Creatinine-clearance	Plasma (in ml) cleared of creatinine per minute by glomerular filtration and secretion. Both serum creatinine and urine creatinine (24h collection) levels are needed.	• Prerenal kidney disease (decreased renal perfusion): e.g. hypovolaemia, hypotension, decreased circulating volume (e.g. congestive heart failure, hepatorenal syndrome), renal artery stenosis, medication-induced
Estimated glomerular filtration rate (eGFR, CKD-EPI)	• Estimation of GFR based on serum creatinine, sex, age, and weight as a marker for muscle mass • Relevant in chronic kidney disease (stages 1-5) • Only reliable in more or less stable kidney function	• Renal kidney disease (reduced clearance due to impaired glomeruli and/or tubules): e.g. acute tubular necrosis (e.g. ischaemia, nephrotoxic drugs), acute interstitial nephritis, diabetes mellitus, medication-induced • Postrenal kidney disease (urinary tract obstruction): e.g. urolithiasis, prostate carcinoma, benign prostatic hyperplasia, urinary retention
Osmolality	• Number of particles dissolved in 1 kg serum (osmolarity: in 1L) • Formula for 'effective osmolality': $2 \times [Na^+]$ + [glucose]	↑ Increased level of osmoles, e.g. Na^+, glucose, urea, or exogenous osmoles, e.g. toxic alcohols ↓ Decreased level of osmoles, e.g. Na^+, glucose, urea
Urea	• Waste product of hepatic protein metabolism • Reabsorbed in the kidneys	↑ • Prerenal, renal, or postrenal kidney disease (if urea/creatinine ratio ↑: prerenal) • Dehydration • Increased protein degradation, e.g. tissue damage, upper gastrointestinal bleeding • High-protein diet ↓ • Haemodilution • Pregnancy • Malabsorption/malnutrition • Severe liver damage

Uric acid/ urate	End product of purine metabolism	↑ • Increased production:
		  - Genetic
		  - Idiopathic
		  - Increased tissue breakdown, e.g. infections, malignancies
		  - Increased nucleic acid metabolism, e.g. leukaemia, lymphoma, haemolytic anaemia
		• Reduced renal secretion, e.g. renal insufficiency
		• Pre-eclampsia/HELLP
		↓ • Xanthine oxidase deficiency
		• Medication-induced

Table 19B // Renal function tests

Acute kidney disease - interpretation

ACUTE KIDNEY DISEASE	PRERENAL	RENAL
Osmolality (urine)	>500 mOsmol/kg	<350 mOsmol/kg
Na⁺ (urine)	<20 mmol/L	>40 mmol/L
Urea/creatinine ratio (serum)	>0.1 mmol/μmol	<0.1 mmol/μmol

Table 20 // Acute kidney disease - interpretation

 The 'effective osmolality' is important because these osmotically active substances cannot pass the semi-permanent cell membrane, and thus can cause water shifts (such as cerebral oedema). Urea, for example, can pass freely through the cell membrane and is unlikely to cause water shifts.

Clotting markers

LAB VALUE	EXPLANATION	INTERPRETATION

International normalised ratio (INR)	· Calculation based on prothrombin time (PT)
	· Measure of the extrinsic and common pathway of the coagulation cascade
	· Monitoring vitamin K anticoagulant therapy
	· Patient plasma PT / normalised plasma PT
		↑ · If prolonged PT + normal aPTT:
		  - Use of coumarines (vitamin K antagonists)
		  - Isolated factor VII deficiency
		  - Coagulation disorders, e.g. coagulopathy or mild vitamin K deficiency
		  - In acute or chronic liver failure. If chronic → progression of advanced liver cirrhosis.
		  - Acute disseminated intravascular coagulation (DIC)
		· If prolonged PT + prolonged aPTT:
		  - Factor I, II, V, X, or fibrinogen deficiency, combined factor deficiencies
		  - Liver failure
		  - Acute disseminated intravascular coagulation (DIC)
		  - Severe vitamin K deficiency
		  - Anticoagulants (e.g. warfarin, direct thrombin inhibitors, others)

Prothrombin test/ time (PT)	Test for the extrinsic and common pathway of the coagulation cascade	Activation of clotting in early disseminated intravascular coagulation ↓

Table 21A // Clotting markers

LAB VALUE	EXPLANATION	INTERPRETATION

Activated partial thromboplastin test/time (aPTT)	• Test for the intrinsic and common pathway of the coagulation cascade
	• Monitoring unfractionated heparin therapy
		↑ If prolonged aPTT + normal PT:
		  • Factor VIII (hemophilia A), factor IX (hemophilia B), factor XI (hemophilia C) deficiency
		  • Factor XII deficiency
		  • Von Willebrand disease
		  • Anticoagulants (unfractionated heparin therapy)
		  • Lupus anticoagulant
		↓ • Strong elevation one or more clotting factors (e.g. factor VIII due to stress)
		  • Activation of coagulation in early disseminated intravascular coagulation (DIC)
		  • Pregnancy (factor VIII ↑ and fibrinogen ↑)

D-dimer	Degradation product of fibrinolysis	↑ • Venous thrombosis (high sensitivity but low specificity)
		  • Pulmonary embolism (high sensitivity but low specificity)
		  • Disseminated intravascular coagulation
		  • Other causes (low specificity):
		    - Pregnancy
		    - Infection
		    - Renal insufficiency
		    - Trauma
		    - Malignancies
		    - Aortic dissection

Fibrinogen	• Coagulation factor produced in the liver
	• Converted into fibrin by thrombin
	• Positive acute-phase protein
		↑ • Inflammatory processes
		  • Trauma
		  • Pregnancy
		↓ • Decreased synthesis, e.g. liver disease
		  • Increased degradation:
		    - DIC
		    - Fibrinolysis
		  • Increased loss, e.g. after bleeding
		  • Medication-induced, e.g. tPA, streptokinase

Table 21B // Clotting markers

Miscellaneous

LAB VALUE	EXPLANATION	INTERPRETATION
Ammonia	Degradation product of proteolysis	↑ Hyperammonaemia: • Congenital urea cycle enzyme defects • Acquired: - Liver cirrhosis (90%) - Infections - Multiple myeloma - Acute leukaemia - Medication-induced
Glucose	• Blood sugar • Main energy source for all cellular processes	↑ Hyperglycaemia: • Impaired glucose tolerance, DM, diabetes gravidarum • Acute stress: trauma, sepsis, myocardial infarction, cerebrovascular accident • Medication: corticosteroids • Endocrinopathy: Cushing's syndrome, acromegaly Hypoglycaemia: ↓ • Medication-induced, e.g. sulphonylurea derivatives, insulin • Insulinoma • Fasting/malnutrition, alcohol • Liver failure • Endocrinopathy: hypocortisolism, panhypopituitarism
Glycated haemoglobin (HbA1c)	• Glycosylated haemoglobin, measure of average blood glucose concentration over the past 6-8 wk • Monitoring adherence and treatment effectiveness	↑ • DM or poorly controlled DM • Erythrocyte lifespan ↓ (falsely lower result), e.g. haemoglobinopathy • Target range in diabetics ≤53 (7%) to ≤64 mmol/mol (8%) depending on age, treatment, and duration of DM
Lactate	• End product of anaerobic glycolysis • Produced by muscle cells and red blood cells, especially in hypoxic state	↑ • Hypoxic states • Dehydration • Shock • Severe anaemia • Severe liver/kidney disease • Medication-induced (e.g. metformin, propofol), toxic (e.g. methanol, carbon monoxide)

Table 22 // Miscellaneous

DIAGNOSTICS

Iron panel

LAB VALUE	EXPLANATION	INTERPRETATION
Ferritin	• Main iron-storage protein • Most important marker for iron deficiency • Correlates with total body iron content • Positive acute-phase protein	↑ • Inflammation or infection • Haemochromatosis or iron-storage disease • Functional iron deficiency (anaemia of chronic disease) • Liver disease • Chronic kidney disease ↓ • Iron deficiency
Iron	• Measure of circulating iron (note: most iron is bound to transferrin) • Not a good parameter for iron-deficiency anaemia due to fluctuating serum levels • Component of heme in haemoglobin and myoglobin • Necessary for cellular energy metabolism, needed for the action of various enzymes (e.g. catalase, cytochrome) and neurotransmitters (e.g. serotonin, dopamine) • Absorption mainly in duodenum and jejunum	↑ • Haemochromatosis • Iron-loading anaemia (thalassaemia, haemolytic anaemia, aplastic anaemia) • Liver disease (hepatitis B or C, alcoholic liver disease) • Excess iron intake (high intake, multiple transfusion, IM/IV iron) • Iron deficiency ↓ • Anaemia of chronic disease (or inflammatory anaemia) • Polycythaemia vera
Transferrin	• Transport protein for iron and zinc • Measure of iron-binding capacity • Negative acute-phase protein	In combination with the other lab results from the iron panel
Transferrin saturation	• Iron-transport protein reflects both protein and iron status • Determination of iron status (deficiency or overload) • Formula: (serum iron level x 100) / total iron-binding capacity (another formula: ratio of serum iron to serum transferrin)	↑ • Iron overload • Sideroblastic anaemia ↓ • Iron deficiency (often in combination with TIBC ↑ and ferritin ↓) • Anaemia of chronic disease (TIBC =/↓) • Chronic infection or inflammation • Extensive malignancy • Kidney disease • Acute bone marrow depression (e.g. in acute inflammation) • Pregnancy

Table 23 // Iron panel

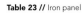

Iron status - interpretation

CONDITION	FERRITIN	MCV	TRANSFERRIN	TRANSFERRIN SATURATION
Iron-deficiency anaemia	↓	↓	↑	↓
Anaemia of chronic disease or inflammatory anaemia	=/↑	=/↓	=/↓	=/↓
Thalassaemia	↓/=/↑	↓	=	↑
Haemochromatosis	↑	=/↑	=/↓	↑ (>45%)

Table 24 // Iron status - interpretation

Nutritional panel

LAB VALUE	EXPLANATION	INTERPRETATION
Vitamin B1 (thiamine)	• Water-soluble vitamin • Involved in carbohydrate, fat and protein metabolism; cellular respiration and oxidation of fatty acids; mitochondrial energy production, protein synthesis, neurotransmitter synthesis	↓ • Poor intake: inadequate diet, chronic alcohol use disorder, bariatric surgery • Poor absorption: malabsorption syndrome, bariatric surgery, short bowel syndrome, vomiting, malnourishment • Increased utilisation: refeeding syndrome, pregnancy, breastfeeding, hyperthyroidism • Increased loss: dialysis, infection, diarrhoea, vomiting, systemic disease, medication-induced (e.g. diuretics)
Vitamin B9/B11 (folic acid or folate)	• Water-soluble vitamin • Necessary for protein and nucleic acid synthesis	↓ • Poor intake: inadequate diet, chronic alcohol use disorder • Poor absorption: diseases involving the jejunum (e.g. celiac disease, short bowel syndrome, amyloidosis), bariatric surgery, elevated pH • Increased loss: dialysis • Medication-induced (e.g. methotrexate, phenytoin, trimethoprim) • Pregnancy • Can cause megaloblastic anaemia

Table 25A // Nutritional panel

LAB VALUE	EXPLANATION	INTERPRETATION

Vitamin B12 (cobalamin)	• Water-soluble vitamin
	• Cofactor in DNA, fatty and amino acid metabolisation, maturation of red blood cells and myelin synthesis
		↑ Hypercobalaminaemia:
		  • Excessive supplementation
		  • Liver disease
		  • Kidney disease
		  • Diabetes mellitus
		  • Haematological malignancy
		  • Solid tumour
		↓ Pernicious (megaloblastic) anaemia
		  • Poor intake: diet lacking of animal products
		  • Poor absorption: bariatric surgery, terminal ileum disease (e.g. Crohn's disease, celiac disease, parasites, intestinal bacterial overgrowth)
		  • Recreational use of nitrous oxide

Table 25B // Nutritional panel

Tumour markers

LAB VALUE	EXPLANATION	INTERPRETATION
AFP	Alpha-fetoprotein: protein produced by a developing fetus that is not found in healthy men or non-pregnant women	↑ • Often in hepatocellular carcinoma • In scrotal or ovarian malignancies
Ca19.9	Glycolipid normally produced in healthy pancreatic tissue and gastric and gall-bladder epithelium	↑ • Often in pancreatic carcinoma or cholangiocarcinoma • In gastric or colorectal carcinoma, pancreatitis, cholestasis, cystic fibrosis
CEA	Carcinoembryonic antigen: protein produced by a developing fetus that is only present in healthy adults in very low concentrations	↑ • Often in colorectal carcinoma • In breast, lung, liver, pancreatic, gastric, and ovarian carcinomas • In smokers
Cancer antigen 125 (CA 125)	Mucine glycoproteïn: protein produced in fetal tissue, specific the epithelial cells of the coeloma	↑ • In ovarian malignancies • In benign diseases (e.g. endometriosis, liver cirrhosis), pregnancy or menstruation
ß-HCG	Hormone produced by trophoblast tissue, found in early embryos and placenta	↑ In ovarian malignancies (choriocarcinoma, germ cell tumours, hydatidiform mole, ectopic pregnancies)
Inhibin B	Peptide hormone produced by growing antral follicles	↑ In ovarian malignancies (granulosa cell tumours)

Table 26 // Tumour markers

Tumour markers are not only used to diagnose malignancies, they are mainly used to monitor the disease process, assess the effect of treatment, estimate metastasis, and monitor recurrence.

Gynaecology diagnostics

Transabdominal ultrasound (TAU)

TAU is used in both obstetric and gynaecological settings. TAU in obstetric patients is used from 12 weeks gestation. In gynaecological patients TAU is used to assess abdominal anatomy or identify macroscopic anatomical abnormalities of the internal genitalia extending beyond the pelvis (i.e. structures beyond the scope of TVU, see Figure 25). In virgin patients TAU is preferred in which a full bladder allows for better visualisation. When performing a gynaecological TAU, assess the following:

- Size and possible abnormalities of the uterus;
- Uterine cavity;
- Adnexa and any cysts/tumours;
- Presence of intra-abdominal free fluid.

In pregnant women, TAU can be used to assess the position, fetal anatomy, growth, location, placental position and possible macroscopic abnormalities (praevia, bilobata, vasa praevia, abruption, retroplacental haematoma), amniotic fluid index (AFI) and fetal movements, cardiac function and circulation (Doppler ultrasound). While performing a routine obstetric ultrasound, assess the following, always interpreting the findings according to gestational age:

- Presence of a fetus/gestational sac in the uterus and the number of fetuses;
- Viability of the fetus;
- In case of multiple fetuses, determine the type of multiple pregnancy;
- Fetal presentation (breech, transverse, cephalic);
- Fetal growth: biparietal diameter (BPD), head circumference (HC), femoral length (FL), abdominal circumference (AC);
- Location and structure of the placenta;
- Single deepest pocket (SDP) or AFI;
- Sex, when allowed according to local laws and requested by the parents.

Transvaginal ultrasound (TVU)

TVU is an ultrasound exam in which the transducer is inserted vaginally (see Figure 25). This exam produces a more detailed view of the cervix, uterus and ovaries because the sound waves have to pass through fewer layers of tissue than in a TAU. TVU is a standard diagnostic tool in gynaecological settings and indications include evaluating IUD placement, assessing uterine size, endometrial thickness and adnexa, early pregnancy detection (intrauterine, ectopic, or molar pregnancy), and suspected abortion. Indications for TVU in pregnant women include determining gestational age in the first trimester, assessing cervical length in suspected cervical insufficiency or premature contractions, localising the placenta and confirming Foley balloon placement.

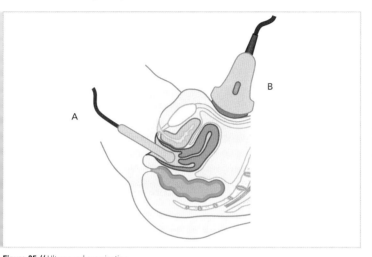

Figure 25 // Ultrasound examination
A: Transvaginal ultrasound (TVU) **B:** Transabdominal ultrasound (TAU)

Hysterosonography

Saline/gel infusion sonography (SIS/GIS), also known as water/gel contrast ultrasound, involves filling the uterus with contrast (water or gel) for improved imaging of intracavitary pathology. Indications for SIS/GIS include suspected intracavitary pathology (e.g. polyp, uterine myoma, uterine niche), abnormal vaginal bleeding, unexplained subfertility/infertility, habitual abortion.

Hysteroscopy

A hysteroscopy is a transvaginal exam in which the vagina, cervix and uterus are examined with a hysteroscope (see Figure 26). If necessary, a diagnostic hysteroscopy can be converted to a therapeutic hysteroscopy to treat certain conditions (e.g. coagulation, polyp or myoma removal, and IUD removal). Indications for diagnostic hysteroscopy include abnormal vaginal blood loss and suspected intracavitary pathology.

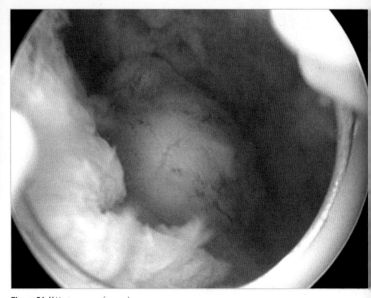

Figure 26 // Hysteroscopy for a submucous myoma

Laparoscopy

A laparoscopy is a diagnostic method in which a laparoscope is inserted into the abdominal cavity through an incision to visualise abnormalities of the uterus, fallopian tubes or ovaries (see Figure 27). If indicated, diagnostic laparoscopy can be converted to therapeutic laparoscopy (adnexectomy, cystectomy, removal of peritoneal, or deep infiltrating endometriosis). Indications for laparoscopy include suspected ovarian torsion, ectopic pregnancy, endometriosis and tumour staging.

Culdocentesis

A culdocentesis is a transvaginal puncture of the pouch of Douglas to sample free fluid to determine the origin. Indications for culdocentesis include analysing abdominal free fluid, ovarian cyst rupture and ovarian carcinoma. It is rarely performed nowadays but may be indicated for intra-abdominal lesions with an inconclusive diagnosis.

Less invasive procedures such as vaginal culture/blood culture (e.g. for suspected PID), and laparoscopy (e.g. for suspected ectopic pregnancy, or ovarian cyst rupture) have come to replace culdocentesis. Culdocentesis can help diagnose free fluid in the pouch of Douglas if other diagnostics remain inconclusive.

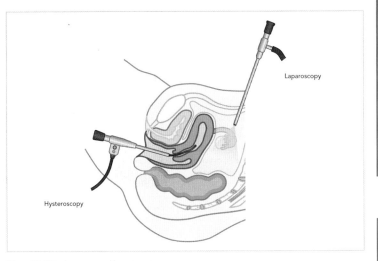

Figure 27 // Hysteroscopy and laparoscopy

Smear test

A smear test is a cytological exam to assess the presence of dysplastic cells. Samples are also examined for structural and functional changes, cell metabolism and nucleus differentiation to detect inflammatory cells and malignant cells. This is a screening test. The examiner inserts a brush into the cervix until it touches the vaginal wall and spins it around clockwise (see Figure 28). Smear test results are classified using PAP scores or the Bethesda system (see Table 27). Samples are also tested for HPV. Divergent samples (≥PAP II and high-risk HPV (hrHPV)-positive, HPV type 16 or 18, ASC-US/ASC-H/LSIL/HSIL, and hrHPV-positive) warrant follow-up colposcopy and possible biopsy or treatment. Indications for cytology include suspected cervical cell dysplasia or malignancy (bleeding on contact, abnormal cervical appearance) and suspected endometrial pathology with postcoital bleeding (pipelle biopsy is preferred in the latter case).

The WHO suggests using either of the following strategies for cervical cancer prevention among the female general population:

- HPV DNA detection in a screen-and-treat approach, screening every 5-10 years at age ≥30 → treat directly after positive HPV screening.
- HPV DNA detection in screen-triage-and-treat approach, screening every 5-10 years at age ≥30 → add partially genotyping HPV, cytology, use of visual inspection with acetic acid, and colposcopy.
- HIV-positive: HPV DNA detection in a screen-triage-and-treat approach, screening every 3-5 years at age ≥25.
- The age to start screening for HPV differs between countries.

LOW GRADE	HIGH GRADE
• Atypical squamous cells of undetermined significance (ASC-US): quantitatively and qualitatively fewer epithelial cell abnormalities than a squamous intraepithelial lesion (SIL). Can be associated with bacterial or yeast infections. • Low-grade squamous intraepithelial lesion (LSIL): epithelial changes that are typically associated with transient HPV infections	• Atypical squamous cells, can't rule out HSIL (ASC-H): cellular changes, high-grade lesions cannot be ruled out. Higher risk of underlying cervical lesions. • High-grade squamous intraepithelial lesion (HSIL): precancerous lesions that are most likely associated with persistent HPV infection; 8% 5-year risk of progression to cervical cancer

Table 27 // Smear test results

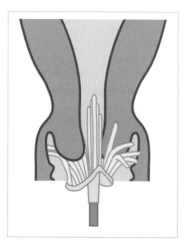

HPV self-collection kits, where people receive the HPV test by mail, can increase the number of participants in cervical cancer screening.

Discuss HPV vaccination with adolescent patients.

Figure 28 // Cervical smear test

Histology

Cervical histology results are given a cervical intraepithelial neoplasia (CIN) or carcinoma in situ (CIS) grade (see Table 28 and Figure 29). Indications for histology include suspected malignancy.

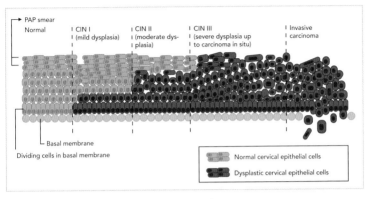

Figure 29 // Evolution of premalignant lesions in histological exams

Cervical intraepithelial neoplasia (CIN):
· Precursor lesion to squamous cell carcinoma.
· Characterised by epithelial dysplasia beginning at basal layer of the squamocolumnar junction and extending outwards.
· CIN I (mild), CIN II (moderate), CIN III (severe).

The **transformation zone** marks the transition from columnar to squamous epithelium and moves with age, starting from a more external location (fertile period) before receding (pre- and postmenopausal). The transformation zone is not visible in postmenopausal women.

RESULT	PAP SCORE	BETHESDA SYSTEM	CIN	SEVERITY OF CELLULAR PROLIFERATION
No result	PAP 0	Insufficient quality for assessment		
Normal result	PAP 1	No dysplasia		
Low-grade cervical dysplasia	PAP 2	ASC-US/LSIL	CIN1	• Mild dysplasia • Changes present in the lower third of the basal epithelium
	PAP 3a1			
High-grade cervical dysplasia	PAP 3a2	ASC-H/HSIL	CIN2	• Moderate dysplasia • Changes present in the lower one-third to two-thirds of the basal epithelium
	PAP 3b		CIN3	• Severe irreversible dysplasia or squamous carcinoma in situ • Changes present in over two-thirds of basal epithelium • Basement membrane still intact
	PAP 4	Endocervical adenocarcinoma in situ		• Adenocarcinoma in situ • Basement membrane still intact
Invasive cancer	PAP 5	Invasive cervical cancer		• Invasion beyond basement membrane of the cervical epithelium • Cervical adenocarcinoma • Endometrial carcinoma • Cervical squamous cell carcinoma

Table 28 // Cytological and histological classifications and findings for cervical neoplasia

Pipelle biopsy

In a pipelle biopsy, a thin tube is inserted into the uterus to take a sample of the endometrium. The main indication for pipelle biopsy is postmenopausal blood loss in conjunction with endometrial hyperplasia (>4 mm to exclude endometrial cancer).

Colposcopy

A colposcopy is a procedure in which the cervix is examined with a stereo microscope. This exam assesses the transformation zone for visual abnormalities. Acetic acid (3%) is often applied to the transformation zone first, followed by lugol, causing atypical cells to stain white/yellow. During a colposcopy, targeted biopsies should be taken from dysplastic areas if necessary. Indications for colposcopy include suspected CIN.

Treatments that can be performed during colposcopy if necessary are a large loop excision of the transformation zone (LLETZ), laser therapy (destruction of dysplastic cells with a laser beam), cryotherapy (freezing of dysplastic cells), thermal ablation (destruction of dysplastic cells by extreme temperature), and cold knife conisation (surgical removal of a cone-shaped inner cervix).

Discharge tests

Amine test

An amine test is performed by adding a drop of potassium hydroxide (POH) to a slide containing vaginal discharge. If an unpleasant fishy odour arises immediately, the test is postive. Indications for the amine test include suspected bacterial vaginosis and, in exceptional cases, *Trichomonas vaginalis*.

 The name 'amine test' derives from the ammonia produced by bacteria that emit a distinctively fishy odour in positive tests.

POH preparation

A drop of discharge is added to a POH preparation, causing the cellular walls to dissolve after a few minutes. This increases visibility under the microscope of hyphae present in a *Candida* infection (see Figure 30).

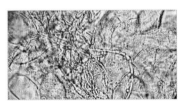

Figure 30 // POH preparation with hyphae

Sodium chloride preparation (0.9% NaCl)

A salt preparation can help identify microbes: mix fluor with a drop of NaCl on a slide. This can be used to visualise trichomonads (moving single-celled organisms with a flagella), clue cells and inflammatory cells under a microscope. Clue cells are suggestive of bacterial vaginosis.

 'Clue'
Clue cells are epithelial cells covered with bacteria and have fuzzy cell walls. This distinctive appearance makes them a key clue for bacterial vaginosis.

Fluoride testing in the NaCl preparation with a pH of 5.0-6.0 is suggestive of *Trichomonas*.

pH test

A pH test is performed by immersing a pH strip into a sample of vaginal discharge (normally 4.0-4.5). Elevated pH may be indicative of disturbed vaginal flora (see Table 29).

RESULTS INDICATIVE OF	AMINE TEST	POH PREPARATION	NaCl PREPARATION	pH TEST
Normal	-	-	No abnormalities	4.0-4.5
Aerobic vaginitis	-	-	Parabasal cells, leukocytes	>6.0
Bacterial vaginosis	+	-	Clue cells	4.0-4.5
Candida albicans	-	Hyphae, pseudo-hyphae and spores	Leukocytes ⊖	4.0-4.5
Trichomonas vaginalis	+/-	-	Trichomonads, leukocytes	5.0-6.0

Table 29 // Vaginal discharge test - indications and interpretation

Pictorial blood assessment chart

A pictorial blood assessment chart (PBAC), or period tracker, is a tool that lets patients chart the amount of menstrual blood loss during menstruation (see Figure 31). This can provide insight into cycle regularity and bleeding patterns and volume. Indications for PBAC include abnormal vaginal bleeding, an irregular cycle, intermenstrual bleeding, menorrhagia and dysmenorrhoea/oligomenorrhoea.

MENSTRUAL PADS	TAMPON	MENSTRUAL CUP	1	2	3	4	5	6	7	8

Figure 31 // Pictorial blood assessment chart, charting number of pads/tampons/cups used

Obstetrics diagnostics

Maternal and infant health can be monitored with various lab and imaging tests, depending on the gestational age (see Table 30).

 Routine Group B Streptococus (GBS) screening for all women from 36+0 to 37+6 weeks gestation, regardless of planned delivery method, unless prophylaxis is already indicated. Urgent screening for women with unknown GBS culture status in labour or with ruptured membranes.

Prenatal screening

Prenatal screening tests are performed prior to delivery to detect diseases and congenital, syndromal or chromosomal abnormalities. The most performed prenatal tests includes obstetric ultrasounds, labs and urinalysis. Indications for these standard tests include evaluating fetal growth, detecting structural fetal abnormalities, and determining or ruling out rhesus antagonism and gestational diabetes mellitus (GDM). The patient can opt to perform screening tests as early as possible in order to detect chromosomal abnormalities. Table 31 contains a list of prenatal screening tests and the gestational age at which they can first be performed. Figure 32 contains the possibilities of invasive prenatal testing.

TEST	1st TRIMESTER	WEEK 18-20	WEEK 26-30	WEEK 36-CHILDBIRTH
Ultra-sound	Gestational age, viability, prenatal screening for congenital abnormalities (nuchal translucency test)	Sex, viability, growth monitoring, structural ultrasound (e.g. screening for congenital heart disease, malformations of limbs, presence of cleft palate)	Viability, fetal position, AFI/SDP, monitoring growth if indicated	
Labs	Blood type, Hb, MCV, rhesus D/c, irregular erythrocyte antibodies (IEA), HbS-Ag, human immunodeficiency virus (HIV), syphilis, toxoplasmosis, CMV, rubella, glucose, TSH, optionally: NIPT (see Table 31)	Oral glucose tolerance test (OGTT) if indicated	Hb, MCV, if mother rhesus D/c-negative: repeat rhesus, IEA and fetal rhesus D antigen, OGTT if indicated	Hb, MCV
Urine	Dipstick, culture, proteinuria, GBS screening if indicated			

Table 30 // Diagnostics for different gestational age categories

TEST	DETERMINE/RULE OUT	TYPE OF TEST
Noninvasive prenatal test (NIPT)	Fetal chromosomal abnormalities (trisomy 13/18/21)	Blood test (see Figure 33)
Combination test (β-hCG + PAPP-A and nuchal translucency test)	Trisomy 13/18/21	Blood test and ultrasound (nuchal translucency test)
Chorion villus sampling	Genetic/chromosomal abnormalities	Needle aspiration of placental tissue
Amniocentesis		Needle aspiration of amniotic fluid
Cordocentesis	Fetomaternal blood group antagonism and treatment of fetal anaemia by transfusion via cordocentesis	Needle aspiration of the umbilical vein
Structural ultrasound	Fetal viability, growth, placental position, screening for congenital abnormalities (e.g. screening for congenital heart disease, malformations of limbs, presence of cleft palate)	Ultrasound
AUS (advanced ultrasound scanning)	Congenital abnormalities, growth monitoring, Dopplers	

Table 31 // Prenatal screening tests

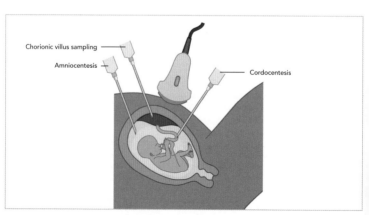

Chorionic villus sampling

Amniocentesis

Cordocentesis

Figure 32 // Invasive prenatal examinations

WHEN	RISKS/DISADVANTAGES
Week ≥11	• Invasive testing is required for confirmation. Only possible with mono-chorial twins, not dichorial twins or vanishing twins. • Placental mosaicism can lead to false-positive test results for common aneuploidies
Weeks 11-14	Provides a risk estimate, not conclusive. Possible for all twins, but not for vanishing twins.
Weeks 11-14	• Risk of abortion ±0.5% • Placental mosaicism → amniocentesis needed for confirmation
Ideally after weeks 16-17	Risk of miscarriage 2%
Week ≥18	Risk of miscarriage 1-2%, 3% procedure related loss and harm to mother
Week 20	Does not reveal all abnormalities
Ideally around week 20	

DIAGNOSTICS

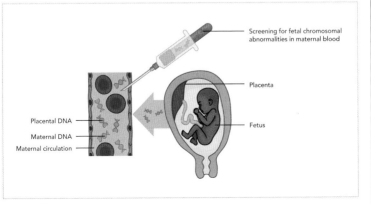

Screening for fetal chromosomal abnormalities in maternal blood

Placenta

Fetus

Placental DNA

Maternal DNA

Maternal circulation

Figure 33 // NIPT

The combined test can also pick up those with a high risk of other genetic syndromes and congenital heart disease.

 The NIPT is a maternal blood test taken from week 11, which screens for trisomy 13, 18, and 21. Maternal blood contains placental DNA, and can be used to screen for fetal chromosomal abnormalities. All women are first asked whether they are interested in receiving information about the test, and the test is always preceded by extensive counseling. The NIPT test can also be positive for maternal malignancies. The mother can decide whether she wants to be informed about such concomittant findings or not.

Oral glucose tolerance test (OGTT)

OGTT serves to determine/rule out GDM. Perform the OGTT when signs of GDM (e.g. macrosomia, polyhydramnios) are suspected. In the second trimester (24-28 weeks pregnant, regular screening), glucose day curves (GDC) are used to screen for GDM. OGTT at 16 weeks (early screening) is indicated for pregnant women with a history of GDM (repeat blood glucose curve/OGTT in second trimester if normal). The OGTT at 24-28 weeks is performed in case of BMI >30, previous child with macrosomia, first-degree family member with DM, certain ethnicities, PCOS, and IUFD. The first step in OGTT is determining the patient's fasted blood glucose level. Next, the patient drinks 75 gr glucose dissolved in 250 ml water and has their non-fasting blood glucose level taken two hours later (see Table 32). Patients with an abnormal OGTT are referred to a diabetes nurse. In principle, an OGTT is not performed in women with a history of bariatric surgery because of risk of dumping syndrome.

TIME	ABNORMAL GLUCOSE LEVEL	NORMAL GLUCOSE LEVEL
Fasted	≥7.0 mmol/L	>5.6-7.0 mmol/L
2 hours after glucose ingestion	≥7.8 mmol/L	<7.8 mmol/L

Table 32 // Diagnostic criteria for GDM after OGTT

Doppler ultrasound

Doppler ultrasonography uses ultrasound to hear and measure the velocity of blood flow in the great vessels. Doppler ultrasound combined with regular ultrasound (duplex) provides an audiovisual representation of blood flow. Doppler can be used to estimate vessel dilation/resistance (usually of the umbilical artery and middle cerebral artery (MCA)). Indications for Doppler ultrasound include fetal growth restriction (FGR), negative discordance and placental insufficiency.

 Brain sparing is a sign of FGR secondary to placental insufficiency. This sign can be detected on Doppler: intracerebral vessel resistance (based on the MCA) will be very low (high flow), resistance in the umbilical artery will be relatively high (low flow).

Cardiotocography (CTG)

CTGs are used to monitor fetal well-being during pregnancy and childbirth by charting fetal heart function (cardiography) and uterine activity (tocogram). A CTG can be performed from 24 weeks gestation, but is of diagnostic value only if it has therapeutic implications. CTGs are interpreted and classified in accordance with the FIGO guidelines, based on baseline heart rate, beat-to-beat variability and accelerations/decelerations (see Table 33). See Figure 34 for a normal CTG and Figure 35 for an abnormal CTG. There are two types of CTG:

- External: two transducers are placed on the mother's abdomen and secured with an elastic belt. One of the transducers records the fetal heart rate and the other records uterine contractility. Effectiveness can be limited by maternal central adiposity, movement, and fetal descent in late 2nd stage of labour.
- Internal: a scalp electrode is attached to the fetal head. This method is possible once the mother's membranes have ruptured, at 1-2 cm dilation. Uterine contractility can still be measured with an external transducer or an intrauterine pressure catheter.

 Contraindications for internal CTG are maternal infectious diseases (e.g. HIV, hepatitis B or C, and fetal coagulopathies/thrombocytopaenia).

Indications for CTG include all maternal and fetal pathology, e.g. suspected abnormal heart sounds, hypertension, FGR, decrease in fetal movement, postterm pregnancy, oligohydramnios, intrapartum analgesia, meconium in amniotic fluid, induced labour and high-risk pregnancies. Treatment is based on CTG findings and FIGO classification:

- Normal CTG: wait-and-see;
- Suboptimal CTG: eliminate possible cause for suboptimal CTG, consider additional diagnostics, change maternal position, monitoring;
- Abnormal CTG: urgently eliminate possible cause for abnormal CTG or proceed to immediate delivery if cause cannot be eliminated.

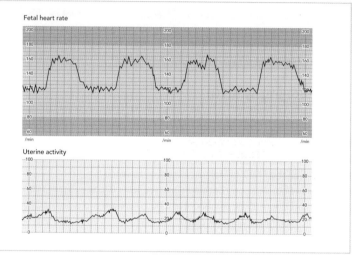

Figure 34 // CTG: baseline heart rate of about 120 bpm, normal variability 5-25, accelerations +, decelerations -, tocogram: 6 contractions/10 min; conclusion: normal CTG

 In situations where no CTG is available (e.g. in home deliveries or in some countries), Doppler is used to check fetal heart rate.

 Use of an intrauterine pressure catheter is not standard practice because of the increased risk of complications (haemorrhage secondary to placental damage). Intrauterine pressure catheters are nonetheless more reliable that external equivalents, and indications include non-progressive dilation in very obese patients unsuited for external monitoring.

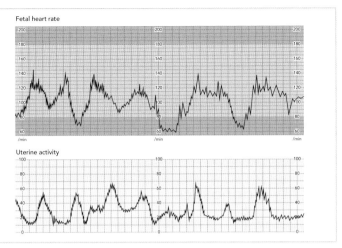

Figure 35 // Abnormal CTG with repeated decelerations

CTG CLASSI-FICATION	BASELINE HEART FREQUENCY	VARIABILITY REACTIVITY	DECELERATIONS
Normal CTG	110-150 bpm	· Accelerations · 5-25 bpm	· Early uniform decelerations · Uncomplicated variable decelerations with duration <60 sec and loss <60 beats
Suboptimal CTG	· 100-110 bpm · 150-170 bpm · Short bradycardia episode (100 bpm or ≤3 min)	· >25 bpm (saltatory pattern) · <5 bpm >40 min with absence of accelerations	Uncomplicated variable decelerations with duration <60 sec and loss >60 beats
	A combination of several intermediary observations will result in an abnormal CTG		
Abnormal CTG	· 150-170 bpm and reduced · variability · >170 bpm · Persistent bradycardia (<100 bpm for >3 min)	· <5 bpm for >60 min · Sinusoidal pattern	· Complicated variable decelerations with duration >60 sec · Repeated late uniform decelerations
Preterminal CTG	Total lack of variability (<2 bpm) and reactivity with or without decelerations or bradycardia		

Table 33 // FIGO classification for intrapartum CTG

Bpm, beats per minute

Intrapartum diagnostics

Maternal and fetal well-being must be monitored regularly during childbirth. General tests, such as the vaginal exam, measuring fundal height, Leopold's manoeuvres and the digital cervical exam should preferably be performed between contractions. In protracted labour, expulsive force can be assessed by performing an exam during a contraction.

 A woman is considered to be in labour when she is having regular, powerful (painful) contractions every 3-5 min for more than 60 min combined with cervical effacement and dilation (3 cm).

Fertility diagnostics

General

In cases of unexplained infertility, fertility testing can be used to gain insight into factors contributing to the woman's or couple's failure to conceive. Exploratory fertility testing includes semen analysis, ovulation testing and ruling out of tubal pathology (see Table 34). Gynaecologists may also examine or test ovulation, ovarian reserve, luteal phase, and tubal and uterine abnormalities (see Table 35). In men, gynaecologists can consider sperm penetration, endocrinological and chromosomal abnormalities, and antisperm antibodies (ASA) (see Table 38).

Basal temperature chart (BTC)

In a BTC, a patient tracks their basal body temperature from the first day of the menstrual cycle to detect ovulation. The patient must take their temperature rectally every day, immediately after waking up. After ovulation, body temperature rises a few tenths of a degree before dropping again after menstruation. Exploratory fertility testing can be an indication for registering a BTC.

Hysterosalpingography (HSG)

An HSG is a contrast X-ray of the uterus (hyster) and fallopian tubes (salpinges). It is used to check the patency of the uterus and fallopian tubes. The use of oil-soluble contrast medium is preferred over a water-soluble contrast medium, because of higher rates of ongoing pregnancy and live births. Indications for HSG include subfertility/infertility (as part of an exploratory fertility exam) and suspected adhesions, tubal damage and uterine damage after an intrauterine infection (e.g. *Chlamydia*) or after intrauterine procedures (e.g. curettage). Consider a lower abdominal X-ray after an HSG to evaluate contrast collection. This may be indicative of adhesions in the lower pelvis.

Chlamydia antibody test (CAT)

The CAT was initially introduced as a screening test for tubal abnormalities in subfertile women. PCR testing is used to detect *Chlamydia trachomatis* (CT) in the acute phase. The CAT targets CT IgG antibodies and is not suitable for determining infection in the acute phase, but can show whether the patient was ever infected with *Chlamydia*. The enzyme-linked immunosorbent assay (ELISA) is becoming increasingly common for *Chlamydia* testing because it is less labour-intensive and easy to standardise. Indications for CAT include suspected tubal pathology due to a possible previous *Chlamydia* infection and differentiates between low and high risk for tubal occlusion.

Exploratory fertility testing

Exploratory fertility testing can be used to assess key aspects of fertility in cases of subfertility of infertility.

EXPLORATORY FERTILITY TESTING	KEY CONSIDERATIONS
Semen analysis	• Volume ≥1.5 ml • Sperm count ≥15 million/ml • Total motility ≥42%, or progressive motility ≥30% • Normal sperm morphology ≥4% • Vitality ≥54%
Ovulation testing	• Symptoms of ovulation • Basal temperature rises 0.3°C/32.5°F due to progesterone ±3 days after ovulation • Growing follicle ultrasound
Luteal phase (unreliable)	• Consider using a BTC to predict ovulation • Midluteal progesterone
Tubal pathology	• CAT for long-term *Chlamydia* infection (IgG) • PCR for short-term *Chlamydia* infection

Table 34 // Exploratory fertility testing

Further fertility testing

If no common cause of subfertility or infertility is found, or if a less common cause is suspected, further fertility testing may be warranted. See Tables 35 and 38 for further fertility testing in women and men, respectively.

Hysterosalpingo-foam sonography (HyFoSy)

HyFoSy is an alternative to the use of HSG as a tubal patency test and can be used as a first-line option in outpatient settings. In HyFoSy foam is created when a solution is pushed through a syringe. The turbulence causes a pressure drop which dissolves the air and creates micro air bubbles. It becomes a foam that maintains echogenicity longer than water. Indications for HyFoSy are subfertility and low risk for tubal and/or uterine disease.

EXAM	SPECIFICATIONS
Ovulation detection	Ultrasound: visible vesicular follicle of max. 22 mm
Ovarian reserve	• FSH test • Ultrasound to check antral follicle count (AFC) in both ovaries, AFC <5 = too low • Optional: AMH
Luteal phase	>11d with midluteal progesterone level >30 mmol/L
Fallopian tube test	HSG and laparoscopy to assess fallopian tube patency and adhesions
Uterine exam	Hysteroscopic exam for uterine abnormalities

Table 35 // Further female fertility testing

WHO CATEGORY	HORMONE STATUS	PREVALENCE	LOCALISATION
1	Hypogonadotropic/ hypo-oestrogenic	10%	Hypothalamic or pituitary gland disorder (anorexia)
2	Normogonadotropic/ normo-oestrogenic	85%	Pituitary-ovarian axis imbalance (PCOS)
3	Hypogonadotropic/ hypo-oestrogenic	5%	Ovarian disorder (POI, chromosomal)

Table 36 // WHO classification of menstrual cycle abnormalities

WHO CATEGORY	HORMONE STATUS	CAUSES
1	Hypergonadotropic hypogonadism (FSH/LH ↑, testosterone ↓/=)	Defective spermatogenesis, testicular failure, Klinefelter syndrome, cytostatics, testis tumour
2	Hypogonadotropic hypogonadism (FSH/LH ↓, testosterone ↓)	Pituitary gland tumour, use of anabolic steroids, Kallman syndrome, morbid obesity
3	Normogonadotropoc azoospermia (FSH/LH =, testosterone =)	Obstruction (e.g. congenital abscence of vas deferens, vasectomy, epididymitis)
Non-WHO classified	Non-obstructive azoospermia	AZF deletions

Table 37 // WHO classification azoospermia

EXAM	SPECIFICATIONS
Endocrinology	FSH, LH, testosterone. If indicated prolactine (e.g. pituitary gland tumour)
Chromosomal	Depends on the father's genetic descent (e.g. Klinefelter syndrome)
Anti-sperm antibodies (ASA)	Mixed antiglobulin reaction (MAR) test: a blood test performed to evaluate the presence of antibodies (often seen after trauma or surgery)

Table 38 // Further male fertility testing

Treatment

🔖 Pharmacological treatment

Analgesics

	MEDICATION	MECHANISM OF ACTION	ADVERSE EFFECTS
	Paracetamol	Analgesic and antipyretic properties via unknown mechanism	Mild adverse effects profile: risk of liver damage at high doses (>150 mg/kg) and in cases of alcoholism and pre-existing liver damage
NSAIDS	**Diclofenac**	Classic non-selective inhibitors of the COX enzyme with analgesic, antipyretic and anti-inflammatory properties	• GI: risk of peptic ulcer • Renal: peripheral oedema, acute/chronic renal insufficiency especially in patients on RAS inhibitors, diuretics, pre-existing renal insufficiency, heart failure, dehydration, sepsis • Cardiovascular: potential ↑ risk especially with COX-2 inhibitors and diclofenac, including risk of heart failure
	Ibuprofen		
	Naproxen		
	Aspirin		
	Celecoxib	Selective COX-2 inhibitor with fewer renal and GI adverse effects	

Table 39 // Analgesics

COX, cyclooxygenase; GI, gastrointestinal; PMHx, past medical history; PPI, proton pump inhibitor; OAC, oral anticoagulation; RAS, renin-angiotensin system; SSRI, selective serotonin reuptake inhibitor

Opioids

	MEDICATION	MECHANISM OF ACTION

OPIOIDS	**Codeine**	• Opioid receptor agonist:
		  - μ receptor: analgesia (main effect)
		  - κ and δ receptor: spinal and peripheral analgesia
		• Fentanyl is more potent than morphine and can be administered transdermally ($t_{1/2}$ 17h), via IV ($t_{1/2el}$ 6-8h) and nasally ($t_{1/2}$ 3-4h)
		• Codeine is a prodrug of morphine that has unpredictable variability in conversion to morphine (10x less potent)
		• Tramadol and buprenorphine are partial agonists. Tramadol also has an SNRI mechanism of action

	Tramadol	
	Morphine	
	Oxycodone	
	Fentanyl	

Table 40 // Opioids. SNRI, serotonin-norepinephrine reuptake inhibitors; TCA, tricyclic antidepressant

 To prevent constipation, always prescribe **opioids** with a **laxative**: e.g. docusate sodium/calcium, bisacodyl, macrogol, lactulose, magnesium sulfate/citrate/hydroxide, methylnatrexone, naloxegol, or enema.

Legend

- ☿ = Additional information
- ● = Indication for prescribing medication
- ⇔ = Interaction with drugs or high-risk groups
- ✖ = Indication for stopping with medication
- ▲ = Intoxication management

NOTES

⇔ Administer lower dose in cases of alcoholism, chronic malnutrition, hepatic insufficiency or dehydration

▲ N-acetylcysteine (cysteine derivative) as an antidote

● Prescribe PPI in patients aged >70, peptic ulcer in PMHx, or age >60 with DM, heart failure or use of corticosteroids, SSRIs, OAC or acetylsalicylic acid

● At low doses of ascal/carbasalate calcium: PPI in patients aged >80, >60 with ulcer in PMHx, or >70 using corticosteroids, OAC, SSRIs or clopidogrel

ADVERSE EFFECTS	NOTES
• CNS: respiratory depression (especially high-risk in COPD), miosis, delirium, sedation, dependence • Pulmonary: bronchoconstriction • GI: motility ↓ (constipation, nausea and vomiting)	⇔ Risk of constipation ↑ due to immobility, poor water and fibre intake, and use of anticholinergics, antidepressants and diuretics ↑ ● So do not forget to prescribe a laxative when starting an opioid ⇔ Risk of respiratory depression and sedation ↑ with alcohol and CNS depressants (anaesthetics, anxiolytics, TCA, hypnotics and sedatives) ⇔ Tramadol combined with SSRIs produces ↑ risk of serotonin syndrome ▲ Naloxone (competitive antagonist) as an antidote for opioid-induced adverse effects ☿ Consider opioid rotation in case of adverse effects or poor effect

STEP 1	Start with paracetamol and add an NSAID if pain relief is insufficient. Diclofenac is 1st choice for colic pain. Consider selective COX-2 inhibitors with CIs for classic NSAIDs.
STEP 2	Add a weak-acting opioid (tramadol) or substitute the non-opioid. Codeine is still used primarily as an antitussive and not for additive pain relief.
STEP 3	Combine a strong oral or transdermal opioid (morphine, fentanyl, oxycodone) with a non-opioid. Fentanyl patches provide relief for nausea, vomiting and small bowel obstruction.
STEP 4	Opt for subcutaneous or IV route.

Table 41 // Treatment of nociceptive pain (World Health Organization (WHO) analgesic ladder)

Anticoagulants

	MEDICATION	MECHANISM OF ACTION	INDICATIONS
PLATELET AGGREGATION INHIBITORS	**Acetylsalicylic acid** (e.g. ASA, aspirin)	ASA irreversibly inhibits the COX enzyme (→ production of platelet aggregation-stimulating thromboxane A2 ↓)	Treatment of ACS, AP and PAD, treatment of MI, CABG, TIA, and ischaemic stroke
	P2Y12 inhibitors (e.g. clopidogrel, prasugrel, ticagrelor)	P2Y12 inhibitors irreversibly inhibits activation via the ADP receptor on the platelet	ACS, TIA or ischaemic stroke. Often used in combination with ASA as dual antiplatelet therapy (DAPT).
	Glycoprotein IIb/IIIa inhibitors (e.g. abciximab, tirofiban, eptifibatide)	Glycoprotein IIb/IIIa receptor inhibition → inhibits binding fibrinogen and von Willebrand Factor → platelet aggregation ↓	Acute coronary syndromes
VKA	**Vitamin K antagonists** (e.g. acenocoumarol, phenprocoumon, warfarin)	Inhibition of vitamin K and with it the synthesis of coagulation factors II/VII/IX/X: • Acenocoumarol has a $t_{1/2}$ of 8-11h, an onset of action of 36-72h and a duration of action of 2d • Phenprocoumon has a $t_{1/2}$ of 160h, an onset of action of 48-72h and a duration of action of 1-2wk	Indicated for: • AF (CHA$_2$DS$_2$-VASc >1) • Mechanical valve prosthesis • Venous thromboembolism (DVT, pulmonary embolism); duration: 3 mo (1st VTE episode provoked by transient risk factor), 6 mo (first idiopathic VTE), >1y (recurring VTE)
HEPARIN GROUP	**Factor Xa inhibitors** (e.g. fondaparinux)	Binding to antithrombin III → factor Xa inhibition	Used to treat venous and arterial thromboembolic disorders before starting OAC, also used as prophylaxis for surgical patients and for bridging. Therapeutic (6 mo) in VTE secondary to malignancy.
	Heparin	Heparin (SC/IV) activates antithrombin (factor III) and thus indirectly inactivates factors Xa and IIa (thrombin)	
	LMWH (e.g. nadroparin, enoxaparin)	LMWHs SC contain fragments of heparin with higher anti-Xa activity and lower anti-IIa activity. LMWHs are renally cleared.	

Table 42A // Anticoagulants
ACS, acute coronary syndrome; ADP, adenosine diphosphate; AF, atrial fibrillation; AP, angina pectoris; CABG, coronary artery bypass graft; DOAC, direct oral anticoagulants; DVT, deep vein thrombosis; LMWH, low-molecular-weight heparin; OAC, oral anticoagulation; PAD, peripheral arterial disease; PCI, percutaneous coronary intervention; Pgp, P-glycoprotein; TIA, transient ischaemic attack; VKA, vitamin K antagonists; VTE, venous tromboembolism

ADVERSE EFFECTS	NOTES
· Hypersensitivity (urticaria, exanthema, angioedema) · Bleeding risk ↑ (haematoma, epistaxis, GI bleeding) · GI (stomach problems)	⇔ Bleeding risk in the elderly and patients using corticosteroids, other NSAIDs and SSRIs ↑ ✖ Prior to procedures with a high risk of bleeding complications, such as neurosurgery: stop ASA/clopidogrel 5-7d in advance. Due to irreversible binding, the duration of action of both drugs is 3-10d.
· Bleeding risk ↑ (haematoma, epistaxis, GI bleeding) · abdominal pain, diarrhoea, dyspepsia	● Perioperative platelet transfusion in case of acute haemorrhage secondary to ASA or clopidogrel use
· Bleeding risk ↑ · Thrombocytopaenia	● Can be indicated after PCI in the case of no/inadequate reperfusion
Bleeding risk ↑	⇔ Bleeding risk ↑ due to: · Corticosteroids and NSAIDs (ulcerogenic) · SSRIs combined with platelet aggregation inhibitor (thrombocytopathy) · Nonadherence · Alcohol consumption · Low vitamin K intake · Febrile illness · Enhanced action of VKA due to cotrimoxazole or after sudden discontinuation of carbamazepine or rifampicin ⚲ For haemorrhage management: see following pages
· Bleeding risk ↑ · Heparin-induced thrombocytopaenia (HIT) type I/II · Anaphylaxis · Transaminases ↑	⚲ Bridging: before any invasive procedure with bleeding risk, a short-acting medication (LMWH/ heparin) is administered to bridge the discontinuation of the OAC ● Following acute haemorrhaging, discontinue heparin/LMWH and administer protamine (partially inhibits anti-Xa activity, less so with LMWH!) IV as an antidote ⚲ For more information on therapeutic blood monitoring, see the following pages

	MEDICATION	MECHANISM OF ACTION	INDICATIONS
DOAC	**Direct IIa inhibitors** (e.g. dagibatran)	Competitive and reversible inhibition of activated factor II	• Prevention of stroke and systemic embolism in non-valvular atrial fibrillation • Treatment of DVT and pulmonary embolism and prevention of recurrent VTE • DOACs can not be used as anticoagulant for mechanical heart valves, and moderate to severe mitral valve stenosis
	Factor Xa inhibitors (e.g. rivaroxaban, apixaban, edoxaban)	Selective inhibition of activated factor X	

Table 42B // Anticoagulants
ACS, acute coronary syndrome; ADP, adenosine diphosphate; AF, atrial fibrillation; AP, angina pectoris; CABG, coronary artery bypass graft; DOAC, direct oral anticoagulants; DVT, deep vein thrombosis; LMWH, low-molecular-weight heparin; OAC, oral anticoagulation; PAD, peripheral arterial disease; PCI, percutaneous coronary intervention; Pgp, P-glycoprotein; TIA, transient ischaemic attack; VKA, vitamin K antagonists; VTE, venous tromboembolism

All antiplatelet drugs require an initial loading dose, often higher, followed by a lower maintenance dose for continued treatment.

The efficacy of **vitamin K antagonists** (coumarin derivatives) depends on the INR. In case of haemorrhage or INR overshoots, vitamin K can be given orally (effect after 8 hours) or intravenously (after 6 hours). Vitamin K treatment lasts 24 hours and must be repeated, certainly with phenprocoumon (long $t_{1/2}$). In life-threatening situations like intracranial haemorrhages a four-factor prothrombin complex concentrate (II, VII, IX, X) should also be administered.

LMWHs have a longer $t_{1/2}$ and more stable serum levels, and no anti-Xa activity monitoring is needed. In case of reduced LMWH renal clearance, the dose should be adjusted based on anti-Xa levels.

DOACs are taken orally and do not require routine INR monitoring, reducing patient burden. DOAC treatment is as effective as VKA treatment, with comparable risk of stroke, cardiovascular death, and other causes of mortality. DOACs are additionally associated with a reduced risk of major bleeding, including intracranial bleeding, compared to VKAs.

ADVERSE EFFECTS	NOTES
• Bleeding risk ↑ • Anaemia • GI: dyspepsia, diarrhoea, nausea, vomiting • Kidney function ↓	⇔ Bleeding risk ↑: • Corticosteroids and NSAIDs • Platelet aggregation inhibitors combined with SSRIs • Thrombolytics • Nonadherence • Alcohol consumption • Febrile illness • Pgp inhibitors such as ciclosporin, itraconazole, ketoconazole, amiodarone and verapamil ⚠ In case of active haemorrhaging on dabigatran, idaruzicimab can be administered as an antidote. In case of direct Xa inhibitors, andexanet alpha can be administered.

INR

The international normalised ratio (INR) is the rate at which blood clots. The physiological INR is 1. An INR of 2 means that blood clots twice as slowly. The target value of INR is between 2.0-3.5, depending on the thrombotic risk.

Bridging

Bridging involves temporarily administering a short-acting agent (LMWH or occasionally unfractionated heparin) to bridge the time without VKA. Coumarin derivatives must be discontinued prior to any invasive procedure with a high bleeding risk. Due to their respective elimination half-lives, acenocoumarol should be discontinued 3-4 days and phenprocoumon 5-7 days prior to surgery. Bridging is indicated in patients with an increased risk of thrombosis. This risk can be estimated with the CHA_2DS_2-VASc score, which uses validated risk factors to evaluate ischaemic stroke risk in patients with AF. Preoperative discontinuation of DOACs is not an indication for bridging because of the short $t_{1/2}$.

Bridging with LMWH is indicated for:
- Very high arterial thromboembolism risk: AF with CHA_2DS_2-VASc score >8, mechanical or bioprosthetic heart valve, or a CVA/TIA <6 months ago.
- Very high venous thromboembolism (VTE) risk: <3 months after first or recurrent idiopathic DVT/pulmonary embolism.

The CHA₂DS₂-VASc score:

Congestive heart failure	1 point
Hypertension	1 point
Age >75	2 points
Diabetes mellitus	1 point
Stroke/TIA/thromboembolism	2 points
Vascular disease	1 point
Age 65-74	1 point
Sex **c**ategory (female = 1, male = 0)	1 point

Antidepressants

<table>
<tr><th></th><th>MEDICATION</th><th>MECHANISM OF ACTION</th><th>INDICATIONS</th></tr>
<tr><td rowspan="2">ANTIDEPRESSANTS</td><td>TCA
(amitriptyline, nortriptyline clomipramine)</td><td>Noradrenaline (NA) and 5-HT reuptake ↓; nortriptyline is more selective for NA, amitriptyline and clomipramine for 5-HT</td><td>· Moderate-severe depression (1ˢᵗ choice for severe depression)
· Neuropathic pain</td></tr>
<tr><td>SSRIs
(fluoxetine, paroxetine, citalopram)</td><td>5-HT reuptake ↓, also has anxiolytic properties</td><td>· Moderate to severe depression
· Anxiety disorders
· Bipolar depression</td></tr>
</table>

Table 43 // Antidepressants

	TREATMENT
STEP 1	· Start with an SSRI or TCA. Wait for 4-6 wk to evaluate the effect. · If patient does not respond: reconsider the diagnosis, check adherence, increase to maximum dose or check blood levels with TCAs.
STEP 2	Switch antidepressants, e.g. by replacing one SSRI for another SSRI or a TCA.
STEP 3	Refer to secondary care.

Table 44 // Medicated treatment for moderate to severe depression

TREATMENT

The **HAS-BLED** Score can be used to assess bleeding risk.

Criterium	Points
Hypertension	1 point
Abnormal renal or liver function	1 point each
Stroke	1 point
Bleeding	1 point
Labile INRs	1 point
Elderly (>65 years)	1 point
Drugs or alcohol	1 point each

ADVERSE EFFECTS	NOTES
· Anticholinergic → dry mouth, dizziness, constipation, micturition disorders, erectile dysfunction, confusion (elderly) · Antinoradrenergic → orthostasis, falls · Antihistaminergic → sedation, weight gain	⇔ CI: recent myocardial infarction and long QT syndrome (conduction disorder = quinidine-like action of TCAs) ⇔ Orthostasis, falls ↑ secondary to dehydration (fever, diarrhoea, vomiting), diuretics, antihypertensives
· Serotonergic → GI symptoms, hyponatraemia (SIADH), thrombocytopathy, sexual dysfunction, serotonin syndrome · Risk of GI haemorrhage with NSAIDs ↑	☼ Watch for anxiety during startup or after dose increase ⇔ Risk of hyponatraemia with thiazide diuretics ↑ ☼ Taper off slowly (agitation, anxiety and sleep problems due to withdrawal)

SSRIs are preferred to TCAs in the 1st step because they have a more favourable adverse effects profile than TCAs while being almost equally effective.

Adjust lithium dose based on plasma levels (narrow therapeutic index between 0.8-1.2 mmol/L). Test thyroid and renal function frequently due to adverse effects profile.

Antiemetics

	MEDICATION	MECHANISM OF ACTION	INDICATIONS
ANTIEMETICS	**Antihistamines** (meclizine)	· Mild sedative and mild anticholinergic effect · Strong antiemetic effect · Reduced excitation of vestibular system	· Motion sickness · Hyperemesis gravidarum (off-label)
	Dopamine antagonists (metoclopramide)	· D2 receptor antagonism in the chemoreceptor trigger zone and the vomiting centre of the medulla · Antagonism of 5HT3 receptors · Agonism of 5HT4 receptors · Proximal gastrointestinal peristalsis ↑, lower oesophageal sphincter tone ↑, pyloric tone ↓	· Prevention of nausea and vomiting secondary to chemotherapy and radiotherapy · Prevention of postoperative nausea and vomiting · Symptomatic treatment of nausea and vomiting
	Dopamine antagonists (domperidone)	· D2 receptor antagonist of chemoreceptor trigger zone of medulla's vomiting centre · Proximal gastrointestinal peristalsis ↑, lower oesophageal sphincter tone ↑, pyloric tone ↓	Nausea, vomiting
	Serotonin antagonists (ondansetron)	· Antagonism of 5HT3 receptors → suppresses vomiting reflex · Antagonism of neurokinin-1 (NK1) receptors	· Prevention of nausea and vomiting secondary to cytotoxic chemotherapy and radiotherapy (treatment >6 mo) · Prevention and treatment of postoperative nausea and vomiting (from >1 mo)

Table 45 // Antiemetics

 If non medicated/diet-specific solutions have insufficient effect in hyperemesis gravidarum, drug treatment can be switched to medication (see Table 46).

 Nearly all drugs are excreted in breast milk to some extent. Careful consideration of drug use or nursing is recommended.

ADVERSE EFFECTS	NOTES
Accommodative dysfunction and miction disorders, dry mouth, dizziness, sedation, drowsiness, blurred vision	◌̣̇ Crosses the placenta ⇔ The central suppressive effect of antihistamines may be exacerbated by other substances such as alcohol
Asthenia, depression, diarrhoea, extrapyramidal disorders, hypotension, drowsiness	◌̣̇ Ineffective in vomiting of vestibular origin ◌̣̇ Use for max. 5d due to risk of neurological adverse effects in mother ⇔ Concomitant use of alcohol should be avoided due to potentiation of the sedative effect ⇔ At the end of pregnancy, extrapyramidal symptoms may occur in the fetus
Dry mouth, anxiety, libido ↓, restlessness, extrapyramidal disorders, headaches, diarrhoea, galactorrhoea, breast tenderness, asthenia	◌̣̇ Max. use 1 wk, possible cardiac adverse effects of mother ⇔ Avoid combination with medication that causes QT interval ↑ ✖ CI: prolactinoma, intestinal bleeding, mechanical obstruction, intestinal perforation, moderate/severe liver insufficiency, disorders with QT interval ↑, electrolyte disorders, heart disease
Headaches, hot flashes, constipation	◌̣̇ Transmitted to child through breast milk ● Use only if strictly indicated due to insufficient data on teratogenesis

TREATMENT	
STEP 1	Antihistamines (e.g. meclizine, promethazine)
STEP 2	Dopamine antagonists (e.g. metoclopramide, domperidone), or serotonin antagonists (e.g. ondansetron)
STEP 3	Corticosteroids (e.g. hydrocortisone) when conventional therapy fails

Table 46 // Antiemetics treatment plan for hyperemesis gravidarum

Antihypertensives

TREATMENT

ANTIHYPERTENSIVES

	MEDICATION	MECHANISM OF ACTION	INDICATIONS
	Central-acting antihypertensives (methyldopa)	• Probable stimulation of central α2-sympathicomimetic receptors • Antihypertensive effect due to peripheral vascular resistance ↓	• Hypertension • Gestational hypertension
	Calcium antagonists/ Dihydropyridines (nifedipine)	Blockade of slow calcium channels (L-type) → coronary and systemic vasodilation	• Hypertension • Stable angina pectoris (AP) • Vasospastic AP • Raynaud's phenomenon • May be used during pregnancy
	Calcium channel blocker (nicardipine)	Dilation of peripheral arterioles with minimal negative inotropic effects	• Severe pre-eclampsia • When other antihypertensive medication fails or is contraindicated
	Direct vasodilators (hydralazine)	Dilation of arterioles with minimal effect on veins and decrease of peripheral vascular resistance	• Hypertension • Pregnancy-induced hypertension (PIH) • Hypertensive crisis • Heart failure (HF)
	Beta blockers (labetalol)	Non selective beta blocker with low sympathomimetic activity	• AP with concomitant hypertension • Hypertension • Gestational hypertension
	Magnesium sulphates (magnesium)	Magnesium downregulates an overstimulated nervous system, peripheral vasodilation	Prophylaxis and treatment of convulsions in severe pre-eclampsia and eclampsia (BP>160/110 mmHg)

Table 47 // Medication for hypertensive treatment

ADVERSE EFFECTS	NOTES
Orthostatic hypotension, (transient) sedation/sleepiness/drowsiness, sleep problems, depression, hallucinations, nausea/vomiting, constipation, oedema	☼ Methyldopa use is associated with liver disease ⇔ Methyldopa use enhances the toxicity of lithium
Hypotension, fall risk, reflex tachycardia, flushing, headache, peripheral oedema	☼ Strictly reserved for pregnant women with severe hypertension who do not respond to standard therapy, requires close monitoring ⇔ Combination with beta blockers can lead to heart failure, hypotension and even myocardial infarction (MI) in high-risk patients (past MI) ⇔ May cause acute pulmonary oedema when combined with a beta blocker, especially when used to suppress contractions ✖ CI nifedipine: secreted in breast milk ✖ Not recommended in 1st trimester due to decreased placental perfusion
Hypotension, severe headache, tachycardia, nausea, vomiting	⇔ Combined with magnesium sulphate: pulmonary oedema or severe hypotension. Pre-hydrate with 500 ml NaCl. ⇔ Combination with beta blocker can lead to severe hypotension ✖ CI: aortic stenosis, compensatory hypertension
Pain (e.g. arms, legs, jaw), chest pain, tachycardia, nausea, dyspnoea, excessive sweating	☼ Transfers to breast milk
Orthostatic hypotension, if administered via injection/ IV: congestive heart failure, hypersensitivity reactions, elevated liver enzyme levels, transient nasal congestion	☼ With maternal labetalol use, the neonate may exhibit symptoms of hypotension, hypoglycaemia, respiratory distress, and bradycardia → 24-48h monitoring indicated ⇔ Avoid combining with calcium antagonists that negatively affect contractility and atrioventricular (AV) conduction due to the risk of hypotension ⇔ Labetalol may enhance the blood glucose-lowering effect of insulin and other oral antidiabetics
Symptoms related to hypermagnesaemia: flushes, hypotension, neuronal blockade → loss of muscle reflexes, muscle weakness, drowsiness	☼ IV magnesium acts immediately and lasts 30 min, IM acts after 1h and lasts 3-4h ⇔ Risk of enhanced hypotension and neuromuscular blockade when combined with nifedipine ✖ Do not administer ≤2h before labour due to risk of fetal hypotension, respiratory distress, and intrauterine hypoxia (secondary to fetal central nervous system (CNS) depression)

Nitroglycerin should be avoided in patients with hypertrophic obstructive cardiomyopathy, because vasodilators can increase left ventricle outflow obstruction by decreasing preload and afterload.

 As soon as pregnancy is confirmed, increase dosage of levothyroxine with approx. 30% for normal fetal cognitive development.

TREATMENT	

STEP 1	💬 Non-pharmacological treatments
	   • Quit smoking and stop drinking alcohol
	   • Limit salt intake
	   • Avoid products containing glycyrrhizin (liquorice)
	   • Avoid specific spices (e.g. ephedra, ma huang)
	   • Physical activity
	   • Stress ↓

STEP 2	✎ Start/adjust pharmacological treatment
	   • Pre-existing hypertension during pregnancy (<20 wk gestation)
	     - Labetalol (first-line option)
	     - Nifedipine
	     - Methyldopa
	   • Pregnancy-induced hypertension (>20 wk gestation)
	     - Labetalol (first-line option)
	     - Nifedipine
	     - Methyldopa
	   • Severe hypertension during critical care during or after pregnancy
	     - Labetalol (oral or IV)
	     - Nifedipine (oral)
	     - Hydralazine or nicardipine (IV)

Table 48 // Treatment plan for hypertensive disorders during pregnancy

TREATMENT

 Labetalol is faster-acting than methyldopa and is preferred in acute situations.

 ACE inhibitors have a teratogenic effect in the 2nd and 3rd trimester, manifesting in neonatal lung hypoplasia, fetal growth restriction (FGR), cranial hypoplasia, persistent ductus arteriosus, and limb contractures.

Benzodiazepines

 Benzodiazepines cross the placenta. Proven teratogenic effect in animals, not in humans. Recommendation: reserved for strict indications, short-term use and lowest dose.

 With maternal use of benzodiazepines in the last month of pregnancy, the newborn should be kept under close paediatric surveillance for at least 24 hours.

 To prevent tolerance and dependence, it is recommended that benzodiazepines be prescribed for <2 weeks and up to 4 weeks. It is recommended to prescribe benzodiazepines as a sleep aid only after other non-pharmacological options have been unsuccessful (e.g. sleep hygiene, cognitive behavioural therapy).

 If a patient develops tolerance and dependence despite taking precautions, the risk of rebound symptoms can be reduced by slowly tapering off and switching to a long-acting benzodiazepine.

INDICATION (CORRELATION WITH $T_{1/2}$)	MIDA-ZOLAM	ZOLPI-DEM	ZOPI-CLON	TEMAZE-PAM	OXAZE-PAM	DIAZE-PAM
Sleep disorders	X	X	X	X		
Anxiety disorders: social phobia / generalised					X	X
Alcohol abstinence					X	X
Epileptic seizure/febrile convulsion/delirium						X

Table 49 // Indications of benzodiazepines

 For the latest information about doses, adverse effects, and more:
- United Kingdom: *www.medicines.org.uk/emc*
- Canada: *go.drugbank.com*
- Netherlands: *www.farmacotherapeutischkompas.nl*

	MEDICATION	MECHANISM OF ACTION
BENZODIAZEPINES	**Midazolam** (ultra-short)	• Benzodiazepines enhance the inhibitory effect of the neurotransmitter GABA, with hypnotic, anxiolytic, anticonvulsant and muscle-relaxant effects • The main differences between the agents are their respective elimination half-lives ($t_{1/2}$=2-3.5h/2-4h/5h/7-11h/4-15h/20-48h, respectively) • Oxazepam is the active metabolite of diazepam • Zolpidem is a benzodiazepine-like hypnotic, which acts rapidly ($t_{1/2}$ 2-4h) and briefly, and mainly has a sedative effect in low doses
	Zolpidem (ultra-short)	
	Zopiclon (short)	
	Temazepam (short)	
	Oxazepam (short)	
	Diazepam (long)	

Table 50 // Benzodiazepines

GABA, gamma-aminobutyric acid; OSAS, obstructive sleep apnea syndrome

Blood glucose-lowering agents

	MEDICATION	MECHANISM OF ACTION
BLOOD GLUCOSE-LOWERING AGENT	**Biguanides** (i.e. metformin)	• Inhibits gluconeogenesis in the liver and glycogenolysis in the liver • Increases peripheral insulin sensitivity
	Sulphonylurea derivatives • Short-acting: tolbutamide, gliclazide • Long-acting: glimepiride	Sulphonylurea derivatives stimulate insulin release through the KATP channels of the pancreas
	Insulin • Short-acting: aspart, lispro • Intermediate-acting: NPH (Humulin N®) • Long-acting: glargine (Lantus®)	There are several types of synthetic insulin, distinguished by their duration of action: short- (4-5h) intermediate- (12-16h) and long-acting (>24h)
	GLP-1 agonists (-glutide)	• Activate GLP-1 receptors, stimulate insulin secretion (glucose-dependent) • Suppress glucagon secretion
	DPP-4 inhibitors (-gliptin)	Inhibits the DPP-4 enzyme, so human GLP-1 ↑
	SGLT2 inhibitors (-gliflozin)	• Reversible inhibition of sodium-glucose cotransporter in the tubular system of the kidneys • Increases glucose (and sodium) excretion via urine

Table 51 // Blood glucose-lowering agents

DPP-4, dipeptidyl peptidase 4 inhibitors; GLP-1, glucagon-like peptide 1; KATP channels, ATP-sensitive K channels; SGLT2, sodium-glucose cotransporter 2 inhibitors

ADVERSE EFFECTS	NOTES
• Drowsiness, alertness ↓ (watch out when driving!) • Muscle weakness (risk of falling) • Anterograde amnesia • Tolerance and dependence • Rebound phenomenon following abstinence (anxiety, sleep problems) • Paradoxical reaction • Respiratory depression	⇔ Risk of adverse effects ↑ in the elderly (greater fat mass/volume of distribution) and patients using alcohol, recreational drugs, opioids and psychotropics (antipsychotics, antidepressants) ⇔ Respiratory depression: COPD and OSAS ⇔ Paradoxical reaction: especially in children ⚠ In case of overdose (respiratory depression), administer IV flumazenil, a short-acting (!) benzodiazepine antagonist

ADVERSE EFFECTS	NOTES
• GI disorders (nausea, vomiting, diarrhoea) • Lactate acidosis (accumulation due to reduced renal excretion)	⇔ Risk of lactate acidosis ↓ in cases of diuretics use, alcohol abuse, heart failure, chronic hypoxaemia (COPD, sepsis) and chronic kidney disease (<30 ml/min/1.73 m²: do not administer; between 30-60 ml/min max. 1000 mg/d)

• Hypoglycaemia (<4 mmol/L; leads to tachycardia, agitation, tremor, sweating and possibly even reduced consciousness), especially with long-acting sulphonylurea derivatives
• Weight ↑
	⇔ Hypoglycaemia: especially in the elderly, with hepatic or renal insufficiency, excessive exertion, skipping meals and reduced intake.
	⊗ Do not give glibenclamide to elderly patients!
	⚠ In cases of hypoglycaemia:
	  • Increase carbohydrate or glucose intake
	  • Administer IV glucose or 1 mg glucagon IM or SC in patients with impaired consciousness (glucagon counteracts insulin)

• Hypoglycaemia (see risk factors in the next column; overdose may also occur) • Weight ↑	
• Gastric emptying ↓ and sensation of satiety ↑ • Lower food intake resulting in weight loss	• No hypoglycaemia due to glucose dependence • GLP-1 agonist initiation can have GI adverse effects. Watch out for dehydration!
• Urogenital infections due to high urinary glucose • Polyuria, pollakisuria	Improves left ventricular function by lowering cardiac pre- and afterload

Hypoglycaemia unawareness: initial symptoms of hypoglycaemia may be masked by non-selective beta blockers (especially in DM1 and 2 with long-term insulin use). Non-selective beta blockers may also delay glucose level recovery after hypoglycaemia.

 It is recommended that women with diabetes discontinue all antidiabetic medications prior to pregnancy and start insulin. Insulin use increases risk of hypertension, pre-eclampsia, prematurity, macrosomia, hyperbilirubinaemia, hypocalcaemia, and polycythaemia. Metformin and SU derivates may be considered as an alternative if the benefits outweigh the risks.

 In patients with atherosclerotic and non-atherosclerotic cardiovascular disease SGLT2 inhibitors and GLP-1 agonists are the first choice for reducing cardiovascular risk.

TREATMENT	
STEP 1	• Start on metformin 2-3x/d 1 tablet. Adjust dosage according to blood glucose and renal function. • In cardiac patients start SGLT2 inhibitors
STEP 2	Add a sulphonylurea derivative, preferably gliclazide 1x/d 1 controlled release tablet (risk of hypoglycaemia and vascular complications ↓)
STEP 3	Add NPH insulin once daily. Insulin isophane is preferred. Switch to insulin glargine or detemir in cases of nocturnal hypoglycaemia or fluctuating glucose levels. Alternative: DPP4 inhibitor or GLP-1 agonist.
STEP 4	Switch to a multi-dose insulin regimen: choose a 1. Mixed insulin regimen 2x/d, e.g. insulin aspart/aspart protamine, or 2. Add a short-acting insulin 3x/d with meals in addition to an intermediate or long-acting insulin. Note: this increases the risk of hypoglycaemia, so the sulphonylurea derivative must often be discontinued.

Table 52 // Pharmacological treatment for DM type 2

Gynaecology

🖊 Pharmacological treatment

Contraception
General

Oral contraceptives (OC) contain hormones that prevent ovulation. There is a wide array of OC, which are either combined oestrogen-progesterone or progesterone-only pills. Combined contraceptives are the most common.

- Progesterone affects the production and composition of cervical mucus, making it impermeable to spermatozoa.
- Oestrogen stabilises the endometrium to maximise cycle regularity.
- Together, progesterone and oestrogen inhibit the release of LH and FSH and thus stop ovulation.

Adverse effects are the main factor in choosing an OC. Second-generation pills are prescribed most often and have the lowest risk of thrombosis. Patients may opt for an alternative pill from the same or another generation if they experience adverse effects. All generations of combined contraceptives increase the risk of thrombosis. Other major adverse effects include:

- First generation: libido ↓, paracyclic symptoms ↓;
- Second generation: libido ↓, paracyclic symptoms ↓, lowest risk of thrombosis, often first choice;
- Third generation: acne ↓ or seborrhoeic skin, adverse effects ↓, relatively high risk of thrombosis;
- Fourth generation: fluid retention ↓, adverse effects ↓, relatively high risk of thrombosis.

When taking OC, it is required to take the pill every day. Long-term use without a pill-free week can cause endometrial atrophy, resulting in spotting. This can be remedied by scheduling a pill-free week or longer if necessary. See Diagram 7 for a roadmap if the patient misses a pill. See Table 53 for a list of contraceptive methods.

CONTRACEPTIVE METHOD	MECHANISM OF ACTION
Combined pill · Oestrogen · Progesterone	Negative feedback on GnRH, FSH and LH → no ovulation, less accessible and permeable cervical mucus and endometrial atrophy
Vaginal ring · Oestrogen · Progesterone	
Transdermal contraception (contraceptive patch) · Oestrogen · Progesterone	
Implanon® Progesterone	Negative feedback on GnRH → no ovulation, less accessible and permeable cervical mucus and endometrial atrophy
Contraceptive injection Progesterone	
Hormonal IUD Progesterone	Local obstruction and thickening of cervical mucus, disrupted endometrial proliferation and motility → and sperm capacitation ↓
Copper IUD	Releases spermicidal agents, obstructive and inflammatory effect → interferes with implantation. Copper also releases prostaglandins → disrupted sperm motility in the uterus and fallopian tubes.
Condom	· Obstructive, sometimes with spermicides · STI prevention
Female condom	Obstructive
Pessary	Obstructive with spermicides
Periodic abstinence	Avoid sexual intercourse 3-5d around ovulation. Ovulation can be estimated using a BTC or a period tracking app.
Coitus interruptus	No fertilisation without sperm cells

Table 53 // Contraceptives

RISKS AND SYMPTOMS	NOTES (INSTRUCTIONS)
· Risk of thrombosis, acne, fluid retention, breakthrough bleeding · Breast cancer risk slightly ↑	· 1 pill daily, monthly 7d pill-free week if necessary · See Diagram 7
Risk of vaginal complaints ↑	· Self-inserted, lasts 3 wk · Can be removed for up to 3h in case of intercourse or defecation difficulties · Insert ≤5 d after the start of period
· Loosening: resorption ↓ · Risk of mastalgia ↑	· Apply to dry, intact skin · Replace every week · One patch-free week after 3 wk · If a contraceptive patch loosens or falls off, apply a new patch within 24h
Can be difficult to remove due to attachment to connective tissue	· Subcutaneous placement · Lasts 3y
Irregular bleeding ⊙, spotting ⊙	IM injection every 3 mo
· Less frequent, shorter-lasting and less blood loss · Risk of spotting in first 3 mo · Risk of perforation/false passage on insertion · Risk of ectopic pregnancy ↑ than with other contraceptives, but lower than without contraception (risk 0.04%) · Risk of expulsion ↑ when using menstrual cups Risk of hypermenorrhoea ⊙	· Intrauterine placement · Lasts 10y (T-shaped copper IUD) · Lasts 8y (Mirena®) · Lasts 6y (Levosert®) · Lasts 5y (Kyleena® and other copper coils) · Risk of PID ↑ → screen for STI first if patient is at risk of STI
N/A	Put on before intercourse
	Insert before intercourse
· Difficult to insert, may be dislocated · Spermicide is effective only once	· Self-inserted · Must be inserted at least 1h before and remain in place for 6h after intercourse for spermicidal effect
Exact ovulation date is difficult to predict → suboptimal reliability	Abstinence from 7d before ovulation to 2d after ovulation
Unreliable, because semen is often emitted before ejaculation	Withdraw the penis before ejaculation

Due to the risk of thrombosis, combined contraceptives are not recommended for women aged ≥35 who smoke.

 Indications for contraception include birth control, menstrual complaints (e.g. hypermenorrhoea, dysmenorrhoea, endometriosis) and possibly menopausal hormone replacement.

 The use of external testosterone or oestrogen as hormone therapy in transgender care is not considered a form of contraception. Individuals may remain fertile while undergoing such treatment.

TREATMENT

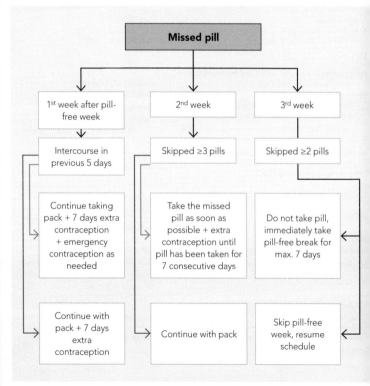

Diagram 7 // Roadmap for missed single-phase combined pill with ethinylestradiol

Emergency contraception

EMERGENCY CONTRACEPTION		
Method	**Gestational age**	**Mechanism of action**

Morning-after pill	<3d after unprotected intercourse	• Contains 1.5 mg levonorgestrel
		• Success rate in unwanted pregnancies:
		  - 95% when taken <24h
		  - 85% when taken <48h
		  - 58% when taken <72h

Progestogen receptor modulator	<5d after unprotected intercourse	Inhibits/delays ovulation
Morning-after intra-uterine device (IUD)	<5d after unprotected intercourse	Prevents nidation, effectiveness approaches 100%

Table 54 // Emergency contraception

Postpartum contraception

After giving birth, women may use the lactational amenorrhoea method (LAM) or other contraceptive methods. LAM is 92.5-99.5% effective if all three of the following conditions are met: <6 months postpartum, exclusively breastfeeding (nobottle feeding), and amenorrhoea. If these three criteria are not met, many women ovulate despite breastfeeding. Non-nursing mothers may start progestogen-only contraception or combined contraceptives three weeks after childbirth (due to thrombosis risk). An IUD can be inserted starting from six weeks postpartum. Nursing mothers often have lactation amenorrhoea and can also opt for alternative forms of contraception, i.e. progestagen-only methods (from two weeks postpartum) and an IUD. Combined pills are not a preferred method of contraception for nursing mothers because they inhibit breastfeeding and may be transmitted via breastfeeding to the child, with potentially adverse effects on brain development in boys and unknown effects in girls. Nursing women who insist on taking combined contraceptives can start from six weeks postpartum.

Not only do rules and regulations, but also beliefs regarding contraception, abortion, and pregnancy termination vary worldwide. Be aware of this before consulting a patient on these topics.

Loop excision/conisation

Loop excision, also called large-loop excision of the transformation zone (LLETZ) or conisation, consists of removing the transformation zone. This procedure is performed when a colposcopy or biopsy results reveal signs of CIN 2/3. In a loop excision or LLETZ, a thin metal loop is used to remove part of the cervix by co-agulation. Conisation involves cutting away a deeper, cone-shaped part of the cervix and is usually performed for an adenocarcinoma in situ or recurrence/ residue after a LLETZ. The specimen obtained during the procedure is then sent to the lab for analysis. Conisation and, to a lesser extent, LLETZ increase the risk of preterm birth.

Female sterilisation

See Table 55 and Figure 36 for an overview of female sterilisation techniques.

 It is important to assess cervical length after LLETZ, as after LLETZ procedures there is a twofold risk ↑ of preterm birth. Repeated procedures further increase this risk.

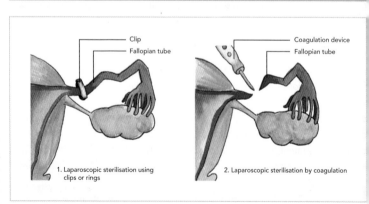

1. Laparoscopic sterilisation using clips or rings

2. Laparoscopic sterilisation by coagulation

Figure 36 // Female sterilisation methods

STERILISATION PROCEDURE	LAPAROSCOPIC STERILISATION USING CLIPS OR RINGS	LAPAROSCOPIC STERILISATION BY COAGULATION OR TUBECTOMY
Technique	• Placing rings/clips on the fallopian tubes • Disrupts fallopian tube continuity	Bipolar coagulation or salpingectomy if mechanical occlusion of the fallopian tubes is not possible
Complications	Serious complications 1-6:1000, mortality 2:100,000	
Chance of pregnancy after surgery	• 10-year chance of pregnancy after sterilisation is ±2:100 • If the procedure is performed in the 2nd half of the cycle, the woman may already be pregnant. • Not 100% protective against pregnancy, e.g. if procedure is performed incorrectly or due to tuboperitoneal fistula	
Reversal surgery possible	Not possible after tubectomy	
Pregnancy after reversal surgery	80% pregnant within 1y of reversal surgery	Coagulation: 65% pregnant within 1y of reversal surgery
Consider	• Convert to laparotomy if laparoscopy proves unfeasible • Tubectomy lowers risk for ovarian cancer	

Table 55 // Female sterilisation

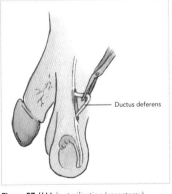

Ductus deferens

Figure 37 // Male sterilisation (vasectomy)

 Vasectomy (severing the ductus deferens) is one of several male sterilisation techniques (see Figure 37).

 Laparotomic sterilisation by coagulation or tubectomy is mainly performed in low-resource settings where no laparoscopy is available or after CS.

Obstetrics

🔗 Pharmacological treatment

See the section Pharmalogical treatment for an overview of e.g. antiemetics, antihypertensives in pregnancy, medication around labour and pregnancy termination.

	TERMINATION OF PREGNANCY	
Method	**Gestation weeks**	**Mechanism of action**
Medication	<12	Mifepristone (antiprogestogen 200 mg once, followed by oral/vaginal misoprostol after 36h (prostaglandin E1 analogue 800 µg). Repeat after 4h with lower dosage as needed
	12-24	Mifepristone (anti-progesterone 200 mg once), followed by misoprostol (prostaglandin E1 analogue 800 µg) 24-48h oral/vaginal/buccal or sublingual. Repeat every 3h with lower dosage
Vacuum aspiration (VA)	<14	After dilation (up to max. 16 mm), the fetus is instrumentally reduced in size and removed. Can be used up to week 15-16
Dilation and evacuation (D&E)	14-24	Dilation of the cervix with osmotic dilators or medication. Evacuation with long forceps and vacuum aspiration with cannulas
Termination of pregnancy on medical grounds	>24	• Usually consists of combined oral mifepristone and vaginal misoprostol • Combined with placenta removal under anaesthesia in 10% of cases

Table 56 // Pregnancy termination possibilities

 Not only do rules and regulations, but also beliefs regarding contraception, abortion, and pregnancy termination vary worldwide. Be aware of this before consulting a patient on these topics.

Analgesia during labour

Not all patients experience the same amount of pain during childbirth. However, childbirth is generally very painful, especially in nulliparas. This pain originates from the uterus and cervix at first and from the back and abdomen in later stages.

When the fetal head descends, it applies pressure on the pelvic nerves, resulting in perineal pain. There are various options for pain relief during childbirth.

Persistent extreme pain can have adverse effects on fetal and maternal well-being. Hyperventilation can cause respiratory alkalosis, which can initiate placental vasoconstriction. As a result, the O_2 affinity of maternal haemoglobin will increase, negatively impacting O_2 transmission to the fetus. In addition, increased blood catecholamine levels may induce placental vasoconstriction. There are various options for pain relief during childbirth:

- Systemic analgesia: usually less effective than neuraxial analgesia and has more adverse effects. The most commonly used analgesics are opioids such as fentanyl, remifentanil (short acting powerful painkiller, lasts 3-5 min), and pethidine. Analgesia can be administered intermittently or via a patient-controlled analgesia pump.
- Neuraxial analgesia: an analgesic can be administered to the epidural and/or spinal space, providing sensory and/or motor block from a specific dermatome. This is the most powerful method of pain relief during labour. Major adverse effects of neuraxial analgesia include a prolonged expulsion phase, hypotension, fever and injection-induced headache. Epidural anaesthesia is also associated with an increased risk of assisted delivery. Contraindications to neuraxial analgesia include coagulation disorders and local infection at the injection site.
- Nitrous oxide: inhaled anaesthetic gas is used in labour to reduce anxiety and diminish pain awareness. It seems more effective than placebo or pethidine (first 30 min), works fast, and can be used in diverse settings.
- Transcutaneous electrical neurostimulation (TENS): non-medicated pain relief treatment during labour. Applying TENS during the active labour phase can reduce labour pain without significant complications. There are indications that TENS can divert the attention of the patient from the heaviest pain. Note that evidence is limited.

 NSAIDs are contraindicated during delivery because they inhibit prostaglandin synthesis, and prostaglandins play an important role in uterine contraction and closure of the ductus arteriosus.

Medication for delivery

MEDICATION	MECHANISM OF ACTION	INDICATIONS
Beta agonists (salbutamol, fenoterol)	Stimulate β2 receptors of myometrial myocytes → reduced intracellular calcium → myometrial relaxation	Imminent preterm birth with contractions in week 24-32
Beta agonists (ritodrine)	Stimulates β2 receptors → cAMP ↑ → activates protein kinase A (PKA) → phosphorylation proteins involved in contraction of smooth muscles → relaxation of smooth muscles	Premature contractions during pregnancy ↓
Calcium antagonists (nifedipine)	Intracellular calcium of myometrial myocytes ↓ → relaxation	Imminent preterm birth with contractions in week 24-32
Nitrates (nitroglycerin)	Converted to nitrous oxide (NO), vasodilator, and smooth muscle relaxation	Fast and short relaxation of cervix and uterus during acute obstetric intervention
NSAIDs (indomethacin)	Prevent release of prostaglandins and cytokines	Imminent preterm birth with contractions before week 30
Oxytocin antagonists (atosiban, sold as Tractocile®)	Competes with oxytocin for oxytocin receptor	Imminent preterm birth with contractions in week 24-32

Table 57A // Medication for delivery

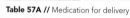

ADVERSE EFFECTS	NOTES
• Maternal: tachycardia, palpitations, tremor, hypotension, hyperglycaemia, flushing, hypokalaemia, pulmonary oedema • Fetal: tachycardia, hyperglycaemia	✖ CI: tachycardia, hyperthyroidism, multiple pregnancies 🔅 Especially as a short-term tocolytic (up to 48h) 🔅 Use during pregnancy reserved for strict indications only due to risk of fetal tachycardia and blood glucose disturbances
Nausea, vomiting, headaches, dizziness, hot flashes, tachycardia, hypotension, hyperglycaemia	Preference for atosiban in cardiovascular risk ↑
Hypotension, flushes, headache, pulmonary oedema, nausea	🔅 Calcium antagonists are as effective as beta agonists but have fewer serious adverse effects 🔅 Strictly reserved for pregnant women with severe hypertension who do not respond to standard therapy, requires close monitoring ✖ Not recommended in 1st trimester due to decreased placental perfusion ⇔ May cause acute pulmonary oedema when combined with a beta blocker, especially when used to suppress contractions
Headache, hypotension, reflex tachycardia or bradycardia	🔅 Effective in 1-2 min, lasts 3-5 min ▲ Available IV access for administration of ephedrine in acute hypotension ⇔ Caution with hypertrophic obstructive cardiomyopathy, aortic or mitral valve stenosis, glaucoma ⇔ Combined with other antihypertensives: severe hypotension ✖ CI: severe hypertension, hypotension, uncorrected hypovolemia, intracranial pressure ↑, insufficient cerebral perfusion, constrictive pericarditis, pericardial tamponade, or sensitivity to nitrates
• Maternal: dizziness, headache, nausea and vomiting • Fetal: cardiac haemorrhage, hypertension, renal problems, jaundice	🔅 Effect differs among women 🔅 Can delay labour between 24h and 7d ● Use during 3rd trimester for premature closure of the ductus arteriosus/Botalli, pulmonary hypertension, clotting disorder causing bleeding, renal impairment/insufficiency, gastrointestinal bleeding/perforation ✖ CI: teratogenic

Local irritation at injection site/entry point	🔅 Atosiban is administered via IV
	🔅 • As effective as beta agonists
	   • No maternal and fetal adverse effects
	   • Disadvantage is high cost
	🔅 Safe for known indications at 24-33 wk gestational age

TREATMENT

	MEDICATION	MECHANISM OF ACTION	INDICATIONS
UTEROTONICS (labour induction)	**Oxytocin agonist** (oxytocin)	Stimulates oxytocin receptor → rhythmic uterine contractions, contraction of myoepithelial breast cells (→ stimulates lactation)	• Induction of labour and stimulation of contractions • Stimulation of uterine contractions for uterine closure after caesarean section (CS) • Prevention/treatment of postpartum haemorrhage
	Progesterone antagonist (mifepristone)	Competes with progesterone for progesterone receptor	• Medical termination of pregnancy • Cervical dilation and softening prior to operative termination of pregnancy • Labour induction in cases of intrauterine fetal demise (IUFD) if prostaglandin or oxytocin have been ruled out
	Prostaglandin agonists (carboprost)	Prostaglandin F2-α analogue, stimulates prolonged uterine contractions	Treatment of third stage of labour when other uterotonics fail
	Prostaglandin agonists (misoprostol)	Stimulate uterine contraction (via prostaglandin receptors) and cervical softening	• Induce labour and stimulate contractions • Postpartum haemorrhage • Termination of pregnancy • IUFD
	Uterotonics, other (methylergometrine)	Strong activating effect on smooth muscle tissue and increase of basal tone, frequency, and amplitude of rhythmic contractions	• Active treatment in postpartum period • Used to treat bleeding after placental delivery, CS, or miscarriage

Table 57B // Medication for delivery

 Use of labour-inducing drugs requires close monitoring of fetal heart rate and uterine activity.

 In case of imminent premature childbirth before week 34, the mother is given an injection of corticosteroids twice over 48 hours (1 every 24 hours) to stimulate lung maturation. Tocolytics are administered to prolong the pregnancy for at least those 48 hours.

 Total spinal anaesthesia is a complication of neuraxial analgesia. It is characterised by acute onset haemodynamic instability, dyspnea, and loss of consciousness.

ADVERSE EFFECTS	NOTES
· Maternal: bradycardia, headache, nausea and vomiting, tachycardia · Fetal: antidiuretic effect	☼ Short $t_{1/2}$ requiring IV or IM administration ⇔ Effect potentiated by prostaglandins ⊗ CI: onset of labour, gestational age <36 wk, suspected/indications of fetal distress before induction, placenta praevia, unexplained haemorrhage <24 wk, anatomical uterine abnormalities, abnormal fetal position, symptoms of chorioamnionitis
Abdominal pain, cervical contractions or cramps, diarrhoea, headache, chills or fever, stomach pain, nausea and vomiting, fatigue	☼ Insufficient data on potential adverse effects. Reported cases of malformations, possibly due to amniotic cord syndrome. ⊗ CI: suspected ectopic pregnancy
Nausea, vomiting, diarrhoea	☼ Do not administer IV ⇔ Monitor blood pressure because of risk of severe hypertension or bronchospasm ⊗ CI: severe hypertension, unstable asthma
Nausea, vomiting, diarrhoea	
Abdominal pain, headache, skin rash, hypertension	⇔ Effect ↑ when combined with prostaglandins ⊗ CI: pregnancy, dilation and expulsion stages until delivery of the anterior shoulder, severe hypertension, pre-eclampsia

◉ Conservative treatment

Labour

Digital cervical exam

During childbirth, dilation can be measured by performing a digital cervical exam. This exam consists of the following steps:

· Cervix: position (posterior/mid position/anterior), length (effacement) and consistency (firm/moderately soft/soft).
· Dilation: estimate dilation in cm by inserting one or both fingers into the open vaginal portion. At 10 cm (full dilation), the edge of the vaginal portion can no longer be felt.
· Membranes: evaluate whether the membranes are intact or have ruptured

- Descent: position of the presenting part relative to the Hodge planes (see Figure 38).
- Presentation: occipital or breech, if neither is palpable → transverse.
- Position (head or breech): fetal head position is described based on the hands of a clock. In an occipital position, the posterior fontanelle is the presenting point (see Figure 39). In a face or sinciput presentation, the presenting point is mentum.

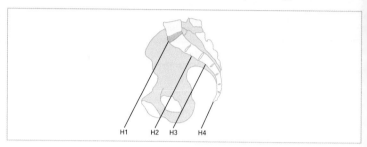

Figure 38 // Hodge planes: represent the different levels of fetal descent
H1: Coincides with the pelvic inlet, through the upper edge of the pubic symphysis **H2:** Parallel to H1, through the lower edge of the symphysis **H3:** Parallel to H1 and H2, through the ischial spines **H4:** Parallel to H1-H3, through the tip of the coccyx (almost coincides with the pelvic floor). When the head of the fetus is just beyond H2, it is at stage H2+.

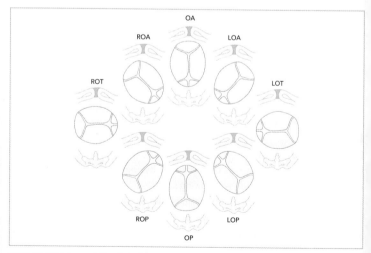

Figure 39 // Fetal presentation during labour
OP: Occiput posterior **ROP:** Right occiput posterior **ROT:** Right occiput transverse **ROA:** Right occiput anterior **OA:** Occiput anterior **LOA:** Left occiput anterior **LOT:** Left occiput anterior **LOP:** Left occiput posterior

When performing a vaginal exam in labour, pay attention to pain, prolapse of the fetal extremities and palpable pulsations from a prolapsed umbilical cord, and assess the bony birth canal, the soft birth canal and the pelvic floor.

Expulsion stage

During the expulsion stage, it is recommended to wait for full dilation and descent of the fetal head before asking the mother to start pushing. During this stage, fetal heart function should be monitored continuously or after each contraction, using a doptone device or CTG. Once the fetal head is crowning, ask the mother to sigh in order to deliver the head slowly and reduce the risk of perineal tears. In order to expedite expulsion local anaesthesia is administered as needed and a mediolateral episiotomy is made. After the fetal head has been delivered, check for a nuchal cord and correct if necessary. The fetus will then complete the external rotation, after which the anterior shoulder is delivered, followed by the posterior shoulder and the rest of the body (see Figures 40 and 41).

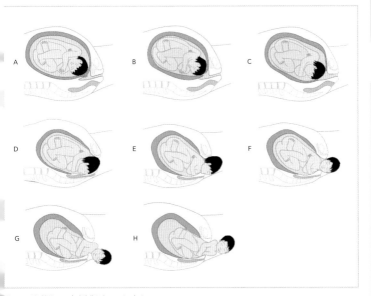

Figure 40 // Normal childbirth, sagittal view
A-D: Head descent and internal rotation from LOT to OA **E:** Head extends in OA **F:** External rotation **G:** Delivery of anterior shoulder **H:** Delivery of posterior shoulder

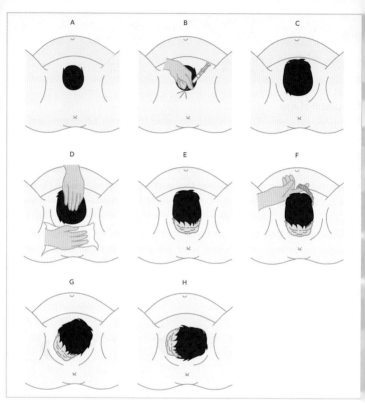

Figure 41 // Delivery of the head, vulvar view

A: Protruding fetal head **B:** Possible indication for episiotomy **C:** Crowning fetal head **D:** Protruding fetal head with perineal support **E:** Head delivered in OA **F:** Correct nuchal cord as needed **G-H:** External rotation

> **Internal rotation:** the longitudinal rotation made by the fetus during the descent and expulsion stage.

Assisted delivery

In case of stagnated labour, maternal exhaustion or fetal distress, the expulsion stage may be accelerated or assisted by using forceps or vacuum extraction (see Table 58 and Figure 42). Forceps are rarely used due to the high risk of pelvic floor damage. However, these risks must be weighed against the significant maternal and fetal morbidity from a full dilation CS.

ASSISTED DELIVERY METHOD	CONTRA-INDICATIONS	TECHNIQUE	COMPLICATIONS
Forceps	Bony part not yet descended (above Hodge 3), feto-pelvic disproportion, unknown fetal head position, fetal demineralising disease	The blades are inserted individually over the baby's ears and then locked together. The dominant hand then moves the forceps horizontally in caudal direction while the non-dominant hand applies downward pressure on the forceps blades.	Maternal pelvic floor damage, fetal damage due to improper blade placement
Vacuum extraction	Hydrocephalus, increased risk of fetal bleeding, fetal gestation <34 wk. Relative contraindication if descent < Hodge 3.	The labia are spread, after which the ventouse (suction cup) is attached to the flexion point (2 cm from the posterior fontanelle). Traction is then applied towards the birth canal, while keeping the fingers on the ventouse for vacuum continuity.	Maternal trauma, cephalic haematoma, fetal intracranial injury

Table 58 // Assisted delivery

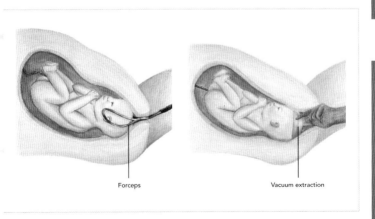

Forceps

Vacuum extraction

Figure 42 // Assisted delivery - forceps and vacuum extraction

Caesarean section (CS)

In the case of fetal distress or a contraindication to vaginal delivery, CS is the preferred method of delivery. See Figure 43 for a quick overview of this surgical technique. See Appendix 1 for a pre-OR checklist.

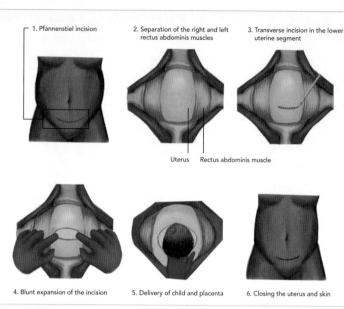

1. Pfannenstiel incision
2. Separation of the right and left rectus abdominis muscles
3. Transverse incision in the lower uterine segment

Uterus   Rectus abdominis muscle

4. Blunt expansion of the incision
5. Delivery of child and placenta
6. Closing the uterus and skin

Figure 43 // Caesarean section

Afterbirth stage
Clamping and cutting umbilical cord
Delayed cord clamping, or allowing the umbilical cord to pulsate prior to clamping with an umbilical cord clamp is preferred. The umbilical cord is cut between the two clamps.

Placental delivery
The placenta is usually delivered spontaneously within ten minutes. Placental delivery can be expedited by administering IV or IM oxytocin after the umbilical cord has been clamped and cut. Oxytocin promotes placental delivery and uterine contraction and reduces the risk of postpartum haemorrhage. The placenta should be delivered within 30 minutes.

Küstner manoeuvre
The Küstner manoeuvre can be used to check if the placenta is in the lower uterine segment and whether it has detached. To perform this manoeuvre, check whether the uterus has contracted, and if so, take the clamp on the umbilical

cord in the dominant hand and apply light traction. If the uterus has not contracted, applying traction to the umbilical cord can cause uterine inversion. Simultaneously, apply caudal pressure to the abdominal wall with the ulnar side of the other hand from the top of the pubic symphysis. If the placenta has failed to detach, the taut umbilical cord will be pulled slightly inward (negative Küstner). In case of a negative result, repeat the Küstner manoeuvre after ten minutes. If the placenta has detached, the umbilical cord will be pulled outward slightly (positive Küstner), see Figure 44.

Baer's manoeuvre

Baer's manoeuvre is used to provide counterpressure at the level of the abdomen. The patient is asked to push during the uterine contraction for placental delivery. The abdominal wall is supported with a flat hand (Baer's manoeuvre). The dominant hand is used to keep the umbilical cord taut without applying traction (see Figure 44).

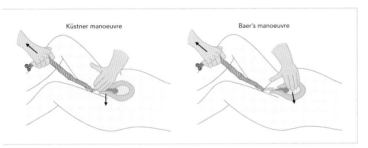

Figure 44 // Küstner manoeuvre and Baer's manoeuvre

Placental exam

When 50% of the placenta has been delivered, grab it with two hands and rotate it without applying traction. Rotating the placenta reduces the risk of torn and ragged membranes. The placenta can be delivered in two ways, by first delivering the fetal side, or by first delivering the maternal side. After expulsion, the placenta should be checked for completeness (membranes, cotyledons, umbilical cord insertion and umbilical vessels). A more detailed placental exam is performed once the mother has stabilised after delivery. If a piece of placenta is missing, the missing part is removed manually, or surgically under anaesthesia.

Postpartum

Newborn care

After childbirth, the child's APGAR score is evaluated after 1, 5 and 10 minutes (see Table 59). A score of 7-10 is normal, a score of 4-7 requires intervention and a score of <3 requires immediate intervention (cardiopulmonary resuscitation (CPR), only when airway and breathing are sufficiently treated by rescue breaths followed by ventilation).

APGAR	0	1	2
Pulse	Absent	<100/min	>100/min
RR	Absent	Gasping, irregular	Vigorous crying, regular
Muscle tone	Limp	Arms and legs flexed	Active movement
Colour	Blue/gray/very pale	Acrocyanosis	Pink
Reactivity	None	Grimaces	Crying, coughing

Table 59 // APGAR score

Maternal monitoring

After childbirth the mother should be monitored, looking for various parameters.
- Vitals
- Perineum, vaginal walls, and sphincter (rectovaginal exam). In case of perineal tears, or an episiotomy, inspect the wound and assess whether sutures are needed. Perineal tears are divided into four grades, depending on the structures involved (see Figure 45).
- Amount of blood loss (postpartum haemorrhage). Administer a blood transfusion if indicated based on baseline Hb and clinical condition.
- Check the 7Bs:
  1 **B**reasts: initiation of lactation, proper latching, nipple fissures
  2 **B**elly/uterus: descending fundal height, lochia (colour, odour), possible blood loss
  3 **B**ladder: urine production, urinary retention
  4 **B**uttocks/pelvic floor: healing of episiotomy/perineal tears, defecation 1-4 days postpartum
  5 Lim**b**s: thrombosis
  6 **B**rain/experience: psyche, maternal depression, mention possibility of dyspareunia
  7 **B**aby: fetal vital signs, fetal movement

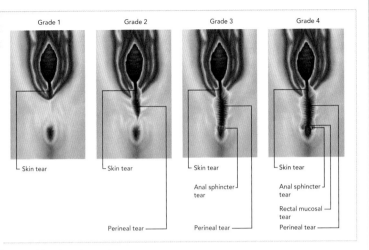

Figure 45 // Grading of perineal tears

Fertility

General

Lifestyle recommendations

Lifestyle can largely influence reproductive health. Modifying lifestyle factors and preventative measures can be beneficial. Important lifestyle factors that can affect fertility:

- Maintaining nutritional health;
- Healthy weight: a BMI <18.5 or >25 is considered to have major effects on health (e.g. infertility, cardiovascular disease, DM);
- Exercise: physical activity has a protective effect on infertility. Vigorous exercise can have a negative effect on the reproductive system through hypothalamic dysfunction;
- Limit stress: stress hormones (e.g. cortisol, adrenaline) have a negative effect on fertility;
- Quit or reduce smoking and use of drugs and/or alcohol;
- Limit caffeine intake;
- Avoid exposure to certain environmental and occupational toxins (e.g. pollution, radiation, chemicals, pesticides, heavy metals).

🔖 Pharmacological treatment

Hormone preparations

	MEDICATION	MECHANISM OF ACTION	INDICATIONS
HORMONE PREPARATIONS	**Oestrogen** (oestradiol)	Most active natural oestrogen	• Climacteric symptoms • Osteoporosis • Persons transitioning to the female gender
	Oestrogen-progestogen combinations (dydrogesterone, lynestrenol, medroxyprogesterone, megestrol, norethisterone, progesterone, tibolone, ulipristal)	Bind and activate progestogens to progesterone receptor → endometrial development	• Climacteric symptoms • Dysfunctional uterine bleeding • Imminent/recurring miscarriage due to progesterone deficiency • Dysmenorrhoea • Endometriosis • Infertility due to corpus luteum insufficiency • Support luteal phase with artificial insemination • Menstrual cycle regulation • Secondary amenorrhoea
	Androgens (testosterone)	Bind to and activate androgen receptor: • Development and maintenance of secondary male sex characteristics and sexual functions • Protein synthesis ↑, protein degradation ↓	• Primary and secondary testosterone deficiency in men • Hypogonadism in men caused by testosterone deficiency • Persons transitioning to male gender

Table 60 // Hormone preparations

Fertility treatment

	MEDICATION	MECHANISM OF ACTION	INDICATIONS
FOLLICLE STIMULATING HORMONE (FSH)	**Aromatase inhibitor** (letrozole)	Inhibits aromatase enzyme competitively → formation of oestrogen from androgen precursors ↓	Anovulation in polycystic ovarian syndrome (PCOS) / WHO II ovulation disorder
	Antioestrogens (clomiphene citrate)	• Binding of oestrogen to receptor and in thalamus ↓ • In thalamus, compensatory secretion of GnRH → FSH/LH ↑	

Table 61A // Medication fertility treatment

ADVERSE EFFECTS	NOTES
Abdominal pain, depression, break-through bleeding, weight changes, headache/migraine, skin rash, nausea, oedema, painful breasts, endometrial carcinoma (with long-term use)	☼ Caution is advised in cases of impaired cardiac/kidney function, as oestrogens can cause fluid retention
Amenorrhoea, breakthrough bleeding, irregular vaginal bleeding	
	⊗ CI: history of idiopathic venous thromboembolism, or active venous thromboembolism ⊗ Discontinue during pregnancy
Gynaecomastia, prostatic hyperplasia, peripheral oedema, exacerbation of hypertension, decreased glucose tolerance, sleep apnoea, altered lipid profile (lower HDL cholesterol)	☼ Concomitant use of adrenocorticotropic hormone (ACTH), or corticosteroids may enhance oedema formation ⇔ May potentiate vitamin K antagonists, possibly requiring a lower dose of vitamin K antagonists and frequent INR monitoring ⊗ Risk of fetal virilisation in pregnant women

ADVERSE EFFECTS	NOTES
Hot flashes, palpitations, nausea, vomiting, headaches, dizziness, hyperhidrosis, diarrhoea, depression, oedema, osteoporosis	⇔ Caution with severe liver insufficiency, as it can increase liver enzymes ⇔ Avoid combination with tamoxifen, other antioestrogens → letrozole efficiency ↓
Hot flashes, nausea, vomiting, abdominal pain, menorrhagia/metrorrhagia, ovary enlargement, risk of ovarian hyperstimulation syndrome (OHSS)	☼ Chances of multiple gestation, gestational diabetes, toxicosis ⇔ Caution with fibromas → fibroma enlargement ⊗ CI: severe liver disease, hormone-dependent malignancies, unknown vaginal bleeding, ovarian cysts, dysfunctional pituitary gland or ovaries

	MEDICATION	MECHANISM OF ACTION	INDICATIONS
FOLLICLE STIMULATING HORMONE (FSH)	**Antioestrogens** (tamoxifen)	• Non-steroid triphenylethylene derivate • Competitive blocking of oestrogen receptor • Oestrogen receptor expression ↓	Controlled hyperstimulation in anovulatory or oligoovulatory patients
	Recombinant human follicle-stimulating hormone (follitropin α)	Stimulates growth and maturations of oocytes	Possibly combined with LH medication in follicle stimulation
	Human menopausal gonadotropin (menotropin)	Production of oestradiol ↑, aromatising androgens	• Anovulation in PCOS and clomiphene citrate failure or resistance • Controlled ovarian hyperstimulation in assisted reproductive treatment – IUI or IVF/ICSI
PULSATILE GNRH	**Gonadorelin-agonist** (gonadorelin diacetate)	Pulsatile release of gonadorelin → FSH and LH production ↑	• Infertility in hypothalamic amenorrhoea • Anovulation with antioestrogens failure / WHO I ovulation disorder
OVULATION INHIBITOR	**Gonadorelin-agonist** (leuprorelin acetate)	Secretion of FSH and LH from pituitary gland ↑ → desensitisation of pituitary gland → FSH and LH ↓	Prevent premature ovulation in controlled hyperstimulation followed by oocyte retrieval by blocking release of LH in IVF/ICSI
	Gonadorelin-antagonist (cetrorelix acetate)	Competitive binding of GnRH-receptors → FSH and LH ↓	
OVULATION TRIGGER	**Recombinant human chorionic gonadotropin** (choriogonadotropin α)	• Replacement of endogen pre-ovulatory LH peak • Induction of last phase of follicle stimulation → ovulation	• Assisted reproductive treatment – IUI or IVF/ICSI • Induction of ovulation and luteinisation after follicle stimulation in anovulatory or oligoovulatory cycles

Table 61B // Medication fertility treatment

ADVERSE EFFECTS	NOTES
Hot flashes, nausea, vomiting, irregular menses, amenorrhoea, eye complaints, thromboembolic events	⇔ Caution with risk factors or history thromboembolic events ⇔ Interaction with oral contraceptives: reduces efficiency (65-75%) ⇔ Antidepressants (e.g. paroxetine, fluoxetine) → tamoxifen ↓ ⇔ Efficiency of vitamin K antagonists ↑
Headache, ovarian cysts, multiple gestation, breast tenderness, skin reactions, mood swings, nausea, vomiting, abdominal pain, OHSS	☼ Risk of multiple gestation ⇔ Caution in patients with asthma because risk of exacerbation ↑ ⇔ Risk of OHSS: monitor follicle development ✖ CI: tumour of pituitary gland or hypothalamus; ovarian, uterine, or breast cancer; enlarged ovaries; unknown vaginal bleeding ⇔ Need for higher dosages with simultaneous use of GnRH agonists for adequate response ⇔ Follicle response enhancement with simultaneous use of clomiphene citrate ✖ CI: tumour of pituitary gland or hypothalamus; ovarian, uterine, or breast cancer; enlarged ovaries; unknown vaginal bleeding; premature ovarian insufficiency; uterine abnormality or myoma
Allergic reaction at injection site, OHSS	☼ Caution with use of levodopa or spironolactone → change in response to gonadorelin
Hot flashes, headaches, mood swings, insomnia, vaginal dryness, breast size ↓, dyspareunia, bone density ↓	⇔ Caution with use: androgen deprivation medication → QT interval ↑ ✖ CI: hypersensitivity leuprorelin, hormone-independent tumours, progressive brain tumour, unknown cause of vaginal bleeding in girls
Allergic reaction or anaphylaxis at injection site, hot flashes, headaches, mood swings, insomnia, vaginal dryness, breast size ↓, dyspareunia, bone density ↓, OHSS	☼ No flare-up effect due to hypoestrogenic status, shortening period cycle, lower dosage needed, immediate effect ⇔ 30 min observation after injection → risk of allergic anaphylactic reaction ⇔ Caution with repetitive use because of limited experience in subsequent cycles ✖ CI: hypersensitivity to GnRH agonists, severe renal insufficiency
Hypersensitive injection site, oedema, headaches, mood swings, OHSS, nausea, vomiting, abdominal pain, breast tenderness	☼ Risk of multiple gestation, thromboembolic event ✖ CI: untreated endocrinological disorders (thyroid disease, adrenal, or pituitary); ovarian, uterine, or breast cancer; primary gonadal insufficiency; uterine anomaly; myoma; unknown vaginal bleeding

	MEDICATION	MECHANISM OF ACTION	INDICATIONS
ORAL ANTI-DIABETIC AGENT	**Biguanides** (metformin)	• Insulin sensitivity ↑, corrects hyperinsulinemia and helps resume ovulation • LH and androgen ↓, FSH ↑	Anovulation in PCOS and clomiphene citrate failure

Table 61C // Medication fertility treatment

 In IVF/ICSI controlled hyperstimulation with gonadotropins is used, combined with gonadorelin agonists or gonadorelin antagonists, depending on the treatment scheme used.

 Luteal phase deficiency consists of insufficient progesterone, failing to maintain a secretory endometrium, and subsequent implantation and growth of the normal embryo. Progesterone luteal phase support can be added to controlled hyperstimulation in IUI.

Invasive, non-pharmacological treatment

Infertility affects 10-15% of the population and is defined as unprotected regular sexual intercourse for twelve months without conception (see Infertility/Subfertility). Causes of irregular menses, semen analysis, and tubal patency can identify the source of the infertility, but 25% of all cases remain unexplained. The Hunault score is used to estimate the chances of spontaneous pregnancy. With a Hunault score >30% there is no indication for assisted reproductive treatment, and expectative management for at least six months is advised. After twelve months, active intervention is preferred for most couples. Ovarian stimulation (OS), intrauterine insemination (IUI), in-vitro fertilisation (IVF), and intracytoplasmic sperm injection (ICSI) are treatment options.

Intrauterine insemination (IUI) with or without controlled ovarian hyperstimulation (COH)

IUI with COH is recommended as a first-choice treatment for unexplained infertility. Give ovulation-stimulating medication (e.g. clomiphene citrate, metformin, letrozole, gonadotropins) and inseminate 24-36 hours after ovulation. There is a risk of multiple gestation.

ADVERSE EFFECTS	NOTES
Diarrhoea, nausea, vomiting, abdominal pain, appetite ↓	✖ CI: acute metabolic acidosis, severe kidney failure, dehydration, severe infection or shock, heart failure (fluid overload), recent myocardial infarction, liver insufficiency, acute alcohol poisoning

Indications for IUI with or without COH are moderate oligoasthenoteratozoospermia (OAT), unexplained infertility with Hunault score <30%, physical disability, or psychosexual problem. Contraindications for IUI with or without COH are bilateral tubal occlusion, amenorrhoea, severe oligospermia, endometritis, cervical atresia, and cervicitis.

In vitro fertilisation (IVF)

IVF is a fertility treatment in which follicle stimulation is enhanced, followed by oocyte retrieval through ultrasound-guided puncture. The acquired oocytes are combined with processed spermatozoa to form embryos. The embryos are incubated, and embryo transfer takes place after 3-5 days.

Indications for IVF are unexplained infertility, endometriosis (ASRM grade IV), ovulation disorders, dysfunctional fallopian tubes, uterine fibroids, genetic disorders, sperm abnormalities, age >38, and unsuccessful treatment with IUI. Contraindications for IVF are significant risk of morbidity and/or mortality for pregnancy, e.g. New York Heart Association (NYHA) class 3 or 4 heart failure, pulmonary hypertension, severe valve stenosis, aortic coarctation, Eisenmenger syndrome, and Marfan syndrome.

🔆 Offer HIV, hepatitis B, and C screening.

Intracytoplasmic sperm injection (ICSI)

ICSI is the treatment of choice for male infertility. With ICSI a single spermatozoon is injected into an oocyte under a microscope. For follicle stimulation and oocyte retrieval, the same procedure is followed as in the IVF procedure.

Indications for ICSI are severe OAT and previous unsuccessful IVF treatments. Contraindications are patients age >44, menopause, uterine anomalies, Asherman syndrome, leiomyoma, unclear ovarian cysts, internal genital tract cancer, severe systemic-progressive genetic disease, and neurotic or psychotic diseases.

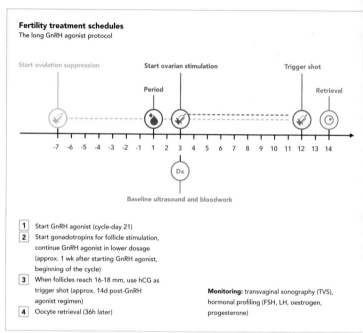

Fertility treatment schedules
The long GnRH agonist protocol

1 Start GnRH agonist (cycle-day 21)
2 Start gonadotropins for follicle stimulation, continue GnRH agonist in lower dosage (approx. 1 wk after starting GnRH agonist, beginning of the cycle)
3 When follicles reach 16-18 mm, use hCG as trigger shot (approx. 14d post-GnRH agonist regimen)
4 Oocyte retrieval (36h later)

Monitoring: transvaginal sonography (TVS), hormonal profiling (FSH, LH, oestrogen, progesterone)

Diagram 8 // Long GnRH agonist protocol

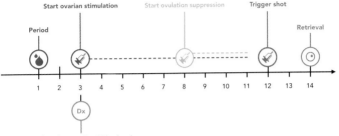

Fertility treatment schedules
GnRH antagonist protocol

1 Start gonadotropins for follicle stimulation (cycle-day 2-3)
2 Start GnRH antagonist for ovulation suppression (cycle-day 7-9)
3 Approx. 6d after start of gonadotropins or when follicles reach 16-18 mm, use hCG as trigger shot
4 Oocyte retrieval (36h later)

Monitoring: transvaginal sonography (TVS), hormonal profiling (FSH, LH, oestrogen, progesterone)
Appropriate for: most patients, particularly useful with high risk of OHSS.
Adverse effects: lower follicular production, lower implantation and pregnancy rate.

Diagram 9 // GnRH antagonist protocol

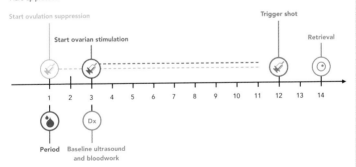

Fertility treatment schedules
Flare-up protocol

1 Start GnRH agonist (cycle-day 1)
2 Start gonadotropins for follicle stimulation (cycle-day 2 or 3)
3 When follicles reach 16-18 mm, use hCG as trigger shot (approx. 14d post-GnRH agonist regimen)
4 Oocyte retrieval (36h later)

Caution in: patients with high risk of OHSS and patients with low ovarian reserve or a history of poor response to previous IVF.

Diagram 10 // Flare-up protocol

Differential diagnosis

 This section lists possible diagnoses you could consider for specific complaints. Important! The diagnoses listed here are not exhaustive and serve only as examples.

Amenorrhoea

Primary amenorrhoea

* Anatomical:
  * Mechanical uterine obstruction (imperforate hymen, transverse vaginal septum)
  * Mayer-Rokitansky-Küster-Hauser syndrome
* Endocrine:
  * Genetic (Turner syndrome, congenital adrenal hyperplasia, androgen insensitivity syndrome, Kallmann syndrome)
  * Hypothalamus (anorexia, excessive exercise, stress, delayed puberty)
  * Pituitary gland (pituitary tumour: prolactinoma, craniopharyngioma, hypothyroidism/hyperthyroidism, hypopituitarism)
  * Ovarian (PCOS, POI)
  * Adrenal gland (androgen-producing tumour)
* Iatrogenic:
  * Medication (including antipsychotics, antidepressants, opioids)
  * Ovarian damage (radiation, surgery)

Secondary amenorrhoea

* Anatomical:
  * Mechanical uterine obstruction (Asherman syndrome, septa)
* Endocrine:
  * Obstetric (pregnancy, breastfeeding)
  * Adverse effect of hormonal IUD (in about 20% of users)
  * Hypothalamus (anorexia, excessive exercise, stress)
  * Pituitary gland (pituitary tumour: prolactinoma, craniopharyngioma; hypothyroidism/hyperthyroidism)
  * Ovarian (PCOS, POI, menopause)
  * Adrenal gland (androgen-producing tumour)

- Iatrogenic:
  - Medication (e.g. antipsychotics, antidepressants, opioids, prior contraceptive injection)
  - Ovarian damage (radiation, surgery)
  - Hysterectomy

Abdominal pain

- Gynaecological causes of abdominal pain (during and outside pregnancy):
  - Adenomyosis, endometriosis
  - Corpus luteum haemorrhage
  - Malignancy (cervical, endometrial, ovarian, uterine)
  - Menstrual pain, ovulation pain (Mittelschmerz)
  - Fibroid necrosis
  - Ovarian cyst (rupture, intracystic haemorrhage)
  - PID (pelvic inflammatory disease)
  - Ovarian torsion (due to ovarian cyst/tumour)
  - Anatomical uterine abnormality
  - Female genital mutilation (FGM)
- Pregnancy (1st trimester):
  - Round ligament pain
  - Ectopic pregnancy
  - Spontaneous or non-spontaneous miscarriage
- Pregnancy (2nd/3rd trimester):
  - Placental abruption
  - Chorioamnionitis
  - Pre-eclampsia/HELLP
  - Immature birth (wk 16-28)/premature birth (wk 28-37)
  - Hydronephrosis (due to uterine pressure)
  - Cystitis (with bladder spasms)
  - Physiological ('hard abdomen', fetal movements)
- Puerperium:
  - Cystitis
  - Endometritis (GAS), parametritis
  - (Infected) haematoma
  - Salpingitis
  - Wound infection

Endometriosis and fibroid necrosis do not cause abdominal pain after menopause because menstrual cycle cessation inhibits endometrial and fibroid growth.

Menstrual cycle disorders

- ◆ Anatomical:
  - · Uterine (adenomyosis)
- ◆ Endocrine:
  - · Genetic (e.g. Kallmann syndrome)
  - · Hypothalamus (anorexia, excessive exercise, stress)
  - · Pituitary gland (hypothyroidism/hyperthyroidism, hyperprolactinaemia)
  - · Ovarian (anovulatory cycle after menarche, PCOS, POI)
  - · Adrenal gland (hyperandrogenism)
- ◆ Bleeding disorder:
  - · Clotting disorders (e.g. Von Willebrand syndrome)
- ◆ Iatrogenic:
  - · Anticoagulants or antiaggregants
  - · Contraceptive (OC, IUD)
  - · Postpilamenorrhoea
- ◆ Idiopathic:
  - · Physiological

Amenorrhoea, polymenorrhoea/oligomenorrhoea, menorrhagia, metrorrhagia, dysmenorrhoea are all symptoms of menstrual cycle disorders with different causes. The differential diagnosis lists the main causes of menstrual cycle disorders.

- · Menorrhagia (cyclical bleeding) is often caused by physiological factors or minor underlying pathology (e.g. fibroids).
- · Metrorrhagia (noncyclic bleeding) is often caused by underlying pathology (e.g. malignant polyps, persistent follicle).

Infertility/subfertility

- ◆ Anatomical:
  - · Uterine (adenomyosis, endometriosis)
  - · Mechanical obstruction (septa, Asherman syndrome)
  - · Tubal pathology (e.g. after *Chlamydia* infection)

- Endocrine:
  - Genetic (oligomenorrhoea/amenorrhoea see Diagram 12 and 13)
  - Hypothalamus (anorexia, excessive exercise, stress)
  - Pituitary gland (hypothyroidism, prolactinoma)
  - Ovarian (PCOS, POI)
- Iatrogenic:
  - Ovarian damage (radiotherapy, surgery, chemotherapy, postinfectious e.g. PID)
  - Tubal surgery (hydrosalpinx, tubectomy after ectopic pregnancy)
  - Medication (e.g. valproic acid, prior contraceptive injection)
  - Sperm quality (oligospermia/azoospermia, obstruction, cystic fibrosis, genetic dysspermatogenesis, varicocele, smoking, cryptorchidia, iatrogenic: e.g. cyclophosphamide, ketoconazole, antiandrogens)

Rotterdam criteria (min. 2 present for diagnosis of PCOS):
- Ultrasound shows ovarian enlargement with >12 follicles in an ovary
- Signs of hyperandrogenism (lab or clinical)
- Oligomenorrhoea or amenorrhoea

PALM COEIU:
- Anatomical or organ abnormalities (PALM): **P**olyps, **A**denomyosis, **L**eiomyomas, **M**alignancy.
- Hypermenorrhoea (COEIU): **C**oagulopathy, **O**vulatory disorders, **E**ndometrial disorders, **I**atrogenic, **U**nclassified.

Hydrosalpinx is a condition of the fallopian tubes caused by dilation and accumulation of serous or clear fluid in the tubes. The uterus and ovaries are disconnected, causing subfertility or infertility. It is characterised by a sausage-shaped tube on TVU.

Hypertension during pregnancy
- Chronic hypertension (pre-existent)
- Gestational hypertension
- Eclampsia/pre-eclampsia, HELLP

Fever

- Peripartum:
  - Chorioamnionitis
  - Epidural anaesthesia
- Puerperium:
  - Thorax (mastitis, pulmonary embolism, pneumonia)
  - Abdomen (cholecystitis, pelveoperitonitis, pyelonephritis, wound infection)
  - Pelvis (endometritis, parametritis, salpingitis, ovarian vein thrombosis, UTI, wound infection)
  - Legs (DVT)

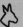 Causes of puerperal fever can be remembered using the acronym **PLAT: P**elvis-**L**egs-**A**bdomen-**T**horax.

Diminished sexual arousal

- Somatic:
  - Pregnancy, breastfeeding
  - Puerperal
  - Pituitary gland (hypothyroidism/hyperthyroidism, prolactinoma)
  - Iatrogenic (e.g. antipsychotics, antidepressants)
- Sexological:
  - Vaginismus
  - Dyspareunia
  - Vulvodynia
  - Orgasm disorder
- Psychological:
  - Stress
  - Relationship problems
  - Fatigue
  - Depression

Vaginal bleeding

- Non-pregnant women:
  - Anatomical (cervical/intracavitary abnormality: carcinoma, cervicitis, cyst, dysplasia, fibroid, polyp)
  - Endocrine (hormonal imbalance: atrophic endometrium with IUD/OC use)

- Pre-menopausal (menstrual bleeding, breakthrough bleeding, withdrawal bleeding: ovulatory bleeding, OC)
- Postmenopausal (atrophic endometrium, use of hormones, endometrial cancer)
- Clotting disorder (e.g. Von Willebrand syndrome)
- Other (ectropion, STI: *Chlamydia, gonorrhoea*)
- Pregnancy (1st trimester):
  - Imminent/complete miscarriage
  - Ectopic pregnancy
  - Implantation bleeding
  - Trophoblastic disease (molar pregnancy)
- Pregnancy (2nd/3rd trimester):
  - Imminent/complete miscarriage
  - Imminent premature childbirth
  - Uterine rupture
  - Placental abnormalities (praevia, circumvallate, abruption)
  - Vasa praevia
  - Peripheral vein haemorrhages
  - Cervical blood loss
- Puerperium:
  - Muscle tone (atonia)
  - Tissue (placental remnant, uterine inversion)
  - Trauma (vaginal/cervical/uterine rupture, bleeding from episiotomy)
  - Thrombosis/clotting disorder (Von Willebrand syndrome, disseminated intravascular coagulation (DIC))
  - Physiological (approx. ≤6 mo postpartum)

Causes of puerperal vaginal bleeding can be remembered using the 4 Ts: **T**one-**T**issue-**T**rauma-**T**hrombosis.

Vaginal itching
- Physiological (atrophic vaginitis)
- Candidiasis
- STI (gonorrhoea, pediculosis pubis, trichomoniasis, scabies)
- Lichen sclerosus et atrophicus (LSEA)
- Lichen ruber planus

Abnormal vaginal discharge

- Infectious:
  - STIs (*Chlamydia, gonorrhoea*, trichomoniasis)
  - Bacterial vaginosis
  - Aerobic vaginitis
  - Candidiasis
- Oncological:
  - Benign (cervical polyp, endometrial polyp)
  - Malignant (vulvar carcinoma, cervical carcinoma)

Conditions

Anatomical abnormalities

Anatomical uterine abnormalities

Ⓓ Anatomical uterine abnormalities result from developmental disorders affecting the Müllerian ducts (see Figure 46).

Ⓔ Overall prevalence 4.3-6.7%. Prevalence of bicornuate uterus 37%, arcuate uterus 15%, incomplete septum 13%, uterus didelphys 11%, complete septum 9%, unicornuate uterus 4.4%

Ⓐe Developmental disorders of the Müllerian ducts

Ⓡ Maternal DES usage

Ⓗx Asymptomatic ⊙, subfertility or infertility, absent menarche (in agenesis)

Ⓟe Bimanual exam: no palpable uterus in case of uterine aplasia

Ⓓx TAU/TVU, MRI, hysteroscopy, laparoscopy: detect anatomical uterine abnormality, and renal abnormalities

Ⓣx 🔪 Metroplasty (reconstruction), be careful of risk of sterility

Ⓟ Treatment cannot cure infertility secondary to a uterine abnormality, but may prevent recurrent miscarriages

⚠ • Often coincides with anatomical abnormalities of the kidneys and ureter (e.g. renal agenesis, horse-shoe shaped kidney, duplex system) due to concurrent development (30-50%), and vertebral abnormalities (up to 29%) (e.g. spina bifida, wedge-shaped vertebral bodies)

• The correct diagnosis is important to prevent pregnancy complications (e.g. malposition of the fetus at term, risk of spontaneous preterm birth, habitual abortion, retained placenta, placenta praevia)

Uterine anomalies result from impaired Müllerian duct development:
• Incomplete fusion → bicorporeal uterus
• Unilateral, incomplete or absent fusion → hemi-uterus, uterine aplasia

Diethylstilbestrol (DES) is a synthetic hormone that was prescribed from the 1950s through the 1980s to prevent miscarriages, and treat bleeding during pregnancy. DES is shown to increase the risk or urogenital birth defects and carcinomas in daughters of mothers who have used DES.

Obstructed hemivagina and ipsilateral renal agenesis (OHVIRA) syndrome:
- Triad of uterine didelphys, unilateral obstructed hemivagina, ipsilateral renal agenesis;
- Incidence: 0.1-3.8%;
- Symptoms: pain, infertility, or complicated obstetrical history.

 With a rudimentary horn: risk of pregnancy in the rudimentary horn.

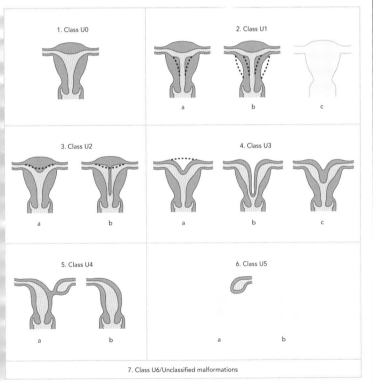

Figure 46 // Overview of uterine anomalies

1: Normal uterus **2:** Dysmorphic uterus **2a:** T-shaped uterus **2b:** Infantile uterus **2c:** Other **3:** Septate uterus **3a:** Partial **3b:** Complete **4:** Bicorporeal uterus **4a:** Partial **4b:** Complete **4c:** Bicorporeal septate uterus **5:** Hemi-uterus **5a:** With rudimentary uterine cavity **5b:** Without rudimentary uterine cavity **6:** Uterine aplasia **6a:** With rudimentary uterine cavity **6b:** Without rudimentary uterine cavity

UTERINE ANOMALY		CERVICAL/VAGINAL ANOMALY	
Main class	**Subclass**	**Co-existing class**	
U0 Normal uterus	No subclass	C0	Normal cervix
U1 Dysmorphic uterus	a. T-shaped b. Infantile c. Others	C1	Septate cervix
U2 Septate uterus	a. Partial b. Complete	C2	Double 'normal' cervix
U3 Bicorporeal uterus	a. Partial b. Complete c. Bicorporeal septate	C3	Unilateral cervical aplasia
		C4	Cervical aplasia
U4 Hemi-uterus	a. With rudimentary cavity (communicating or not horn) b. Without rudimentary cavity (horn without cavity/no horn)	V0	Normal vagina
		V1	Longitudinal non-obstructing vaginal septum
U5 Aplastic uterus	a. With rudimentary cavity (bilateral or unilateral horn) b. Without rudimentary cavity (bilateral or unilateral uterine remnants/aplasia)	V2	Longitudinal obstructing vaginal septum
		V3	Transverse vaginal septum and/or imperforate hymen
U6 Unclassified malformations		V4	Vaginal aplasia

Table 62 // ESGE classification of uterine, cervical, and vaginal anomalies (UxCxVx).

Vaginal agenesis

D Vaginal aplasia or agenesis is a congenital defect involving the partial or complete absence of a vagina (see Figure 46). It often occurs in conjunction with uterine agenesis (Mayer-Rokitansky-Küster-Hauser (MRKH) syndrome).

E Incidence 20:100,000/year

Ae Developmental disorders of the Müllerian ducts (MRKH syndrome)

Hx Primary amenorrhoea, abdominal pain, no penetration possible

PE In agenesis, spreading the labia minora does not reveal an introitus

Dx · TAU/TVU: detect vaginal aplasia
· Pelvic MRI: detect vaginal aplasia/agenesis

Tx ✐ Vaginoplasty

P Vaginoplasty, the creation of an artificial vagina, has a 70% success rate

⚠️ Often accompanied by renal agenesis, spinal abnormalities, Klippel-Feil syndrome, and hearing disorders

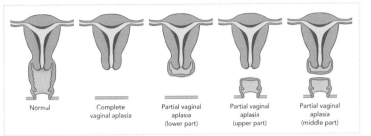

Figure 47 // Vaginal aplasia

Imperforate hymen

Ⓓ An imperforate hymen is the closure of the hymenal opening. This can lead to the accumulation of menstrual blood in the vagina and uterus.

Ⓔ Incidence 0.05-0.1%

Ⓐₑ Embryonic hymen fails to regress

Ⓗₓ Primary amenorrhoea, cyclic abdominal pain

Ⓟₑ • Normal secondary sexual features
  • External inspection of the vulva: spreading the labia minora reveals a bulging, translucent blue hymen resulting from the accumulation of menstrual blood → haematocolpos (see Figure 48)

Ⓓₓ No added value

Ⓣₓ 🔪 Incision of the hymen

Ⓟ Very good

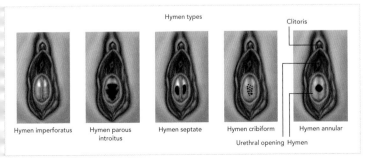

Hymen types

Clitoris

Hymen imperforatus Hymen parous introitus Hymen septate Hymen cribiform Hymen annular

Urethral opening Hymen

Figure 48 // Imperforate hymen

Female genital mutilation (FGM)

(D) FGM is the partial or total excision of the external female genitalia or other harmful practices to the female genitals for non-medical reasons mostly in girls under age 15.

(E) Prevalence ♀ 200 million, incidence 3 million, mostly in Africa (e.g. Somalia, Sierra Leone), Asia (Indonesia, Malaysia), Middle East (Egypt, Yemen), and South America (Colombia, Peru)

(Ae) • Short-term: extreme pain, excessive blood loss, infection, shock, or death
 • Long-term: dysmenorrhoea, prolonged menstruation, chronic pain, sexual dysfunction, obstetric complications, anxiety disorders, depressive disorders, posttraumatic stress disorder (PTSD)

(PE) Abnormal female genitals, different types of FGM

(Tx) 💬 Psychological support, education, risk assessment, early detection, photographs for legal purposes

🖊 Reconstructive surgery: de-infibulation, clitoral reconstruction

(P) Obstetric complications: de-infibulation during vaginal birth

(!) Type 4 FGM includes all other harmful procedures to the female genitalia in which physically small procedures could go unnoticed after healing

General gynaecology

Adenomyosis

(D) Adenomyosis is the presence of endometrial glandular tissue in the myometrium.

(E) Peak age 35-50, incidence unknown

(Ae) Idiopathic

(R) Multiparity, age >40, previous CS, or uterine surgery

(Hx) Menorrhagia, dysmenorrhoea

(PE) Bimanual exam: diffuse uterine enlargement and tenderness

(Dx) • TVU: asymmetric myometrium with possible cysts surrounded by hypertrophic myometrium (see MUSA criteria, see Figure 49)
 • Pelvic MRI: asymmetric uterine wall thickening
 • Definitive diagnosis requires pathology (PA) after hysterectomy

(Tx) 🖊 Induced amenorrhoea with continuous OC, progesterone, and GnRH analogues

🖊 If medication is ineffective: hysterectomy or embolisation of the uterine artery

(P) Unknown

(!) Definitive diagnosis requires hysterectomy and subsequent histology

Globular

Asymmetrical thickening

Cysts

Hyperechoic islands

Fan-shaped shadowing

Echogenic subendometrial lines and buds

Translesional vascularity

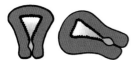

Irregular junctional zone

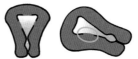

Interrupted junctional zone

Figure 49 // MUSA criteria for adenomyosis

 With familial metrorrhagia, always consider a genetic coagulation disorder (e.g. Von Willebrand disease).

Bartholin cyst

(D) A Bartholin cyst, also called bartholinitis, is an inflammation of Bartholin's gland (see Figure 50). Bartholin's gland is about 5 mm in size and drains mucus through ducts at 4 and 8 o'clock of the vulvar vestibule just behind the hymenal ring. A cyst or abscess can develop if one of these ducts is blocked.

(E) Lifetime risk of a cyst or abscess ±2%, highest risk in fertile life stage

(Ae) Duct exit obstruction

(Hx) Days since onset of swelling: pain, discomfort, mucus/pus discharge, fever (25% of patients with an abscess present with fever), past medical history (PMHx): vulvar problems

(PE) · Cyst: largely non-tender swelling that is soft to the touch
   · Abscess (bartholinitis): soft or fluctuating, very painful swelling, often surrounded by erythema and sometimes oedema, T ↑

(Dx) · Cervical swab: suspected STI (chlamydia, gonorrhoea)
   · Biopsy in postmenopausal women: to rule out malignancy

(Tx) 💬 Asymptomatic: no treatment
   💊 Symptomatic: analgesics as needed until marsupialisation, consider AB
   🔪 Symptomatic: marsupialisation or incision followed by drainage and Word catheter insertion. The wound should be left partially open to allow the cyst to drain.

(P) Risk of recurrence (0-17%)

(!) Watch out for vulvar intraepithelial neoplasia (VIN) or vulvar carcinoma, especially in postmenopausal women

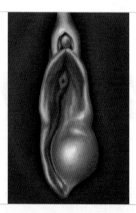

Figure 50 // Bartholin cyst

Endometriosis

(D) Endometriosis is the presence of functional endometrial tissue (stroma and glandular ducts) outside the uterine cavity (rectovaginal septum, peritoneum, intestinal or bladder wall, outside the abdominal cavity ⊖), see Figures 51 and 52. For internal endometriosis, see adenomyosis.

(E) ±10% of the fertile female population, peak incidence at age 25-40

(Ae) Hypothesis: retrograde menstruation, haematogenous/lymphatic spread, metaplasia from mesothelium

(R) Endometriosis in 1st-degree relative, nulliparity (pregnancy and lactation → endometriotic lesions regress due to progesterone), no contraception for menstrual suppression

(Hx) Asymptomatic (25%), secondary dysmenorrhoea, chronic abdominal pain, dyspareunia, subfertility, fatigue, nausea, bloating, headache, site-dependent complaints (dysuria, rectal blood loss, painful defecation (dyschezia))

(PE) • Speculum exam: translucent blue endometriotic lesions in the posterior fornix
• Bimanual exam: nodules at the level of the uterosacral ligament, ovarian mass, thickening in posterior vaginal wall/rectovaginal septum
• Rectovaginal exam: swollen rectovaginal septum

(Dx) • TVU: presence of adenomyosis or endometriomas, sliding viscera bladder and rectosigmoid (sign of deep infiltrating endometriosis)
• Pelvic MRI (without contrast): deep infiltrating endometriosis, extension of endometriosis before surgery, imaging modality of choice in virgin patients
• Labs: CA125 ↑
• Laparoscopy with biopsy in negative imaging results and/or where empirical treatment was unsuccessful or inappropriate: macroscopic black/brown lesions with red papules, blisters and white discolouration

(Tx) ✎ Analgesics, hormonal (ovulation and menstruation suppression: continuous OC, continuous progestogen (medroxyprogesteron acetate, norethisteron acetate, desogestrel, or dienogest), hormonal IUD, GnRH analogue)

✎ Laparoscopic resection, cystectomy, adhesiolysis

(P) • No correlation between severity of symptoms and number or size of lesions
• Symptoms often disappear in the absence of periods (menopause, contraception, pregnancy)
• Symptoms frequently recur after resection or upon discontinuation of hormonal therapy

(!) Hormonal treatment does not improve fertility in subfertile women. Surgery can improve fertility, but not to normal levels. Depending on the severity of endometriosis, consider IUI/IVF.

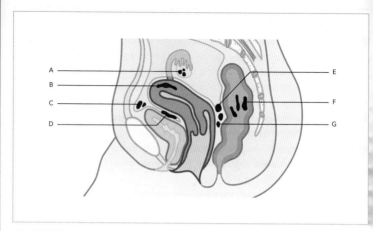

Figure 51 // Common sites of endometriosis
A: Ovaries **B:** Myometrium (adenomyosis) **C:** Abdominal **D:** Between uterus and bladder **E:** Pouch of Douglas **F:** Intestinal wall **G:** Rectovaginal septum

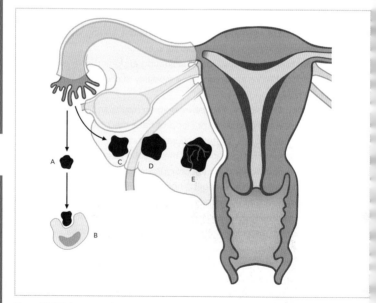

Figure 52 // Endometriosis: hypothetic pathogenesis
A: Retrograde menstruation **B:** Clearance by macrophages **C:** Quantity ↑ or clearance capacity ↓ allowing peritoneal microfoci to form **D:** Slow growth **E:** Angiogenesis

Lichen sclerosus et atrophicus (LSEA)

(D) LSEA is a chronic skin disorder of the vulva and perianal region in women and of the foreskin and glans penis in men. LSEA also has anogenital and extragenital presentations.

(E) • Prevalence <2% of women
  • ♂:♀ = 1:6, peak ages prepubertal girls (7-8 yr), and perimenopausal/postmenopausal (>52 yr)

(Ae) Idiopathic, strong evidence of underlying autoimmune disorder

(R) Skin trauma, menopause

(Hx) Asymptomatic (30%), vulvar/anal itching, dysuria, stranguria, vaginal/rectal blood loss, pain (on defaecation), dyspareunia

(PE) Epithelial atrophy, hypopigmentation, hyperkeratosis, erosions, altered anatomy (e.g. labial fusion), figure of eight (vulvar/perineal/anal), burying of the clitoris under preputium, narrowing vaginal introitus (speculum exam may be painful)

(Dx) Biopsy (if diagnostic uncertainty): epithelial atrophy (narrow epidermis, possibly with hyperkeratotic lesions), subcutaneous hyalinisation (loss of fibrillar structures), and thinning squamous epithelium

(Tx) 🖊 Non-medicated agents (preferably ointments), topical class 3-4 corticosteroids on a taper schedule, topical immunomodulators

(P) Possible progression to VIN I with risk of developing squamous cell carcinoma ↑, lifetime risk of vulvar carcinoma ±5%

(!) Extragenital skin pathology resulting from LSEA (15%) can manifest anywhere on the skin and in the mouth

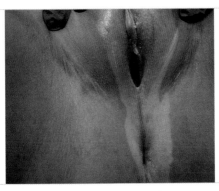

Figure 53 // Visible anatomical changes in lichen sclerosus et atrophicus

Lichen planus (LP)

(D) LP, also called lichen ruber planus, is an inflammatory disease of the mucosa (mouth, oesophagus, nose, ear canal, tear duct, and conjunctiva), skin, and anogenital region. The latter can be classified into three types: erosive, classic, and hypertrophic.

(E) Prevalence of cutaneous lesions 0.2-1.0%, oral lesions 1-4%, anogenital lesions unknown, peak age 25-70

(Ae) Idiopathic, possibly autoimmune-related

(R) Autoimmune disorder (e.g. DM, thyroid disorders, vitiligo, inflammatory bowel disease, systemic lupus erythematosus (SLE)), positive FHx

(Hx) Pain ⊙, itching, severe eruptions: nail abnormalities, cicatricial alopecia, dysphagia (oesophageal passage complaints), odynophagia (painful swallowing)

(PE) (P) Oral mucosa, flexing side elbows, lower arms, back of the hand, lower legs, sacral region, glans penis

   (A) Mostly annular grouping, sometimes solitary or generalised

   (S) One or more lesions, miliary or lenticular

   (S) Polygonal

   (O) Sharply defined

   (N) Purple/red with white stripes/marks at the surface (Wickham's striae)

   (E) Papules and plaques

- Vulvar inspection: typical erythema with sometimes Wickham's striae, superficial erosions at vaginal introitus of penis, with pain
- Speculum examination: for suspected erosive vaginal lichen planus with typical erythema with sometimes Wickham's striae, superficial erosions at vaginal wall

(Dx) Biopsy (if diagnostic uncertainty): lymphocytic infiltrate with cytotoxic T-lymphocytes applying the epidermis

(Tx) ✎ • Itching: systemic antihistamines. Genital lichen planus: local corticosteroid (class 3 or 4) combined with vaseline. Vaginal lichen planus: suppository with hydrocortisone. Alternative: local calcineurin inhibitor (tacrolimus).

   • Mostly spontaneous recovery in 1-2y, risk of vulvar carcinoma ↑

(!) Other different types of LP: drug-induced LP (NSAIDs, angiotensin-converting enzyme (ACE) inhibitors, beta blockers), LP of nails, LP of hair (lichen planopilaris), verrucous LP

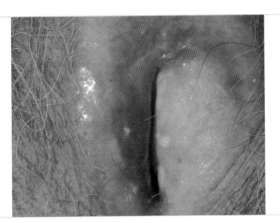

Figure 54 // Vaginal lichen planus

 PASS ONE can be used to systematically assess dermatological conditions: **P**osition, **A**rrangement, **S**ize, **S**hape, **O**utline, **N**uance/colour, and **E**fflorescence.

Ovarian torsion

(D) Ovarian torsion is the complete or partial twisting of an ovary around the adjacent ligaments, causing severe restriction of the blood supply (see Figure 55). The fallopian tubes may also be involved (adnexal torsion).

(E) • Occurs in patients of all ages but especially of childbearing age, in patients undergoing ovulation induction for infertility and in patients with ovarian tumours
  • Prevalence unknown

(Ae) Twisting of the suspensory ligaments of the ovaries → restricted blood supply → ischaemia → pain

(R) Ovarian cyst/tumour (>5 cm), fertile age, pregnancy, ovulation induction, ovarian torsion in PMHx

(Hx) Acute abdominal pain, nausea, vomiting, fever, vaginal bleeding

(PE) • Vitals: T ↑, pulse ↑, BP ↑
  • Abdomen: possible guarding (muscular defense), possible palpable abdominal mass
  • Bimanual exam: possible palpable ovarian mass, ovarian tenderness

(Dx) TVU with Doppler: enlarged ovary, ovarian perfusion ↓, whirlpool sign

Tx • Premenopausal, functioning ovaries: laparoscopic detorsion

• Postmenopausal, tumour-induced torsion and/or non-functioning ovary: salpingo-oophorectomy/oophorectomy

P Ovarian torsion secondary to ovarian cyst/tumour has high risk of recurrence if cyst/tumour is not surgically removed

! Assess presence of cysts/tumours during surgery

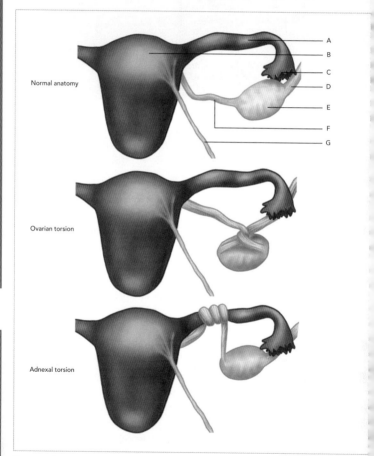

Figure 55 // Ovarian torsion and adnexal torsion
A: Fallopian tube **B:** Uterus **C:** Fimbriae **D:** Infundibulopelvic ligament (suspensory ligament of the ovary) **E:** Ovary **F:** Ovarian ligament **G:** Round ligament of the uterus

CONDITIONS

Urinary incontinence

	STRESS INCONTINENCE	URGE INCONTINENCE	OVERFLOW INCONTINENCE
D	Involuntary leakage of urine during exercise and/or increase in intra-abdominal pressure (coughing, sneezing, etc.).	Characterised mainly by a strong urge to urinate, which can lead to unwanted urine leakage.	The patient is unable to void completely, causing the bladder to overfill and leak or dribble urine.
E	Prevalence ♀ 10-17:100, 1-2:10 of non-pregnant ♀ aged >20, ♂ aged 19-44 1:21, ♂ aged 45-64 1:9, ♂ aged >65 1:5		
Ae	Dysfunctional/deficient sphincter mechanism (see Figure 56)	Often idiopathic, sometimes caused by detrusor overactivity, secondary to obstruction, neurological disorders (see Figure 56)	Impaired bladder emptying (see Figure 56)
R	♀, vaginal deliveries, chronic obstructive pulmonary disease (COPD), radical prostatectomy, or prostate radiotherapy	Adiposity, constipation, advanced age, PMHx: pregnancy, idiopathic, pelvic radiotherapy, neurological disorders	♂
HX	Urine leakage when coughing, laughing and/or exercising (intra-abdominal pressure ↑)	Urinary incontinence, patient never wants to be too far from a toilet	Urinary incontinence, especially at night, dribbling throughout the day
PE	Stress incontinence test +	Stress incontinence test -	
DX	· Urine sediment to rule out UTI · Uroflowmetry and measurement of postvoid residual volume: residual urine in bladder after urination · Urodynamic test (UDT): bladder dysfunction		
TX	🗨 Lifestyle advice: weight loss and smoking cessation, pelvic floor physical therapy 💊 Oestrogens 🔪 Surgery (tension-free vaginal tape surgery (TVT)/trans obturator tape (TOT))	🗨 Neuromodulation, transcutaneous electrical neurostimulation (TENS), or posterior tibial nerve stimulation (PTNS), pelvic floor physical therapy 💊 Parasympathetic inhibition with antimuscarinics, sympathetic stimulation with beta-3 agonist 🔪 Intravesical botox, sacral neuromodulation	🗨 Treat underlying obstruction or neurogenic bladder 🔪 Catheterisation
P	Good recovery after treatment		

Table 63 // Types of urinary incontinence

CONDITIONS

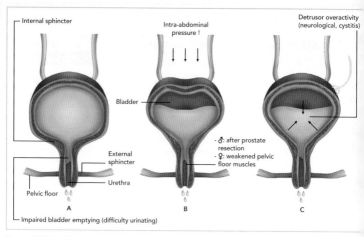

Figure 56 // Overflow, stress and urge incontinence
A: Overflow incontinence **B:** Stress incontinence **C:** Urge incontinence

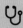 The typical patient with stress incontinence is a multiparous woman who leaks urine while laughing and running and therefore avoids social activities.

 The typical patient with urge incontinence is a 75-year-old patient who is hesitant to leave the house because they often feel sudden and strong urges to urinate and cannot make it to the toilet in time.

CONDITIONS

182

Prolapse

(D) A prolapse is a condition in which pelvic floor dysfunction or increased intra abdominal pressure cause the vagina to sag, usually accompanied by one o more of the following structures: uterus, bladder, urethra, rectum, small in testine.

(E) Prevalence 3:500, prevalence age >65 12:500

(Ae) Pelvic floor dysfunction, increased intra-abdominal pressure. See Figure 5 for the pathophysiology of the different types of prolapse.

(R) Parity (decreased pelvic floor function), aging, adiposity, posthysterectomy increased intra-abdominal pressure (coughing, sneezing), connective tissue disease

(Hx) 'Ball feeling' in the vagina or rectum, constipation, dyspareunia, incontinence (miction/defecation), lower back pain, complaints progress during the day

PE · Atrophy/lesions of the external genitals, standing exam
· Speculum exam: vaginal atrophy, signs of prolapse with/without Valsalva manoeuvre
· Vaginal exam/rectal exam: strength and coordination of the levator ani muscle, palpate possible prolapsed organ
· Classification according to POP-Q (see Figure 58)

Dx · TAU/TVU: organs involved, extent of prolapse (see Table 64)
· Dynamic rectovaginal examination (DRE): extent of prolapse on dynamic contrast X-ray

Tx Pelvic floor physical therapy, pessary if posterior wall allows it (1st choice due to recurrence risk after OR)

🔪 Surgical correction/resection:
· Anterior/posterior wall prolapse: anterior and/or posterior wall surgery (anterior/posterior colporrhaphy), implant for recurrent prolapse
· Sagging middle compartment: sacrospinal fixation, hysterectomy as last resort/if co-indicated

P 30% need repeat surgery

! · Watch for decreased muscle tone on pushing: hypertonia can cause prolapse symptoms, because the patient has to overcome considerable resistance when pushing
· Hysterectomy may increase the risk of prolapse in another compartment

---

🔆 Prolapses are caused by multiple factors that can be divided into four categories:
· Predisposing factors (e.g. genetics)
· Promoting factors (e.g. vaginal delivery, high birthweight, age, BMI, levator hiatal area, levator defect, hysterectomy, lung disease, constipation)
· Decompensating factors (e.g. menopause, medication)
· Protective factors (e.g. caesarean delivery, smoking)

🔆 **Prolapse types:**
· Anterior compartment: urethra and bladder (urethrocele/cystocele)
· Middle compartment: uterus or vaginal apex if uterus is absent (uterine/vaginal apex prolapse)
· Posterior compartment: small intestine and rectum (enterocele/rectocele)

1. Anterior compartment prolapse

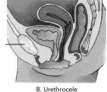

Pubic symphysis

Labium minus

A. Cystocele

B. Urethrocele

2. Middle compartment prolapse

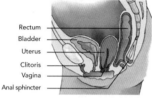

Rectum
Bladder
Uterus
Clitoris
Vagina
Anal sphincter

A. Uterine prolapse

Normal uterus

I. Uterus drops into the vagina

II. Uterus drops down to introitus

III. Uterus drops beyond the introitus

Procidentia

B. Grading system for uterine prolapses

3. Prolapse of the rear compartment

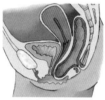

A. Rectocele

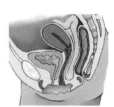

B. Enterocele

Figure 57 // Prolapse: pathophysiology

STAGE	MEANING
0	No prolapse
1	The most distal portion of the prolapse is >1 cm above the hymen
2	The most distal portion of the prolapse is <1 cm above or below the hymen (inside or outside the vagina)
3	The most distal portion of the prolapse is >1 cm below the hymen
4	Complete eversion of the uterus and vagina or complete protrusion of the total length of the vagina by ≤2 cm

Table 64 // Stages of vaginal prolapse

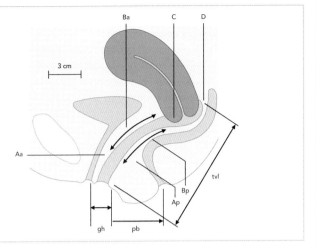

igure 58 // POP-Q reference chart

a: Reference point on anterior vaginal wall **Ba:** Most prolapsed point on the anterior vaginal wall **C:** Most istal point of the vaginal apex/cervix **D:** Most distal point of the posterior fornix **Ap:** Reference point on osterior vaginal wall **Bp:** Most prolapsed point on the posterior vaginal wall **gh:** Genital hiatus: distance om the middle of the urethral meatus to the middle of the posterior hymenal ring **pb:** Perineal body: dis-nce from the posterior limit of the gh to the midanal opening **tvl:** Total vaginal length: distance from hy-en to D, with D at its original position

Sexology

Dyspareunia

Dyspareunia is genital pain associated with intercourse. There is a superficial type, with pain near the introitus during penetration, and a deep type, with pain higher up in the vagina or abdomen caused by thrusting or friction.

Prevalence 10-20%, in primary care practices 45%

- Somatic: pelvic floor hypertonia, vaginal atrophy, vulvar infection, vulvar mass, LSEA, provoked vulvodynia (PVD), allergy (latex condoms), infection, endometriosis, anorectal pathology (fissures, haemorrhoids), anatomical abnormalities (e.g. ovarian cyst), insufficient lubrication
- Psychological: stress, negative sexual experience
- Relational: relationship problems, inadequate stimulation

Anxiety (e.g. before penetration), depression, relationship problems, decreased libido, PMHx: sexual abuse, perimenopausal and postmenopausal, infections

Continuous genital pain associated with intercourse, situational/generalised pain, vaginismus symptoms (e.g. difficulty using tampons)

(PE) Anogenital redness (especially between the 4 and 8 o'clock position of the vulva), haemorrhoids, vestibular/introital fissure, signs of LSEA, speculum exam (haemorrhage, inflammation), vaginal exam (pelvic floor hypertonia, mass, endometriosis, anatomy, cervical motion tenderness), touch test +

(Dx) TVU: to rule out anatomical anomalies

(Tx) 💬 Counselling on dyspareunia (physiological cycle of arousal, importance of lubrication, origin of sexual problems, factors that prolong or exacer bate symptoms)

👁 Cognitive behavioural therapy (CBT), pelvic floor physical therapy, sex therapy

🔗 Topical lidocaine cream, estriol vaginal suppositories/cream (post menopausal)

(P) No improvement if aetiology is left unaddressed

(I) Vicious circle: libido ↓ → lubrication ↓, vaginal relaxation ↓ → pain → libido ↓, pelvic floor hypertonia ↑

> 🔆 Dyspareunia, vaginismus, and vulvodynia have now also been sub-
> sumed under the term 'genitopelvic pain/penetration disorder', em-
> phasising triggering factors, treatment, and prevention.

Vaginismus

(D) Vaginismus is characterised by spasms of the pelvic floor muscles and upper leg adductors that obstruct vaginal penetration (intercourse or insertion of e.g. a finger or cotton swab).

(E) Prevalence is unclear, differs between countries, secondary vaginismus has its peak prevalence at postmenopausal age

(Ae) • Primary: present from first attempt at intercourse (rarely somatic)
• Secondary: pelvic floor hypertonia, somatic (infection, inflammatory der matitis), psychological (e.g. negative sexual experience in PMHx)

(R) Stress, pain on penetration (vicious circle)

(Hx) Continuous muscle spasms, pain on penetration

(PE) Speculum exam if possible: to rule out vaginal abnormalities

(Dx) Consider STI test: to rule out STIs

(Tx) 💬 • Primary: referral to sexologist and pelvic floor physiotherapy
• Secondary: see dyspareunia

CONDITIONS

P Unknown

! Closely associated with PVD: many women with vaginismus also meet the criteria for PVD

Provoked vulvodynia (PVD)

D PVD is a syndrome with vulvar pain present for at least three months without somatic cause. PVD is the main cause of superficial dyspareunia. Differentiate between local and generalised vulvodynia.

E Prevalence 7-13% in premenopausal patients

Ae · Non-infectious: allergic, granulomatous (Crohn's disease, sarcoidosis), lichenoid, psoriatiform, vesiculobullous, vasculopathy
· Infectious: *Candida*, spirochetes (*Treponema pallidum* (syphilis)), bacterial (*Staphylococcus aureus*, *Neisseria gonorrhoeae*), parasites (*Trichomonas vaginalis*), viral (*Herpes simplex*), non-specific (bartholinitis)
· Possible nerve fibre proliferation due to local inflammatory response

R · Pelvic floor hypertonia, psychosocial problems, PMHx: infection (especially bacterial vaginosis and *Candida albicans*), trauma, allergy (latex condoms)

Hx Genital rash, painful intercourse, arousal/libido ↓, vestibular pain (burning sensation)

PE Focal vulvar redness, rash (especially between the 4 and 8 o'clock position of the vulva), speculum exam (atrophy), vaginal exam (pelvic floor hypertonia, possible prolapse), touch test +

Dx TVU: to rule out anatomical abnormalities

Rx 💬 Acute: avoid irritation (soap), emollient cream, topical anaesthetics, temporary abstinence from intercourse

👁 Chronic: all of the above in combination with pelvic floor physical therapy, sexological/psychosocial therapy

✏ Consider vestibular resection (Woodruff vulvoplasty) as a last resort

P Unknown

! Pain associated with menses is not typical of vulvodynia, but is typical of a hormone-dependent pain syndrome

💡 **Friedrich's triad:** pelvic floor hypertonia, positive touch test and localised redness (especially between the 4 and 8 o'clock position of the vulva).

Orgasm disorder

D An orgasm disorder is the repeated delayed occurrence or absence of orgasms or markedly diminished intensity of orgasms with adequate sexual arousal and stimulation.

E Prevalence ♀ 5-10%

Ae Idiopathic, drug-induced, psychological, relational, somatic

R Depression, psychiatric disorders, poor health status

Hx Inadequate arousal/stimulation, situational/generalised, past orgasms, absent/delayed/weak orgasm, medication use

PE Inspection of the external genitalia and TVU for internal genitalia if needed to rule out anatomical abnormality as underlying cause

Dx Consider hormone blood test: to rule out underlying cause

Tx 💬 · Remove underlying cause
- · Psychosocial behavioural therapy: CBT, masturbation training, intimacy exercises for couples

P Directed masturbation training provides the best outcome for both primary and secondary orgasm disorders

Diminished libido

D Diminished libido is the decreased desire or interest in sexual activity.

E Prevalence ♀ 20-50%

Ae Idiopathic, androgens ↓ (libido, sexual interest), hormonal contraception, oestrogen levels ↓ (menopause → lubrication ↓, vasocongestion)

R Stress, psychiatric disorders, endometriosis, prolapse, PMHx: childbirth

Hx Genital sensation ↓, sexual interest and fantasies ↓, painful intercourse

PE Vaginal exam: pelvic floor hypertonia

Dx Consider hormone blood test: to rule out underlying cause

Tx 💬 Sexological evaluation and counselling, psychological counselling
     🔗 Vaginal atrophy: topical oestrogens

! Androgen and oestrogen blood level testing has no added value in evaluating a decreased libido

Gender dysphoria (GD)

D GD is a disorder associated with an inconsistency between personal gender identity and physical gender or assigned gender.

E Prevalence 1%, onset at age 3-4 years

Ae Complex interaction of unknown biological and environmental factors

R Exposure to large quantities of sex hormones in utero and parental influence

Dx • DSM-5: persistently identifying as the opposite gender; preference for cross-dressing or imitating the clothing style of the opposite gender; aversion to one's own clothing style; inclination towards toys, games, or stereotypical activities of the opposite gender with a strong aversion to those of the same gender; preference for playmates of the opposite gender; dislike of one's own sexual characteristics; and a desire for the physical gender characteristics of the experienced gender
  • ≥6 of the symptoms for >6 mo

Tx 🗨 Coaching
   • Tanner M/G stadium ≥2: pubertal suppression hormones (GnRH agonists)
    • Patients age >16: cross-sex hormonal therapy (male-to-female: oestrogen therapy, female-to-male: testosterone)
   >16y: mastectomy, >18y gender-affirming surgery

P Gender-affirming treatment in childhood: socially and psychologically indistinguishable from peers. In adults, the outcome for this treatment is less favourable.

🔆 Individuals who have undergone medical and/or surgical interventions for gender affirmation or confirmation (formerly known as sex reassignment) are historically referred to as transexual. While some transsexual individuals may also identify as transgender, many predominantly identify with the male or female gender they have transitioned to.

🔆 It is crucial to distinguish between gender identity and gender expression. Gender identity pertains to an individual's psychological understanding of their gender, while gender expression relates to how a person outwardly presents their gender to the world.

Menstrual cycle disorders

Menstrual cycle disorders are characterised by abnormal blood loss during menstruation or by an abnormal cycle length (see Table 65). A normal menstrual cycle lasts 21-42 days, with ovulation occurring around days 12-14. In 95% of women menopause occurs between ages 44-56. Cycle abnormalities can manifest in different ways and are categorised by the associated symptoms. The causes of amenorrhoea and oligomenorrhoea are classified according to WHO categories, which can serve as an aid in the differential diagnosis process (see Table 36).

- **Primary amenorrhoea:** complete absence of menses.
- **Secondary amenorrhoea:** absence of menses after previous menses.

In case of amenorrhoea or oligomenorrhoea, consider:
- Disorder of sex development (primary amenorrhoea).
- Contraceptive use: hormonal contraception can cause spotting and breakthrough bleeding, but withdrawal bleeding can also be absent. Progesterone causes endometrial atrophy (hormonal IUD). Thin mucous membrane can lead to the absence of menses, but is also fragile and can therefore lead to spotting.
- PCOS: a common cause of menstrual cycle abnormalities caused by oligomenorrhoea in response to androgen overproduction (due to various causes).

DISORDER	MENSES LENGTH	AMOUNT OF BLOOD LOSS	CYCLE LENGTH
Menorrhagia	↑	↑	Normal
Metrorrhagia	↑	↑	Unpredictable
Hypermenorrhoea	↑/normal	↑	Normal
Hypomenorrhoea	↓	↓	Normal
Oligomenorrhoea	↓/normal	↓/normal	↑

Table 65 // Types of abnormal menstruation

For more information about primary and secondary amenorrhoea, see the sections on Differential diagnosis and Clinical reasoning.

Premenstrual syndrome (PMS)

D PMS is characterised by physical and/or psychological symptoms that disturb daily life and occur cyclically during the luteal phase of menstruation. Time of onset ranges from two days to one week before the onset of menstruation (see Figure 59). Premenstrual dysphoric disorder (PMDD) is a more severe variant of PMS, with severe mood swings and behavoural changes.

E Prevalence PMS 12% onset from age 20-30, PMDD 5-8%

Ae Idiopathic, possible imbalance between oestrogen and progesterone → relative progesterone deficiency

Hx Headache, abdominal pain, breast tenderness, back pain, bloating, oedema, weight ↑, mood disorders, emotional imbalance, agitation, fatigue, depression, panic disorders

PE No added value

Dx • Period tracker: cyclical, recurring symptoms
   • Trial with GnRH analogue (diagnostic if symptoms disappear)

Rx 💬 Lifestyle advice: coffee, nicotine, salt and hot spices ↓, exercise ↑, stress ↓, CBT
   💊 • OC (drospirenone-ethinylestradiol), GnRH analogues, SNRIs, SSRIs (fluoxetine, sertraline, paroxetine)
   • For mastodynia: consider bromocriptine

P Unknown

! Hysterectomy does not resolve symptoms

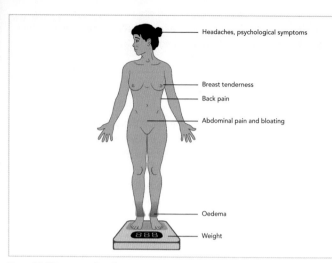

Figure 59 // Premenstrual syndrome

Adolescent metrorrhagia

(D) Adolescent metrorrhagia is characterised by heavy, prolonged and/or unpre dictable bleeding in the years following menarche that does not occur in regu lar cycles. Bleeding associated with adolescent metrorrhagia is almost alway anovulatory.

(E) Incidence unknown, usually the first two years after menarche

(Ae) Hormonal imbalance during puberty, often familial

(R) Positive family history

(Hx) Severe, prolonged menses

(PE) Speculum exam: to rule out other causes of blood loss. There is no need t perform a speculum exam in virgins, given the low risk of vaginal and cervi cal pathology

(Dx) • Diagnostic treatment with norethisterone (bleeding stops within 2-3 day or OC

• Period tracker: irregular and/or prolonged cycle

• Labs: to rule out clotting disorders

• TVU: thick and irregular endometrial structure, rule out congenital and in trauterine abnormalities

(Tx) 💊 OC (regulates the menstrual cycle), consider iron supplementation

(P) The menstrual cycle usually stabilises after 2 years

Premature ovarian insufficiency (POI)

(D) POI, formerly called premature ovarian failure (WHO 3), occurs when menopause starts before age 40 (see Figure 60).

(E) Prevalence 3,700:100,000

(Ae) Auto-immune diseases, infections, radiotherapy, or chemotherapy, idiopathic (60%), abnormal karyotype

(R) Familial, infections, radiotherapy or chemotherapy

(Hx) Menopausal symptoms before age 40, subfertility

(PE) Speculum exam: vaginal atrophy

(Dx) Labs: FSH ↑, oestrogen ↓

(Tx) 💊 Oestrogen replacement to prevent osteoporosis and cardiovascular disease, always in combination with progesterone to reduce risk of endometrial carcinoma

(P) Chance of pregnancy after diagnosis 5-10%

(!) Pregnancy only possible with oocyte donation

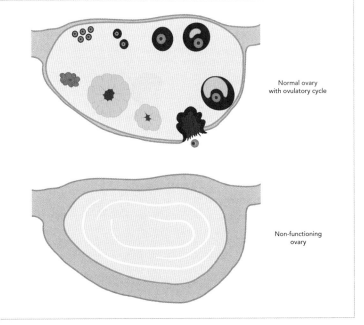

Normal ovary with ovulatory cycle

Non-functioning ovary

Figure 60 // Premature ovarian insufficiency

Menopause

(D) Menopause is the permanent cessation of menstruation.

(E) • In 95% of women, menopause occurs between ages 44-56
   • 50% of women experience menopause by age 51

(Ae) No more functional follicles (physiological, genetic)

(R) Hormone therapy for treatment of oncological diseases

(Hx) Menopausal symptoms (see Figure 61): night sweats, irritability, hot flashes, sexual dysfunction, vaginal dryness, fatigue, mood disorders

(PE) Speculum exam: vaginal atrophy, possible labial atrophy

(Dx) Labs: hypergonadotropic, oestrogen ↓

(Tx) 💊 • For severe symptoms, consider short-term hormone substitution (lowest dosage for the shortest period of time), aim to discontinue treatment after 6 mo
   • Hormonal oestrogen substitution combined with progesterone when uterus in situ, start with dermal estradiol

(P) Irreversible

(!) Aging and menopause are associated with a risk of: osteoporosis ↑, cardiovascular events ↑, urogenital atrophy ↑, breast carcinoma ↓ due to loss of oestrogen

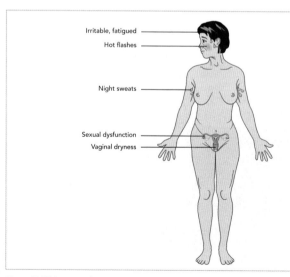

Irritable, fatigued
Hot flashes
Night sweats
Sexual dysfunction
Vaginal dryness

Figure 61 // Menopausal symptoms

Menopause is the date of a patient's final menstrual period and can only be diagnosed 12 months after the fact. **Postmenopause** is the time after menopause. **Perimenopause** or menopausal transition is the time when menopausal symptoms may occur.

Genital infections

Aerobic vaginitis

(D) Aerobic vaginitis is a disruption of the vaginal flora characterised by a lack of lactobacilli and an increase in aerobic bacteria.

(E) Unknown

(Ae) *Escherichia coli*, *Staphylococcus aureus*, group B *streptococcus* (GBS)

(R) Unknown

(Hx) Burning sensation, dyspareunia, malodorous discharge (not an amine smell)

(PE) Speculum exam (see Figure 62 for cervicitis as seen during speculum exam): inflamed/red/oedematous vagina, ulcers, white, malodorous discharge

(Dx) Discharge test: parabasal cells secondary to inflammation, leukocytes, lactobacilli ↓, pH >6

(Tx) 🔗 Symptomatic: ABx, topical oestrogens in postmenopausal women

(P) High risk of recurrence despite ABx

(!) • Rule out disruptive factors first (e.g. washing with soap, continuous use of pantyliners) to avoid further disruption of vaginal pH and flora
   • In very rare cases, the symptoms are caused by a carcinoma

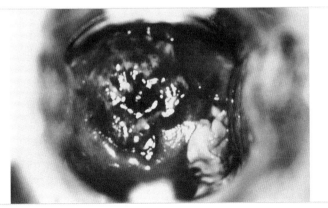

igure 62 // Cervicitis as seen during speculum exam

Bacterial vaginosis

(D) Bacterial vaginosis is a disruption of the vaginal flora characterised by a lack of lactobacilli and an increase in anaerobic or facultative anaerobic bacteria.

(E) Incidence 1,500:100,000/year, 22-29% of patients with vaginal discharge complaints have bacterial vaginosis

(Ae) *Gardnerella vaginalis* (50%)

(R) Disruption of vaginal flora

(Hx) Asymptomatic (50-75%), amine smell, abnormal discharge

(PE) Speculum exam: thin, white, homogeneous discharge, amine smell

(Dx) · Direct preparation: pH >4.5, amine smell in POH preparation, clue cells in NaCl preparation
  · Gram staining: *Gardnerella vaginalis* gram-positive

(Tx) 💊 If symptomatic: ABx

(P) Recurrence 30-50% within 1 year

(!) Pregnancy: risk of prematurity ↑

 Bacterial vaginosis is not considered an STI due to the lack of an unequivocal causative agent and male equivalent.

 Amsel criteria: homogeneous (greyish white) discharge, discharge pH >4.5, positive amine test and visible clue cells on NaCl preparation. If ≥3 criteria are met: diagnose bacterial vaginosis.

Vaginal candidiasis

(D) Vaginal candidiasis is a yeast infection but is not considered an STI.

(E) Incidence 2,500:100,000/year, 17-39% of patients with vaginal discharge complaints have candida vaginalis

(Ae) *Candida* species, especially *Candida albicans* (85-90%)

(R) DM, AB use, oestrogen ↑, immunosuppression

(Hx) Vaginal discharge, vulvar/vaginal itching, burning sensation, dyspareunia, sometimes dysuria

(PE) · Vulvovaginal erythema, vulvar oedema
  · Speculum exam: discharge is thick and white (like cottage cheese), and concentrated near the vaginal wall

(Dx) · Discharge pH test: 4.0-4.5
  · Discharge microscopy: pseudohyphae, ±50% false negative

- Culture
- Tx 🔖 Vaginal or oral antimycotics
- P Considered a recurrent infection if ≥4 infections/y (25%), consider determining resistance pattern
- ! Neonatal: thrush, watch out for mortality due to sepsis attributed to *Candida* infection

Listeriosis

- D Listeriosis is an infectious disease caused by a bacterium. *Listeria monocytogenes* does not belong to the resident flora of the vagina.
- E Prevalence (perinatal period) 1:37,000-100,000 births
- Ae *Listeria monocytogenes* (gram-positive rod) → possible transmission from unwashed vegetables and cheeses made from unpasteurised milk
- R Elderly patients, immunocompromised patients, pregnant women
- Hx • Maternal: asymptomatic ⊕, tightness, gastrointestinal symptoms, fever ⊖
  - Fetal: IUFD, neonatal meningitis, rash with pink papules, sepsis with multiple organ failure
- PE Green amniotic fluid, T ↑ ⊖
- Dx • Amniotic fluid/blood culture in case of an unexplained intrauterine infection, or IUFD: gram-positive rod
  - Placental biopsy: granulomatous micro-abscesses in the placenta
- Tx 🔖 ABx
  🖊 After 32 wk of amenorrhoea: proceed to delivery with abnormal CTG, CS if needed
- P Morbidity and mortality ↑, especially with infections in the 3rd trimester
- ! Risk of IUFD

Pelvic inflammatory disease (PID)

- D PID is an acute inflammation of the uterus, fallopian tubes, ovaries and/or nearby organs.
- E Lifetime prevalence 4.5% in women of reproductive age, peak age 15-25
- Ae Infection of the upper genital tract, usually caused by an ascending STI (*Chlamydia* ⊙, *gonorrhoea* ⊙)
- R Multiple sexual partners, PMHx: PID, IUD
- Hx Lower abdominal pain (worsens with intercourse), vaginal bleeding (intermenstrual, menorrhagia, postcoital), duration of pain, abnormal discharge, malaise, fever

- PE Possible signs of an acute abdomen (peritonitis), peristalsis, T ↑, lower abdominal pressure pain, right upper quadrant tenderness in perihepatitis, speculum exam (abnormal discharge volume/colour/odour), vaginal exam (adnexal and cervical motion tenderness)
- Dx · Labs: infection parameters ↑
  - · Smear test/culture: STI (gonorrhoea, chlamydia)
  - · TAU/TVU: rule out other causes, and tubo-ovarian abscess (TOA)
- Tx 💬 Contact tracing for underlying STIs
  - 🔗 Broad-spectrum oral ABx, consider hospitalisation with IV AB depending on severity
- P Risk of subfertility or infertility depending on duration, severity and possible recurrences
- ! · Complications: pelveoperitonitis, TOA, Fitz-Hugh-Curtis syndrome (see Figure 63)
  - · Risk of chronic lower abdominal pain, dyspareunia, ectopic pregnancy and infertility ↑

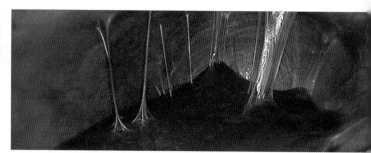

Figure 63 // Fitz-Hugh-Curtis syndrome with perihepatic adhesions

 The **Fitz-Hugh-Curtis syndrome**, also known as perihepatitis, is an inflammation of the liver capsule and/or diaphragm caused by an ascending infection from the pelvis. This can cause perihepatic adhesions and upper right quadrant abdominal pain, possibly radiating to the right shoulder.

 Adnexitis and salpingitis are often used as synonyms for PID and refer to inflammation of the fallopian tube and ovary, usually occurring in fertile life stage.

CONDITIONS

Sexually transmitted infections (STIs)

Chlamydia

(D) Chlamydia is a urogenital bacterial STI caused by *Chlamydia trachomatis*.

(E) ♀>♂, prevalence 3.7-4.7%, particularly during reproductive life stage, peak age 15-24

(Ae) *Chlamydia trachomatis*: intracellular gram-negative bacteria, incubation period 1-3 wk

(R) Multiple sexual partners, unprotected intercourse, PMHx: *Chlamydia* infection, age <25

(Hx) • Asymptomatic (♀ 60-70%, ♂ 50%)
- ♀: discharge ↑, dysuria, abnormal vaginal bleeding, lower abdominal pain
- ♂: watery discharge or dysuria

(PE) • Asymptomatic ☺, abdominal tenderness and rebound tenderness on palpation, muscular defence
- Speculum exam: cervicitis
- Vaginal exam: adnexal and cervical motion tenderness pain (indications of salpingitis/pelvic inflammatory disease (PID))

(Dx) • Labs: *Chlamydia* antibody test (CAT) + (only if previously infected with *Chlamydia*)
- PCR *Chlamydia* (plus *gonorrhoea*): ♂ on first-catch urine sample, ♀ on intracervical swab
- Culture: ♀ intracervical or ♂ urethral swab (test for both *gonorrhoea* and *Chlamydia* due to increased risk of co-infection)
- Rectal culture if anal sex, anal complaints, or vulnerable sexual behaviour
- Oral culture if unsafe oral sex

(Tx) 💬 Contact tracing (all sexual partners over the past 6 mo)
- 💊 Azithromycin, doxycycline (1st choice for ♀)
  - Alternatives (e.g. due to allergy): amoxicillin, levofloxacin, ofloxacin

(P) • Frequent recurrent infection
- Untreated: 20% chance of complications e.g. chronic pelvic pain, subfertility/infertility, ectopic pregnancy, Fitz-Hugh-Curtis syndrome (perihepatitis) with PID

(!) • Pregnancy: risk of prelabour rupture of membranes (PROM), and premature birth
- Possible vertical transmission to fetus with risk of neonatal conjunctivitis and pneumonia

- Risk of ascending infection secondary to undertreated asymptomatic manifestation

> 🔔 In patients with frequent breakthrough bleeding with proper contraceptive use or postcoital bleeding, consider an underlying *Chlamydia* infection.

> 🔔 *Chlamydia trachomatis* is an intra-cellular bacteria, so remember to rub thoroughly when collecting the culture sample.

Gonorrhoea

(D) Gonorrhoea, also known as 'the clap', is a bacterial STI caused by *Neisseria gonorrhoeae*.

(E) Prevalence♀ 0.9%, ♂ 0.6%, peak age 15-49

(Ae) *Neisseria gonorrhoeae* (gonococcus), intracellular gram-negative diplococcus, incubation period 2-14 d

(R) *Chlamydia* infection, multiple sexual partners, unprotected intercourse, anal sex, prostitution, ♂:♀ = 4:1

(Hx) Asymptomatic ☺, abdominal pain, dysuria, fever ⊖, pharyngitis ⊖, ♀ vaginal discharge ↑ (30-60%), ♂ urethritis (with purulent dribbling), or proctitis

(PE) Speculum exam: red irritated cervix, cervicitis

(Dx) • PCR *gonorrhoeae*: ♂ on first-catch urine sample, ♀ on intracervical swab, test for both *gonorrhoeae* and *Chlamydia* due to increased risk of co-infection
- Culture (♀ intracervical or ♂ urethral swab)
- Rectal culture if anal sex, anal complaints, or vulnerable sexual behaviour
- Oral culture if unsafe oral sex

(Tx) 💬 Contact tracing (all sexual partners over the past six mo)
🗝 Single-dose IM ceftriaxone

(P) Untreated: risk of subfertility/infertility, ectopic pregnancy, Fitz-Hugh-Curtis syndrome with PID (perihepatitis)

(!) Many patients are asymptomatic, resulting in delayed treatment

> 🔔 Neonates may be exposed to vertical transmission, possibly causing neonatal conjunctivitis.

Genital herpes

D Genital herpes is a herpes simplex virus (HSV) infection in the genital region (see Figure 64). There are two types of HSV: HSV-1, and HSV-2.

E ♂:♀ = 1:2, prevalence 400,000,000, each year 100,000,000 new infections, 70% of the population has a positive HSV serology

Ae HSV-2 (80%), HSV-1 (20%)

R Reduced immunity: increased risk of infection and exacerbation, multiple sexual partners, unprotected intercourse

Hx Asymptomatic ⊕, irritation, burning sensation, pain, fever ⊖

PE **P** Genital area

    A Grouped

    S Miliary

    S Round

    O Sharp borders

    N Red

    E Blisters and ulcers

- Primary infection: regional lymph node swelling, urethritis symptoms, vaginal discharge (♀)
- After 6-7d: clear fluid-filled blisters that burst open, followed by ulcers
- Location: glans, foreskin and shaft of the penis (♂), vulva, perineum or cervix (♀), skin pathology around the anus or proctitis

Dx Labs: HSV blood test (pregnant women), PCR on ulcer swab

Tx 💊 • Symptomatic: zinc oxide ointment or zinc sulfate cream
- Local analgesia: lidocaine and zinc oxide ointment or systemic analgesia with paracetamol or NSAID
- Antivirals (e.g. valaciclovir): shorter duration, reduced severity of symptoms, shorter contagion period

P • Up to 90% of patients experience >1 recurrence, 20% experience >10 recurrences, higher recurrence risk with HSV-2 infection, absence of visible ulcers does not rule out infection
- Lesions heal in 7-28d without scarring, during recurrences herpetiform blisters appear that produce non-indurated painful ulcers

! Extragenital complications: aseptic meningitis, urinary retention (lumbar radiculopathy: Elsberg's syndrome), skin pathology elsewhere on the body

🔔   **Kiss of death**: kissing a neonate while having a cold sore may result in a potentially fatal neonatal herpes infection.

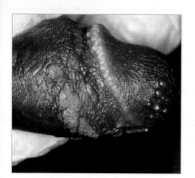

 Risk of maternal-fetal transmission:
- Low (1-3%) when patient has PMHx of genital herpes
- High in primary genital herpes. If acquired at time of labour or <6 weeks prior to delivery: indication for CS.

Figure 64 // Genital herpes

Condylomata acuminata/human papilloma virus (HPV)

(D) Condylomata acuminata, or anogenital warts, are caused by HPV, a DNA virus with >100 serotypes. It is a sexually transmitted infection of the mucous membranes in the anogenital region (see Figure 65).

(E) Incidence 1:1,000/year, peak prevalence: ages 15-29. >90% of people infected with HPV do not develop warts. 50% of women with vulvar warts also have cervical HPV infection.

(Ae) HPV type 6 and 11, incubation period: 1-8 mo

(R) Multiple sexual partners, unprotected intercourse, anal sex, ♂, smoking, oropharyngeal HPV, immunocompromised patients

(Hx) Itching ⊖, irritation ⊖, discharge with urethral and vaginal infection

(PE) For internal infections: speculum exam, proctoscopy, urethroscopy

  (P) Anogenital area, cervix, urethra

  (A) Solitary or multiple

  (S) Miliary to lenticular

  (S) Verrucous, papillomatous

  (O) Sharp borders

  (N) Skin-colour, pinkish red or brown

  (E) Papula

(Dx) • Biopsy if in doubt: histology and/or HPV test. Histology shows typical koilocytes that may harbour viruses, usually accompanied by hypergranulosis

  • Cytology on smear test: CIN

  • Colposcopy with 3-5% acetic acid staining and lugol: atypical and damaged cells stain white/yellow

(Tx) 💬 Prevention: condom use (does not provide full protection, virus can often be transmitted near the base of the condom)

🔖 Genital warts: podophyllotoxin, imiquimod, sinecathechin

🔪 Excision, electrocoagulation, cryotherapy

P Spontaneous remission in 20% after 3 mo and 90% after 2y. Risk of developing cervical carcinoma in oncogenic serotypes after 10-15y.

> 🔆 Immunocompromised patients may develop very large and difficult-to-treat genital warts, known as giant condylomata acuminata of Bushke-Löwenstein.

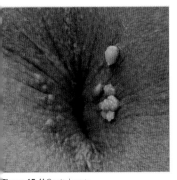

Figure 65 // Genital warts

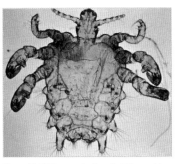

Figure 66 // Microscopic view of phthirus pubis

Pediculosis pubis (phthiriasis pubis)

D Pubic lice infestations are caused by *Phthirus pubis*, a blood-sucking louse that feeds on human blood. Pubic lice are found in the pubic area and can spread to other areas with body hair by scratching (armpits, chest hair, eyebrows, eyelashes).

E Incidence 500:100,000/year, prevalence unknown

Ae • Transmission: physical intimacy, sharing clothes
   • Incubation time: >5d
   • Nymphs and mature lice feed on blood → allergic reaction to bites → itching

R • Infection risk: multiple sexual partners, travellers (sleeping on used sheets)
   • More severe course: corticosteroids → lice count ↓

Hx Itching 😀, secondary bacterial skin infections ☹

PE Lice on skin or at the base of unshaven pubic hair, excoriations, impetigo

(Dx) Microscopy or magnifying glass: detect lice (see Figure 66), nits

(Tx) 💊 Dimeticone lotion (silicone base), permethrin 5% cream, possibly with malathion 0.5% lotion in case of co-infection with head lice

(P) • Treatment most effective way to control nymphs and mature lice
• Frequent use of pediculicides results in persistent itching

(!) Pediculosis pubis is usually sexually transmitted → deploy diagnostics for other STIs

Scabies

(D) Scabies is a highly contagious infestation of the epidermis by the *Sarcoptes scabiei* mite (see Figure 67). The mite burrows into and lives in the area between the stratum corneum and stratum granulosum. Transmission occurs through prolonged or frequent direct contact. The mites can also be spread by fomites (inanimate objects).

(E) Prevalence 0.2-71.4%, incidence in general practice 3:1000/year, endemics occur regularly

(Ae) Intense itching due to an allergic reaction to enzyme production, faeces and parasitic antigens

(R) Poor hygiene, multiple sexual partners, living in a care facility or dorm room, immune disorder

(Hx) Intensely itchy lesion, especially at night, incubation period 2-6 wk

(PE) (P) Interdigital space, flexed side of wrists, lateral part of the foot, head is unaffected in adults, ♂ penis, ♀ around the nipples (see Figure 68)

(A) Grouped, symmetrical

(S) Several to dozens of lesions

(S) Round, raised, sometimes linear (burrows)

(O) Highly variable

(N) Skin-coloured to red

(E) Polymorphic with papules, papulovesicles, crusts and scratch marks

(Dx) • Dermatoscopy: larger mites can look like small black triangles (V's, delta sign)
• POH preparation: detect mites or nits

(Tx) 💬 Wash textiles based on laundry label, also treat partners or roommates

💊 Apply permethrin or benzyl benzoate to whole body or take oral ivermectin. Reapply benzyl benzoate after first 24h and repeat after a week. Repeat permethrin and ivermectin treatment after a week.

(P) Complete eradication very likely with adequate treatment

(!) Scabies crustosa or norvegica is a very severe, contagious form of scabies that occurs especially in immunocompromised or elderly people in care facilities and is characterised mainly by hyperkeratosis, papules and nodules on the extremities

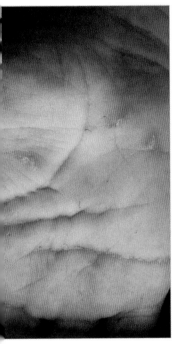

Figure 67 // Scabies

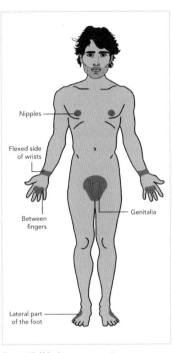

Figure 68 // Scabies: common sites

Labels in figure: Nipples, Flexed side of wrists, Between fingers, Genitalia, Lateral part of the foot

Syphilis

(D) Syphilis is a bacterial STI caused by *Treponema pallidum* ssp. *pallidum*. Syphilis has two stages: early syphilis, with an infection duration <1 year (contagious) and late syphilis, with an infection duration >1 year (non-contagious). Syphilis can be systemic and often occurs in combination with HIV.

(E) ♂:♀ = 8:1, prevalence 0.5%, incidence US: 13.5:100,000/year

(Ae) Treponema pallidum ssp. pallidum, a spirochete that invades the skin through small lesions produced during sexual activity or pre-existing lesions

(R) Vulnerable sexual behaviour, prostitution, persons from endemic areas, multiple sexual partners, unprotected intercourse

(Hx) Painless skin lesions, ulcer, fever, general malaise, weight ↓, muscle and joint pain

(PE) · Early syphilis:
  (P) At contact site (genitals, cervix, anal, mouth)
  (A) Solitary
  (S) Miliary to lenticular
  (S) Round or oval
  (O) Sharp borders
  (N) Red
  (E) Macula, papule, later ulcer

· Secondary syphilis: many different manifestations including palmar and plantar roseoles (red maculae), non-itching exanthema on extremities and trunk, condylomata lata, syphilitic alopecia (noncicatricial alopecia), ulcers over the body
· Neurological exam: to rule out neurosyphilis
· Vitals: T ↑

(Dx) · Labs: antibodies + (TPPA, TPHA), if TPHA + → rapid plasma reagin (RPR) assay
· Darkfield microscopy: direct fluorescent antibody (DFA) visible on exudate from suspicious lesions
· Eye exam: possible reduced vision in ocular syphilis
· Cardiac ultrasound: thoracic aortic dilation, aortic valve insufficiency ('cardiovascular syphilis')
· Lumbar puncture (LP): lymphocytic pleiocytosis, protein ↑

(Tx) 🖊 · Standard treatment for early and late syphilis: single IM injection benzathine benzylpenicillin. Latent syphilis: 3x IM injections.
  · 2nd choice for patients with a penicillin allergy: doxycycline

(P) Good after adequate therapy, follow up anti-treponemal therapy with 2y of serological screening and consider LP, ECG and chest X-ray after 1y

(!) · Possibility of transplacental transmission with risk of premature childbirth and fetal bone, kidney, and skin abnormalities, previous infection does not confer immunity
· Test for co-infection with HIV, treatment with benzathine benzylpenicillin can spark Jarisch-Herxheimer reaction due to endotoxins released by dead spirochetes

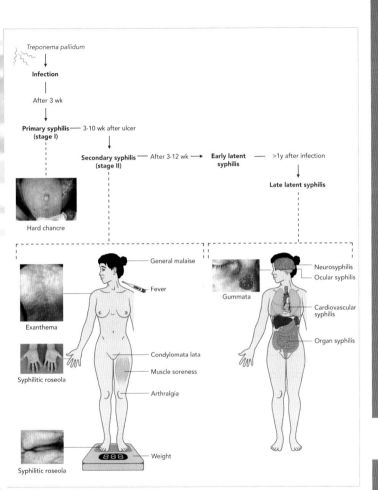

Treponema pallidum

Infection

After 3 wk

Primary syphilis — 3-10 wk after ulcer
(stage I)

       Secondary syphilis — After 3-12 wk → **Early latent** — >1y after infection
       (stage II)   **syphilis**

                                            Late latent syphilis

Hard chancre

General malaise

Fever

Exanthema

Syphilitic roseola

Condylomata lata

Muscle soreness

Arthralgia

Syphilitic roseola

Weight

Gummata

Neurosyphilis
Ocular syphilis

Cardiovascular syphilis

Organ syphilis

Figure 69 // Syphilis: stages

Syphilitic skin abnormalities may resemble other skin pathology, earning syphilis' nicknames of 'the copycat disease' and 'the great pretender'.

Stages of syphilis (see Figure 69):
- 1st stage (primary syphilis): after ±3 wk, a papule (painless, firm, round or oval ulcer (hard chancre) develops at the site of infection → heals in 3-6 wk.
- 2nd stage (secondary syphilis): the 2nd stage usually occurs 3-10 wk after the hard chancre, following haematogenous spread and bacterial proliferation. General symptoms (e.g. fever, general malaise, weight ↓, muscle and joint pain) and skin symptoms (e.g. erythrosquamous plaques) develop in this stage. Symptoms often spread to the palms. Syphilis is also accompanied by condylomata lata, flat, shiny papules or plaques that are red to grey in colour and mainly occur in the anogenital region. These lesions contain many spirochetes and are therefore highly contagious.
- Early latent syphilis: after 3-12 wk, 2nd stage symptoms may disappear spontaneously. Symptoms may recur within a year.
- Late latent phase: the immune system response has eliminated most bacteria from the body. Skin abnormalities disappear, but ±66% remain in this latent phase and clearance of all bacteria is unlikely. Granulomatous nodules and nodular/ulcerative gummata, neurosyphilis and cardiovascular syphilis may occur at this stage.

Trichomoniasis

(D) Trichomoniasis is an infection of the vagina caused by the parasite *Trichomonas vaginalis* (see Figure 70).

(E) Prevalence 0.4-0.6%, peak age 45-55

(Ae) *Trichomonas vaginalis*: protozoa, flagellar locomotion, colonises vagina and urethra

(R) Prostitution, multiple sexual partners, unprotected intercourse

(Hx) Asymptomatic (50-85%), ♂: occasional urethritis, prostatitis, or epididymitis, ♀: malodorous, green, foamy vaginal discharge

(PE) Speculum exam: strawberry cervix (erythematous papules on cervix/vagina wall with pinpoint haemorrhages), discharge (10-30% visible trichomonads)

(Dx) • Labs: PCR on swab (to rule out other STIs), pH ↑
- Microscopy: vaginal discharge, trichomonads, leukocytosis

(Tx) 🖊 One-time 2 g oral metronidazole or 2x/d 500 mg for 1 wk (for recurrent infections), also treat partner

(P) • ♀: asymptomatic infection (carry parasite for a long time)

- ♂: heals spontaneously
- Rare complications: prostatitis, balanitis, epididymitis, infertility

! Higher risk of prematurity, dysmaturity, PROM in pregnant patients

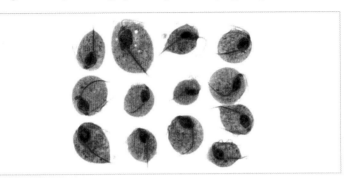

Figure 70 // *Trichomonas vaginalis*

Disorders of sex development

Androgen insensitivity syndrome (AIS)

D AIS is a syndrome in which the body does not respond to androgens in the blood due to a gene mutation. Typical characteristics include the 46XY karyotype, and genital development marked by male internal genitalia and female external genitalia (see Figure 71).

E Incidence 2:100,000/year

Ae Mutation in androgen receptor gene on X chromosome → androgen insensitivity → testosterone ineffective → no external virilisation

Hx Primary amenorrhoea, normal breast development, no pubic hair, dyspareunia

PE Normal height, normal clitoris and labia, no pubic hair, inguinal mass (testis), inguinal herniations, short, dead-end vagina

Dx • Labs: DHT =/↑
   • TAU/TVU: absent uterus and ovaries
   • Karyotype: 46XY

Tx ✎ Oestrogen supplementation
   ✐ Postpubertal orchidectomy due to risk of malignancy

P Pregnancy impossible

! Patients with partial AIS can have a female or male phenotype and may be infertile

DHT is the biologically active variant of testosterone and is responsible for the differentiation of the urogenital tract, external genitalia, urethra, and prostate.

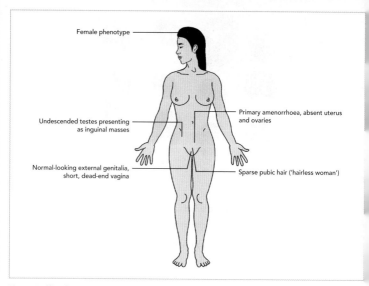

Female phenotype

Undescended testes presenting as inguinal masses

Normal-looking external genitalia, short, dead-end vagina

Primary amenorrhoea, absent uterus and ovaries

Sparse pubic hair ('hairless woman')

Figure 71 // Androgen insensitivity syndrome

Ovotesticular disorder of sex development (hermaphroditism)

(D) Hermaphroditism is an ovotesticular disorder of sex development in which a patient has both male and female internal genitalia.

(E) 60% 46XY, 30% 46XX, 10% mosaicism

(Ae) Exposure to maternal, exogenous or fetal androgens → both the Müllerian ducts and Wolffian ducts are fully/partially developed

(Hx) Dysmorphic external genitalia

(PE) Ambiguous genitalia with varying degrees of virilisation (underdeveloped vagina, uterus always present), see Figure 72

(Dx) • Labs: DHT ↓

• Karyotype: 46XY, 46XX, mosaic

(Tx) 🖊 DHT substitution (if DHT ↓)

✎ Surgical correction of external genitalia

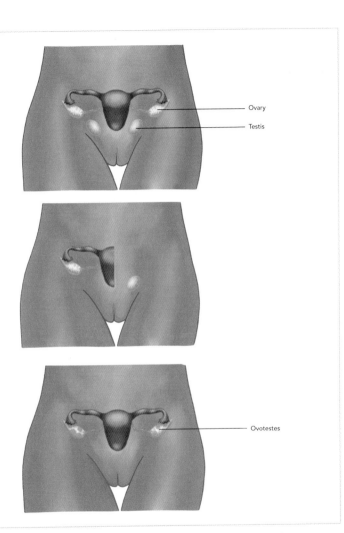

Figure 72 // Ovotesticular developmental disorder: manifestations of the internal genitalia

  · **Hermaphroditism:** male and female external and internal genitalia.
· **Pseudohermaphroditism:** male and female external genitalia, but male or female internal genitalia.

Kallmann syndrome

(D) Kallmann syndrome is caused by a gene mutation and is characterised by the development of primary sex characteristics and the absence of secondary sex characteristics.

(E) Prevalence ♂ 10:100,000, ♀ 1.5:100,000, mostly X-linked recessive → lower incidence in women

(Ae) Gene mutation → olfactory bulb and tract aplasia → no migration of GnRH neurons from the olfactory plate to the hypothalamus → no GnRH → no sex hormones

(Hx) · Hyposmia/anosmia, absence of pubertal growth spurt, sparse pubic hair (see Figure 73)
 · ♀: primary amenorrhoea, little breast development, no secondary sexual characteristics
 · ♂: little beard growth, no voice break, micropenis, small scrotum

(PE) · Normal primary and absent secondary sexual characteristics, ♂ micropenis and small scrotum
 · Speculum exam: to rule out other causes for primary amenorrhoea

(Dx) · Labs: GnRH ↓, oestrogen ↓, androgens =
 · Brain MRI: absent olfactory nerve, olfactory bulb and olfactory sulcus

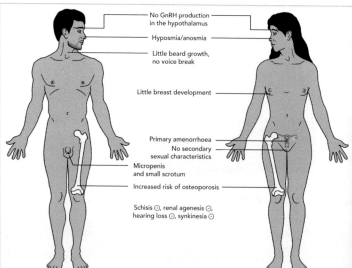

No GnRH production in the hypothalamus

Hyposmia/anosmia

Little beard growth, no voice break

Little breast development

Primary amenorrhoea
No secondary sexual characteristics

Micropenis and small scrotum

Increased risk of osteoporosis

Schisis ⊖, renal agenesis ⊖, hearing loss ⊖, synkinesia ⊖

Figure 73 // Kallmann syndrome

Tx 💊 Hormone replacement (♂ testosterone, ♀ oestrogen), pulsatile GnRH for women who want to have children

P Ovulation induction has a 95% success rate, spermatogenesis induction has a 75-90% success rate

! • Sometimes associated with schisis, renal agenesis, hearing loss and synkinesia
  • Risk of osteoporosis ↑

Adrenogenital syndrome (AGS)

D AGS is an autosomal recessive genetic disorder that disrupts enzymes involved in glucocorticoid production, resulting in insufficient cortisol production and therefore increased ACTH release. This leads to androgen overproduction and adrenal hyperplasia (congenital adrenal hyperplasia, CAH). Increase in androgen and/or mineralocorticoid synthesis depending on enzyme deficiency type and mutation penetrance.

E Incidence 1:15,000/year

Ae 21-hydroxylase deficiency (90%), other deficiencies in cortisol synthesis (see Diagram 11)

R Unknown

Hx Depends on sex, age of presentation and type (see Table 69)

PE In all women, virilisation and severity depend on the time of onset of androgen elevation

Dx Heel prick: detect 17-OH-pregnenolone ↑

Tx 💊 • Glucocorticoid supplementation → inhibits hypothalamic-pituitary axis → stops excessive androgen production
  • Mineralocorticoid supplementation

🔪 Ambiguous external genitalia: reconstructive surgery

P If left untreated, the salt-wasting type can be fatal within weeks

! Addison crisis/shock at birth

> 🔆 **Adrenoleukodystrophy**: X-linked adrenal cortex insufficiency (mutation in ABCD1 gene on Xq28) with neurological degeneration due to segmental demyelination and axonal degeneration. The clinical picture manifests mainly in males (peak age 10-20), 4% of female carriers are symptomatic (peak age 20-40). Symptoms are similar to those of acquired adrenal cortex insufficiency with accompanying mixed polyneuropathy, spastic paraplegia and myeloneuropathy. Treatment is identical to treatment for primary adrenal cortex insufficiency.

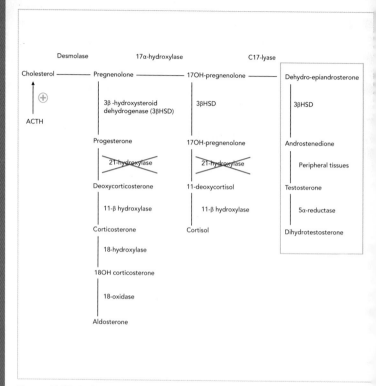

Diagram 11 // Pathophysiology of adrenogenital syndrome

	SALT-WASTING TYPE		**NON-SALT-WASTING TYPE** (simple virilising)
D	Cortisol and aldosterone deficiency.		Cortisol deficiency.
PE	♀: virilisation		
	♀ and ♂: vomiting, dehydration		♂: precocious puberty
Dx	Labs: cortisol ↓, ACTH ↑, genetic diagnostics		
	Labs: aldosterone ↓, sodium ↓, potassium ↑, hypoglycaemia		Labs: aldosterone ↓

Table 66 // Two subtypes of AGS

5α-reductase deficiency

D 5α-reductase deficiency is a disorder of sex development that occurs in individuals with a 46,XY karyotype.

E Unknown

Ae Mutation in SRD5A2 → conversion of testosterone to dihydrotestosterone ↓ autosomal recessive inheritance

Hx Ambiguous external genitalia, fertility problems, gynaecomastia ☉

PE Female/ambiguous external genitalia, gynaecomastia ☉

Dx · Genetic diagnostics: fluorescence in situ hybridization (FISH), karyotype or array comparative genomic hybridisation (aCGH) (for sex chromosomes), DNA testing for SRD5A2 gene
   · TAU/TVU: male internal urogenital system
   · Labs: testosterone/DHT ratio following hCG stimulation ↑, urine steroid profiling

Tx 💊 Exogenous testosterone
   🔪 Consider surgical correction

Klinefelter syndrome

D Male sex-linked chromosomal abnormality characterised by one or more additional X chromosomes (see Figure 74). Karyotype is 47XXY.

E Prevalence ♂ 200:100,000

Ae · 50% additional X from father
   · 50% additional X from mother
   · 15% mosaicism

Hx · Mild learning disability, mainly speech, and language difficulties
   · Infertility

PE Gynaecomastia, no chest hair, wide hips, small testes, height ↓ with long limbs

Dx · Genetic diagnostics: karyotype
   · Labs: testosterone ↓, LH ↑, FSH ↑
   · TAU/TVU: male internal genitals
   · Genomic test: detect Klinefelter syndrome

Tx 💬 Lifestyle counselling, symptomatic (e.g. physical therapy, speech therapy)
   💊 Exogenous testosterone (Testicular Sperm Extraction (TESE)/ICSI)

P No impact on life expectancy, mainly psychological and fertility problems

! Pay attention to osteoporosis → DEXA scan in adulthood

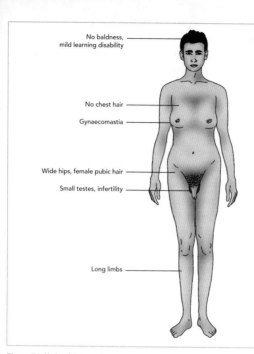

No baldness, mild learning disability

No chest hair

Gynaecomastia

Wide hips, female pubic hair

Small testes, infertility

Long limbs

Figure 74 // Klinefelter syndrome

Mayer-Rokitansky-Küster Hauster syndrome (MRKH syndrome)

D MRKH syndrome is a disorder of sex development in individuals with a 46XX karyotype, resulting in abnormal internal genitalia.

E Prevalence 20:100,000

Ae Disrupted Müllerian duct fusion during embryonic development, combination of unknown genetic and environmental factors

Hx Primary amenorrhoea, cyclical abdominal pain, fertility problems

PE Vaginal agenesis, normal development of secondary sex characteristics

Dx • TAU/TVU/pelvic MRI: uterine and vaginal malformations, sometimes rudimentary uterus (possibly with functioning endometrium), normal ovarian development, renal abnormalities (e.g. solitary kidney)

• Consider confirming diagnosis with laparoscopy

Tx ✎ Consider vulvoplasty/neovagina

! Pregnancy through surrogacy only

Turner syndrome

D Female sex-linked chromosomal abnormality in which one X chromosome is fully or partially missing (see Figure 75). Karyotype is 45X.

E Prevalence ♀ 10-50:100,000

Ae • 60-80% missing X due to loss in paternal meiosis
• Mosaicism
• Deletion of X chromosome

Hx Infertility

PE • Congenital cardiac and renal abnormalities
• Discrepancy in blood pressure between upper and lower limbs: aortic co-arctation
• Gonadal dysgenesis, no secondary sexual characteristics, high hairline, short, wide neck with skin folds, wide thorax with widely spaced nipples, cubitus valgus, short stature

Dx • Genetic diagnostics: karyotype
• TAU/TVU, cardiac ultrasound: gonadal dysgenesis, congenital cardiac or renal defects

Tx 💬 Lifestyle counselling, symptomatic (e.g. physical therapy, speech therapy)
💊 Exogenous oestrogen, growth hormone
🔪 Consider correction of cubitus valgus or aortic coarctation

P No impact on life expectancy, mainly psychological and fertility problems

! Pay attention to severe congenital heart defects

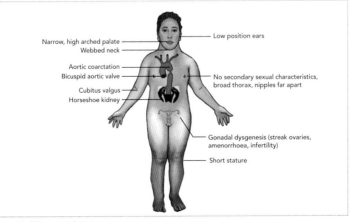

Narrow, high arched palate
Webbed neck
Aortic coarctation
Bicuspid aortic valve
Cubitus valgus
Horseshoe kidney

Low position ears

No secondary sexual characteristics, broad thorax, nipples far apart

Gonadal dysgenesis (streak ovaries, amenorrhoea, infertility)

Short stature

gure 75 // Turner syndrome

Swyer syndrome

(D) Swyer syndrome is a disorder of sex development in individuals with a 46XY karyotype, resulting in disrupted embryonic differentiation characterised by a female phenotype and male sex.

(E) Prevalence 1-2:100,000

(Ae) Mutation in e.g. MAP3K1 (18%), SRY (15%), DHH or NR5A1 that usually arises de novo but is sometimes passed on through Y-linked, X-linked, autosomal dominant, or autosomal recessive inheritance

(Hx) Primary amenorrhoea, fertility problems

(PE) Female internal and external genitalia

(Dx) • Genetic diagnostics: DNA testing for gene mutations
   • TVU: gonadal dysgenesis (streak gonads: absence of ovaries or testes)

(Tx) 🖉 Exogenous oestrogen and progesterone
   🔪 Streak gonad removal

(!) Risk of malignant gonad degeneration ↑, pregnancy only possible with oocyte donation

Fertility

Female subfertility

(D) Female subfertility is caused by absent ovulation, inability of the egg to reach the sperm, implantation failure, or genetic problems. Subfertility is the inability to achieve pregnancy despite twelve or more months of regular well-timed intercourse and a normal cycle.

(E) Prevalence 2.2:100, incidence ♀ age 25-44: 900:100,000/year

(Ae) • Functional: ovarian dysfunction (21-25%), tubal dysfunction (14-20%), hormonal imbalance, PCOS, POI, genetic (carrier translocation, mosaicism), anorexia, hypothalamic amenorrhoea (stress), hyperprolactinaemia, hyperthyroidism/hypothyroidism
   • Anatomical: abnormal genitalia (10-13%), endometriosis, adhesions (Asherman syndrome)/damage from surgery/infection

(R) Adiposity/anorexia, alcohol, occupation and surroundings (exposure to harmful substances), drugs, smoking, age >35

(Hx) Presence/absence of previous pregnancies, irregular cycle, dysmenorrhoea, genital development disorder, past gynaecological or abdominal infections. PMHx: abdominal surgery

(PE) Complete gynaecological exam to rule out possible underlying cause

- **Dx** • TVU/HSG: to rule out anatomical aetiology
  - Labs: FSH (↑ in POI/menopause), LH, oestrogen and progesterone to rule out hormonal problems, TSH ↑ and T4 ↓ to rule out hypothyroidism, prolactin to rule out prolactinoma
  - CAT: to differentiate between low or high risk for tubal pathology and the need for a HSG
  - Ovarian reserve test (ORT): to determine ovarian aging
- **Tx** 💊 Hormonal ovarian stimulation, IUI, IVF, ICSI

  🔪 Hysteroscopy and removal of endometriosis, fallopian tube surgery in case of obstruction
- **P** Couples with long-term subfertility and advanced maternal age → poorer prognosis
- **!** IVF/ICSI comes with a risk of multiple births and OHSS, characterised by e.g. peripheral oedema and risk of thrombosis

 Even fertile couples only have a 15-25% chance of getting pregnant per cycle. In the first year, ±75% of women become pregnant.

- Hunault score: probability of a spontaneous ongoing pregnancy <1 year.
- Hunault score <30%: intervention may lead to better results than watchful waiting.

- **Primary subfertility:** the couple has never achieved pregnancy together.
- **Secondary subfertility:** the couple has previously achieved pregnancy.

🔆 **Infertility** is the inability to conceive.

Male subfertility

- **D** Male subfertility is the inability to achieve spontaneous pregnancy after one year of regular and well-planned intercourse.
- **E** 30% male contributing factor
- **e** • Functional: hormonal (hypergonadotropic hypogonadism, hyperprolacti-

naemia), sperm production ↓ (cytostatics, radiotherapy), genetic disorders (see Table 37)

- Anatomical: obstructive, testicular abnormalities, anomalous seminal vesicles

Ⓡ Adiposity, alcohol, occupation (exposure to harmful substances, sedentary occupation), drugs, smoking, testicular heating/compression (e.g. varicocele). PMHx: surgery, mumps

ⓅⒺ Secondary sex characteristics (hair distribution, testicular volume)

Ⓓˣ Labs: DHT =/↓, semen analysis (oligoasthenoteratozoospermia (OAT), combinations are common

Ⓣˣ Hormone replacement (testosterone), surgical treatment of varicocele, vaso-epididymostomy for vasectomy reversal

Ⓟ Cause often goes undiagnosed

> In men, the chances of recovering fertility after vasectomy reversal decrease after a longer infertility period.

> Semen quantity and quality can be described as: oligo (low sperm count), astheno (low motility) and terato (abnormal morphology).

> Varicocele is esp. frequent on the left side, as the left testicular vein drains via the left renal vein. This leads to more back-flow compared to the right side, where the testicular vein drains directly into the inferior vena cava.

> Varicocele is present in around 25% of subfertile men and in around 10-15% of fertile men. This means that varicocele can lead to subfertility, but the patient still has a good chance of being fertile.

> The quality of sperm has decreased drastically over the past decades. What was considered subnormal 50 years ago is now considered better than normal. Research suggests this decline may be due not only to our current lifestyle but also to the use of agricultural fertilizers and pesticides.

Polycystic ovarian syndrome (PCOS)

Ⓓ PCOS is a syndrome characterised by an irregular menstrual cycle, possibl combined with reduced fertility and insulin resistance. The diagnosis is mad

if at least two of the Rotterdam criteria are present:
- Oligo-ovulation and/or anovulation;
- Clinical and/or biochemical signs of hyperandrogenism (biochemical: total testosterone >70 ng/dl, androstenedione >245 nl/dl, DHEA-S >248 μg/dl; clinical: acne, hirsutism, acanthosis nigricans);
- Polycystic ovaries (≥12 follicles of 2-9 mm diameter per ovary or ovarian volume >10 ml).

E Prevalence 10-13%, 20-40% of women with a 1st degree relative with PCOS

Ae Probably multifactorial: hereditary factors, aromatase deficiency of granulosa cells, androgen overproduction

R Adiposity, hyperinsulinaemia, positive family history, use of antiepileptics

Hx Oligomenorrhoea or amenorrhoea (>3y post-thelarche), hirsutism, acne, hyperinsulinaemia ⊝ (see Figure 76 and 77)

PE • Inspection: signs of hyperandrogenism (acne, hirsutism), adiposity, acanthosis nigricans
- Bimanual exam: bilateral ovarian enlargement

Dx • Labs: hyperandrogenism, insulin ↑, FSH =, LH ↑, testosterone ↑, glucose ↑
- TAU/TVU: polycystic ovaries (see Figure 78)

Tx 💬 Lifestyle advice: weight loss, exercise, lower intake of carbohydrates and fats, smoking cessation

💊 • OC (preferably combined pill), metformin
- For women who want to have children: OC (preferably combined pill), ovulation induction with FSH, letrozole (off-label), or clomiphene citrate

🔪 For women who want to have children: consider surgical electrocoagulation of ovarian cysts → androgen milieu ↓

P Risk of developing cardiovascular disease, DM type 2, metabolic syndrome, and endometrial carcinoma (due to continuous oestrogen stimulation)

! • Most common cause of oligomenorrhoea/amenorrhoea, and subfertility in women
- Adviced to generate 3-4 menstruations a year because of the risk of endometrial carcinoma
- Pregnancy complications (miscarriage, hypertension in pregnancy, preeclampsia, higher gestational weight gain, GDM, FGR, preterm delivery, small for gestational age babies and low birth weight, CS)

💡 In PCOS, excess androgen production prevents selection of a dominant follicle → failure to ovulate.

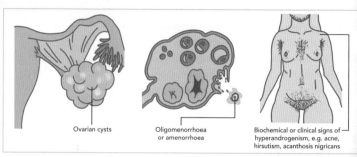

Figure 76 // PCOS: Rotterdam criteria

Ovarian cysts

Oligomenorrhoea or amenorrhoea

Biochemical or clinical signs of hyperandrogenism, e.g. acne, hirsutism, acanthosis nigricans

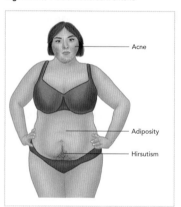

Figure 77 // Symptoms of PCOS

Acne

Adiposity

Hirsutism

Ovarian cysts

Figure 78 // Transvaginal ultrasound in PCOS

CONDITIONS

Asherman syndrome

(D) Asherman syndrome is characterised by secondary amenorrhoea due to intrauterine adhesions.

(E) 7% of all menstrual cycle disorders, incidence unknown

(Ae) Intrauterine adhesions after surgical procedures or past infections

(R) Intrauterine operations (e.g. curettage), intrauterine infections

(Hx) Secondary amenorrhoea/hypomenorrhoea, subfertility/infertility

(PE) Speculum exam/vaginal exam: to rule out other causes of secondary amenorrhoea

(Dx) • Labs: normogonadotropic (LH =, FSH =), oestrogen =
 • STI test: to rule out *Chlamydia*
 • Diagnostic hysteroscopy: possible intrauterine adhesions

Tx 🖋 Hysteroscopic resection of adhesions followed by applying barrier agents to prevent new adhesions

P No optimal treatment, women remain subfertile

! • Risk of recurrence 3.1-23.5%
• Neither IUD placement nor estrogen treatment have proven effective to prevent intrauterine adhesions or facilitate pregnancy

---

Ovarian hyperstimulation syndrome (OHSS)

D OHSS is a potentially life-threatening complication of ovulation induction. The exogen hCG causes luteinisation of granulosa cells with growth of multiple follicles and corpus luteum cysts, causing the ovaries to grow. Release of vascular endothelial growth factor (VEGF) induces capillary permeability and ascites.

E Severe OHSS prevalence 0.1-2%

Ae Administered exogenic hCG in fertility treatment

R Ovulation induction, age <35, polycystic ovaries, history of OHSS

Hx Abdominal pain, bloating, nausea, vomiting, dyspnoea, weight gain, syncope, oliguria/anuria, thromboembolic event

PE Weight ↑, presence of ascites and/or pleural effusion

Dx • TVU: enlarged ovaries, presence of ascites
• Labs: see Table 67

Tx 🖊 Avoid administering hCG
Mild/moderate OHSS (outpatient):
💬 Limit activities, daily weighing, and measurement of abdominal circumference
🖊 Paracetamol, rehydration (1-2L/d)
🖋 Ascites drainage
Severe OHSS:
💬 Admit patient, fluid balance, daily weighing, and measurement of abdominal circumference
🖊 Rehydration until Ht >0.40, antiemetics, paracetamol, thromboprophylaxis, consider albumin suppletion
🖋 Ascites drainage

P Symptoms disappear slowly after rehydration

! Risk of complications (e.g. ovarian torsion, thromboembolic events, sepsis, pericardial effusion, arrhythmias, acute respiratory distress syndrome (ARDS), and acute kidney failure)

SEVERITY OF OHSS	CLINICAL FEATURES	BIOCHEMICAL FEATURES
Mild	• Mild abdominal discomfort • Bloating • Ovarian size usually <8 cm²	• Haematocrit <0.45 • Serum albumin normal • White cell count <15,000/ml • Kidney function normal • Liver function normal
Moderate	• Moderate abdominal pain • Nausea and/or vomiting • Ascites on ultrasound • Ovarian size usually 8-12 cm²	• Haematocrit <0.45 • White cell count <15,000/ml • Kidney function normal • Liver function normal
Severe	• Clinical ascites (and/or hydro-thorax) • Ovarian size usually >12 cm² • Oliguria (<300 ml/d or 30 ml/h)	• Haematocrit >0.45 • Hyponatraemia (Na <135 mmol/L) • Hypo-osmolality (osmolality <282 mOsm/kg) • Hyperkalaemia (P >5 mmol/L) • Hypoproteinaemia (serum albumin <35 g/L) • White cell count >15,000/ml • Kidney function normal • Liver function ↓
Critical	• Tense ascites/large hydrothorax • ARDS • Thromboembolism • Oliguria/anuria	• Haematocrit >0.55 • Hyponatraemia (Na <135 mmol/L) • Hypo-osmolality (osmolality <282 mOsm/kg) • Hyperkalaemia (P >5 mmol/L) • Hypoproteinaemia (serum albumin <35 g/L) • Hypoproteinaemia (serum albumin <35 g/L) • White cell count >25,000/ml • Kidney function ↓ • Liver function ↓

Table 67 // Classification of OHSS

CONDITIONS

Abnormalities in pregnancy

 Abnormalities are grouped by the first trimester in which they usually occur or present for the first time, but may still arise or persist in subsequent trimesters.

Abnormalities in the first trimester

Ectopic pregnancy

Ⓓ An ectopic pregnancy is a pregnancy (blastocyst) that nestles outside the uterine cavity.

E · Prevalence: 1-2% of all pregnancies
   · Extrauterine implantation: fallopian tube (±95%), mainly in the ampulla (70%), ovary (±3%), cervix (<1%), abdomen (1-2%) or a CS scar (see Figure 79)

Ae Difficult passage to endometrium due to tubal adhesions or ciliary damage after infection, surgery or endometriosis

R PID (especially gonococcal infection), fertility disorder, endometriosis, age (>30), IUD, PMHx: ectopic pregnancy, or abdominal surgery (tubal and uterine surgery, sterilisation, complicated abdominal surgery), IVF

Hx Asymptomatic, amenorrhoea, unilateral abdominal pain, vaginal blood loss, collapse/near collapse

PE · Consciousness ↓, pulse ↑, BP ↓, capillary refill =/prolonged
   · Abdominal palpation: varying from painless to acute abdomen (in a ruptured ectopic pregnancy)
   · Speculum exam: uterine bleeding

Dx · Labs: serum/urine β-hCG lower than expected. Serial β-hCG test every 2d: <50% increase in 48h, Hb =/↓
   · TAU/TVU: localisation ectopic mass (>35 mm separated from the ovary), free abdominal fluid in intraperitoneal haemorrhage, no visible intrauterine gestational sac (despite β-hCG >2,000 IU/L), possible pseudogestational sac without fetal pole, endometrial thickening
   · Abdominal MRI: can be used in the diagnosis of caesarean scar or interstitial pregnancies

Tx 🗨 · If asymptomatic with low and decreasing β-hCG level (<1,500 IU/L): active β-hCG monitoring to rule out persistent trophoblast
   · Abstinence from intercourse due to rupture risk
   · In ectopic pregnancies without present ectopic mass (or ectopic mass <35 mm) and β-hCG <5,000 IU/L, or ectopic pregnancies located in an area with poor surgical access (CS scar/intramural duct/cervix): methotrexate
   · In RhD-negative women: anti-rhesus D (RhD)

🔪 Laparoscopy, convert to laparotomy in case of complications, insufficient visibility, or unstable patient:
   · Tubectomy: for major rupture or ectopic pregnancy. Preferred in healthy contralateral side
   · Tubotomy: spares fallopian tube, preferred for fertility reasons. Can be considered in affected contralateral side.
   · Additional methotrexate treatment if insufficient decrease in β-hCG.

- (P) • Mortality mainly due to hypovolaemic shock following fallopian tube rupture
- • Recurrence risk 10%
- (I) • Pregnancy of unknown location (PUL): positive pregnancy test with unknown location of pregnancy
- • Consider presence of heterotopic pregnancy (mainly after IVF): simultaneous intrauterine AND extrauterine pregnancy → contraindication to drug treatment
- • Monitor hepatic and renal function before and during methotrexate therapy

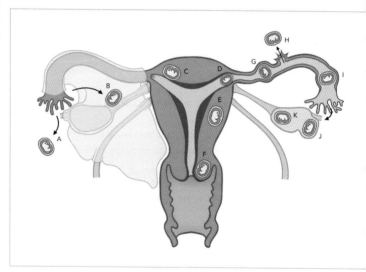

Figure 79 // Ectopic pregnancy: locations
A: Primary abdominal or secondary abdominal after tubal abortion **B:** Intraligamentary **C:** Interstitial **D:** Cornual **E:** Intramural **F:** Cervical **G:** Isthmic **H:** Secondary abdominal after rupture **I:** Ampulla **J:** Secondary ovarian **K:** Primary ovarian

 Every patient of childbearing age with symptoms of abdominal pain should receive a pregnancy test.

 In ectopic pregnancy, life-threatening haemorrhage may occur due to contact with maternal circulation or tubal rupture. Avoid vaginal exam and perform TAU in case of a suspected ruptured ectopic pregnancy.

A woman of childbearing age in hypovolaemic shock with a positive β-hCG and ultrasound with free abdominal fluid/blood has a ruptured ectopic pregnancy until proven otherwise.

Hydatidiform mole

D A hydatidiform mole or molar pregnancy occurs when an improperly fertilised egg implants in the uterus and is followed by abnormal trophoblast tissue proliferation. A molar pregnancy is a premalignant condition. A distinction is made between complete molar pregnancy, which is the most dangerous and can be malignant, and partial molar pregnancy, which is often less dangerous.

E Incidence in Europe 100:100,000 pregnancies, ±2% of miscarriages are moles

Ae Two types are distinguished (see Figure 80):
  • Complete mole (80%): an egg lacking maternal chromosomes is fertilised by a diploid sperm or a single sperm with genetic duplication after fertilisation. Abnormal placenta, absent fetus
  • Partial mole (20%): genotypically normal egg fertilised by two sperm cells resulting in triploidy. Possibly presence of normal or abnormal fetus

R Very low or advanced maternal age, PMHx: molar pregnancy

Hx Pelvic tenderness and pressure, vaginal bleeding (reddish-brown), hyperemesis gravidarum

PE • Fundal height: positive discordance
  • Bimanual exam: uterus larger than expected, bilateral ovarian masses

Dx • Labs: β-hCG ↑ for gestational age
  • TVU: typical grape-like structures
    - Complete: central heterogeneous mass, abnormal placenta, no embryo or fetus
    - Partial: abnormal placenta with cystic structures, amniotic fluid =/↓, fetus may be present (often with asymmetric growth restriction), transverse gestational sac diameter ↑

Tx Anti-RhD immunoglobulins in RhD-negative mother, chemotherapy for persistently high β-hCG, contraception during follow-up

  • Curettage or hysterectomy (age <40, not trying to conceive, exceptional circumstances)
  • Follow-up: weekly β-hCG test until β-hCG is negative, followed by monthly β-hCG test for 6 mo. Patient should not get pregnant again during follow-up

P · Recurrence risk in subsequent pregnancy: 1%
· Risk of choriocarcinoma: 15-20% in complete mole, 1-5% in partial mole
  risk of lung metastases (see Figure 81)

! Mole may be associated with anaemia, early-onset pre-eclampsia, hyperthy-roidism and thecalutein cysts → risk of ovarian rupture or torsion

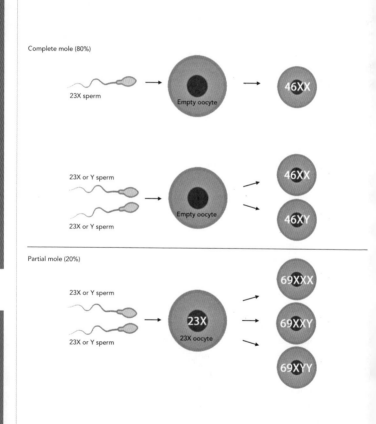

Figure 80 // Complete and partial hydatidiform mole

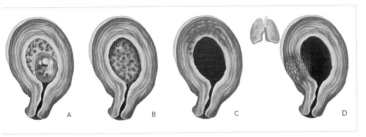

Figure 81 // Partial/complete hydatidiform mole, persistent trophoblast and choriocarcinoma
A: Partial hydatidiform mole **B:** Complete hydatidiform mole **C:** Persistent trophoblast **D:** Choriocarcinoma

 A mole (and occasionally a miscarriage or ectopic pregnancy) may be followed by a persistent trophoblast or the cells may mutate and develop into a choriocarcinoma. These patients generally respond well to chemotherapy.

Multiple pregnancy

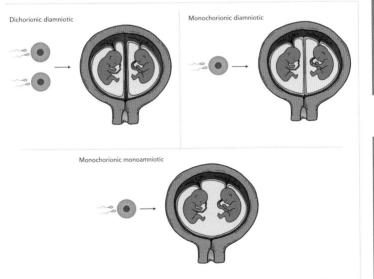

Dichorionic diamniotic

Monochorionic diamniotic

Monochorionic monoamniotic

Figure 82 // Multiple pregnancy

	MONOZYGOUS	**DIZYGOUS**
D	· Formed by cleavage of a fertilised ovum (see Figure 82) · Dichorionic diamniotic (DCDA): 1/3 of monozygotes · Monochorionic diamniotic (MCDA): 2/3 of monozygotes · Monochorionic monoamniotic (MCMA): rare	· Formed by polyovulation (see Figure 82) · Always a DCDA placenta
E	Incidence <0.5% of spontaneous pregnancies	Incidence 0.7% of spontaneous pregnancies
Ae	A fertilised ovum splits → initially identical children, mutations and environmental factors may spark differences	Polyovulation → multiple ova fertilised by different sperms, need not be from the same man → two non-identical children
R	Ovarian stimulation, IVF	Age, parity, IVF, genetics and predisposition, iatrogenic factors (e.g. ovulation stimulation)
Hx	Pregnancy symptoms (e.g. nausea and vomiting) are more common in twin pregnancies	
Dx	TAU: · MCMA: no visible septum, MCDA: T-sign · Regular monitoring of fetal growth · Screen voor TTTS: umbilical artery pulsatility index (UAPI), MCA peak systolic velocity (MCA PSV), AFI/SDP	TAU: · DCDA: Lambda sign · Regular monitoring of fetal growth
Tx	🖉 · During pregnancy: 200 mg iron, 1 mg folic acid, high-calorie diet · Before childbirth: always take a blood sample for crossmatching, and insert precautionary IV line due to increased risk of postpartum haemorrhage · Imminent preterm birth: corticosteroids for fetal pulmonary maturation	
P	· The average twin pregnancy ends in wk 37, triplet pregnancies in wk 34, quadruplet pregnancies in wk <31 · Indication for caesarean delivery: monochorionic-monoamniotic twin pregnancies ends in wk 32–34 · Risk of maternal complications, infant morbidity and mortality ↑ (esp. pregnancy-induced hypertension (PIH), pre-eclampsia, preterm birth and FGR)	
!	· Puerperal complications are almost identical to those of singleton pregnancies, but are more severe and frequent. · Monoamniotic twins have higher risk of mortality due to congenital abnormalities and umbilical cord entanglement	

Table 68 // Multiple pregnancy

Twin-to-twin transfusion syndrome (TTTS)

D TTTS occurs exclusively in monochorionic twins and is characterised by placental vascular anastomoses that cause unequal blood flow between the two fetuses (see Figure 83).

E Prevalence 9-15% of monochorionic diamniotic pregnancies

Ae · Unbalanced vascular anastomoses → cardiovascular instability
· Donor: hypovolaemia → renal dysfunction → stuck twin with olighydramnios
· Acceptor: hypervolaemia → cardiac hypertrophy, macrosomia, urinary output ↑ → polyhydramnios → eventual hydrops fetalis (due to cardiac decompensation)

Hx Asymptomatic, sudden increase in fundal height, abdominal discomfort

PE Fundal height: positive discordance

Dx TAU: monochorionic placenta, polyhydramnios/oligohydramnios. The septum seems to disappear as it is stuck against the donor child, called 'stuck in twin'. Quintero's five stages represent the severity of TTTS.

Tx 🗣 Frequent ultrasound monitoring of fetal growth and amniotic fluid
✎ Laser coagulation of anastomoses, amniodrainage in child with polyhydramnios

P · If left untreated, 90% end in miscarriage
· If one twin dies, the other usually follows. The acceptor usually dies first from cardiac decompensation due to volume overload.

! Mirror syndrome: generalised maternal oedema (including pulmonary oedema) in hydrops fetalis 'mirrors' fetal and placental oedema

---

🔅 **The Quintero staging system distinguishes five stages of TTTS based on ultrasound testing**:
· Stage **1**: one fetus with oligohydramnios and one with polyhydramnios, donor bladder visible
· Stage **2**: one fetus with oligohydramnios and one with polyhydramnios, no donor bladder, normal Doppler
· Stage **3**: one fetus with oligohydramnios and one with polyhydramnios, no donor bladder, abnormal Doppler
· Stage **4**: signs of hydrops in one or both fetuses
· Stage **5**: death of one or both fetuses

CONDITIONS

Twin anaemia polycythaemia sequence (TAPS) is characterised by small placental anastomoses, causing one twin to develop anaemia and the other to develop polycythaemia without amniotic fluid volume abnormalities (as opposed to TTTS). TAPS occurs spontaneously in ±5% of monochorionic multiple pregnancies and in up to 15% after laser coagulation.

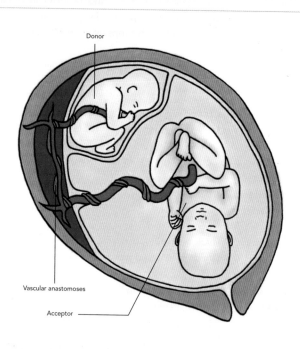

Donor

Vascular anastomoses

Acceptor

Figure 83 // Twin-to-twin transfusion syndrome

Substance abuse during pregnancy

Intrauterine and postpartum tobacco exposure both increase the risk of IUFD.

SUBSTANCE	COMPLICATIONS
Alcohol	• The impact of fetal alcohol exposure is cumulative with the dose • Obstetric: IUFD, FGR, prematurity • Neonatal: fetal alcohol syndrome (FAS), psychoneurological damage, neonatal abstinence syndrome
Amphetamines (including MDMA)	• Obstetric: placental abruption, hypertensive complications, FGR, IUFD, malignant hyperthermia • Neonatal: congenital defects, prematurity
Cannabis	The effect of cannabis during pregnancy is unclear. The limited number of studies on the topic show no direct adverse obstetric effects. Adverse effects seem to arise mainly from concomitant tobacco use and other substance abuse.
Cocaine	• Obstetric: placental abruption, FGR, placenta praevia, fetal and placental vasoconstriction → fetal hypoxia → prematurity, cerebral infarctions • Neonatal (first days): congenital defects (various), high-pitched crying, hyperactivity, hyperarousal, irritability, tremor, tachypnoea/apnoea • Neonatal (long-term): behavioural difficulties
Opioids (including heroin)	• Obstetric: anaemia, multiple pregnancy, FGR, IUFD, preterm contractions • Neonatal: neonatal abstinence syndrome (autonomic dysfunction, vomiting, circadian rhythm disorders, diarrhoea, high-pitched crying, hypertonicity, tremor, feeding problems with failure to thrive (FTT))
Tobacco	• Obstetric: placental abruption, FGR, IUFD, placenta praevia, preterm prelabour rupture of membranes (PPROM), prematurity • Neonatal: asthma, congenital defects (especially schisis), behavioural problems, microcephaly, IUFD

Table 69 // Risks of substance abuse during pregnancy

Hyperemesis gravidarum

D Hyperemesis gravidarum is excessive/persistent vomiting during pregnancy with risk of dehydration.

E • Prevalence 1.1-3.6%, especially in 1st half of pregnancy
   • ±75% of all pregnant women experience nausea, half of which also experience vomiting

Ae Idiopathic ⊙, linked to somatic/psychogenic disorders and high serum β-hCG (e.g. multiple pregnancy, hydatidiform mole, trisomy 21)

R High β-hCG level (multiple pregnancy, molar pregnancy), motion sickness, FHx: hyperemesis gravidarum

Ix Nausea, vomiting (morning or all day long), abdominal pain, pallor, signs of dehydration, dizziness, weight ↓, palpitations, headache

PE · Pulse ↑, BP =/↓, acetone breath
  · Volume status: dry eyes/mucosa, sunken eyes, skin turgor ↓

Dx · Blood gas test: metabolic alkalosis
  · Labs: potassium ↓, chloride ↓, magnesium ↓, calcium ↓, haematocrit ↑, liver enzymes ↑, urea ↑, possible hyperthyroidism
  · Urine: ketonuria

Tx 🖉 · Vomiting without hypovolaemia: eat small bites, supplement vitamins and potassium, avoid triggers, start workday later, antiemetics as needed
  · Vomiting with hypovolaemia: hospitalisation with rehydration and vivitamin supplementation, potassium and antiemetics, enteral nutrition if indicated

P · Physiological vomiting disappears after 10-12 wk of amenorrhoea
  · Recurrence risk: 15-20%

I · Complications: cardiac arrhythmia (hypokalaemia), dehydration, Mallory Weiss tears, Wernicke encephalopathy (vitamin B1 deficiency)
  · Pay attention to other causes of vomiting, like diabetic ketoacidosis in DM

Miscarriage

D Spontaneous miscarriage, is a (spontaneous) expulsion of the fetus before week 16. In some countries a distinction is made between early (week 12) and late (weeks 12-15) miscarriage. See Figure 81 for several types of miscarriages

E · Prevalence: 10-20% of all pregnancies (5% of multiparas), 80% in first trimester
  · After week 8: 0.6% risk of spontaneous miscarriage

Ae Congenital defects in embryos/fetuses, chromosomal abnormalities, placental insufficiency, maternal clotting disorders, subclinical hypothyroidism

R Chromosomal abnormalities, subclinical hypothyroidism, DM, clotting disorders, maternal age

Hx Vaginal bleeding (spotting to heavy bleeding), abdominal pain

PE · Monitor vitals: pulse =/↑, BP =/↓, T =/↑
  · Abdominal palpation: peritoneal stimulation (intra-abdominal haemorrhage)
  · Speculum exam: origin and volume of blood loss
  · Bimanual exam: uterine size and consistency

Dx · Labs: β-hCG fails to rise (usually doubles in 48h), Hb =/↓, blood group test
  · TAU/TVU: yolk sac possibly still present, fetal vital signs: no heartbeat, no fetal/yolk sac growth, blighted ovum (embryonal sac with diameter >25 mm

without fetal parts)

Tx 🔵 Before wk 12: repeat ultrasound after 1-2 wk

💊 • Oral mifepristone (uterine sensitisation to prostaglandins) followed by
vaginal misoprostol after 36-48h to induce fetal expulsion
• Anti-RhD in rhesus D-negative women

 Surgical abortion (curettage), especially in partial miscarriage and heavy
blood loss

P 95% chance of successful expulsion with misoprostol

> 🔅 Criteria for miscarriage:
> • Crown-rump length (CRL) ≥7 mm, no heartbeat
> • Mean sac diameter 25 mm, no embryo
> • Absent embryo 14d after gestational sac without yolk sac
> • Absent embryo 11d after gestational sac with yolk sac

> 🔅 **Induced abortion** is the deliberate termination of pregnancy. It can
> be performed until 24 weeks gestation. The terms and guidelines re-
> garding termination of pregnancy differ between countries.

Imminent miscarriage and incipient miscarriage

D Imminent miscarriage is an impending miscarriage. Incipient miscarriage is
an inevitable miscarriage.

Hx Minor mucus-like blood loss, minor lower abdominal cramps, vaginal bleeding

PE • Vaginal exam (only when ectopic pregnancy is ruled out): closed external
os, uterus feels weak, mobile, slightly enlarged, very slightly tender
• Speculum exam: minor blood loss from external os possible

Dx TAU/TVU: yolk sac (pay attention to pseudo-ring formation in ectopic pregnancy), fetal cardiac function ↓ from 6-8 wk

Tx 🔵 Watchful waiting

Incomplete miscarriage

D Incomplete miscarriage is characterised by incomplete fetal expulsion, as
opposed to complete miscarriage.

Hx Increased vaginal bleeding, lower abdominal pain

PE • Speculum exam: possible visible tissue debris
• Vaginal exam: finger can often be inserted into external os

Dx TAU/TVU: tissue debris in the uterine cavity or cervix

Tx 🖊 Surgical abortion (curettage) with prophylactic antibiotics or manual removal of products of conception from cervix if possible

💊 Consider misoprostol if bleeding is acceptable

Missed abortion

D Missed abortion is an asymptomatic miscarriage in which the embryo is still in utero.

Tx 💬 Wait for spontaneous expulsion of fetal parts

💊 Misoprostol, mifepristone

🖊 Surgical abortion (curettage) with prophylactic antibiotics

- Uterine size <14 wk: mifepristone 200 mg orally 24-48h before misoprostol. Misoprostol 400 µg sublingually, buccally, or vaginally, or 600 µg orally.
- Uterine size 14-24 wk: mifepristone 200 mg orally 24-48h before misoprostol. Misoprostol 400 µg sublingually, buccally, or vaginally every 3h.

Septic miscarriage

D A septic miscarriage is an infection of the uterine cavity in spontaneous abortion or following an induced abortion.

Ae Gram-negative bacteria 😶

Hx Fetid odour/discharge, fever, malaise, abdominal pain, vaginal bleeding

PE • T ↑, pulse=/↑, RR =/↑

- Speculum exam: dilated cervix
- Bimanual palpation: weak, tender uterus

Dx STI risk assessment

Tx 💊 AB

🖊 Curettage, if life-threatening: hysterectomy

! Endotoxic shock with few symptoms in gram-negative bacterial infection

Recurrent miscarriages

D Recurrent miscarriages are defined as two consecutive spontaneous miscarriages.

Ae Genetic abnormalities, uterine abnormalities, maternal clotting disorders, DM, subclinical hypothyroidism

Dx Diagnosis of underlying cause

> Following the removal of a fetus or fetal remains, an ultrasound must be performed to check if the uterine cavity is empty.

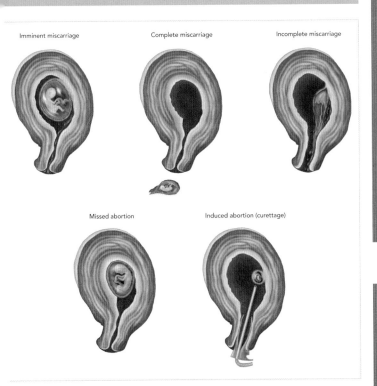

Imminent miscarriage   Complete miscarriage   Incomplete miscarriage

Missed abortion   Induced abortion (curettage)

Figure 84 // Types of miscarriage

Abnormalities in the second trimester

Gestational diabetes mellitus (GDM)

(D) DG, also called gestational diabetes mellitus (GDM), is a type of DM that develops during pregnancy.

(E) Prevalence 5-9% of all pregnancies

(Ae) β cell hypertrophy during pregnancy

(R) • DM in family, BMI >30, descent (Indo-Surinamese, South Asian, Middle Eastern, Moroccan, Egyptian, Afro-Caribbean), PCOS
  • PMHx: GDM, impaired glucose tolerance (IGT)/prediabetes, macrosomatic infant

(Hx) Asymptomatic ☺

(PE) Fundal height: positive discordance in macrosomia

(Dx) • TAU: macrosomia, polyhydramnios, evaluate congenital abnormalities
  • Labs: glucose ↓, OGTT as needed 4-point glucose curve after inconclusive OGTT, 24-28 wk, early OGTT at 16 wk in case of previous GDM

(Tx) 💬 • If abnormal glucose day curve (GDC):
      - Step 1: diet (30-35 kcal/kg, spread throughout the day) and exercise
      - Step 2: insulin, target blood glucose between 3.0-7.0 mmol/L (55-126 mg/dl)
  • Regular monitoring, ultrasound (with fetal growth measurement), GDC
  • CTG monitoring during labour
  • Postpartum: monitor neonatal glucose levels (risk of hypoglycaemia) breastfeeding is recommended, test fasting maternal glucose and HbA1c after 6 wk
  🖊 Childbirth: consider inducing labour before week 40 in patients using insulin or in case of macrosomia

(P) • Recurrence risk: 60%
  • Maternal risk of developing DM type 2 within 5-10y ↑↑

(!) • Maternal: risk of pre-eclampsia ↑, polyhydramnios ↑, infections (especially urogenital) ↑
  • Fetal: macrosomia, birth trauma, shoulder dystocia, organomegaly, postnatal hypoglycaemia (possible brain damage if left untreated)

Prolonged and increased fetal exposure to glucose via the umbilical cord results in fetal hyperglycaemia and subsequent pancreatic islet hyperplasia → chronic hyperinsulinaemia → risk of postpartum hypoglycaemia ↑ and DM type 2 later in life ↑.

Cervical insufficiency

D Cervical insufficiency is structural cervical weakness during pregnancy, causing dilation without contractions.

E Prevalence ±0.5%

Ae Low collagen level in the cervical connective tissue

R Cervical trauma (curettage, LLETZ, or other gynaecological procedures), congenital cervical abnormalities (maternal DES use), PMHx: cervical insufficiency

Hx Asymptomatic ☺, cramps, back pain, abnormal vaginal discharge (consistency, colour, volume)

PE Speculum exam: possibly shortened or open cervix or visible fetal membranes

Dx • TAU/TVU: cervix <25 mm, funnelling followed by cervical dilation, during Valsalva method ↑
   • Tocogram: normal, no contractions
   • Urine/amniotic fluid culture: normal (to rule out infection)

Tx 🗨 Follow-up every 1-2 wk until 24 wk: detect further shortening
   🖊 Vaginal progesterone until 36 wk if cervical length ≤25 mm before 24 wk
   🖌 Cervical cerclage: cervix <10 mm despite vaginal progesterone, and no contraindications. Abdominal cerclage can be considered.

P High recurrence risk in subsequent pregnancy

! Contraindications to cerclage: active haemorrhage, active preterminal contractions, intrauterine infection, IUFD, PPROM, vaginal blood loss, and multiple pregnancies

 If cervical insufficiency symptoms occur in the 2nd trimester, it is between 14-20 weeks.

 Monitor cervical length with TVU in patients with a history of unexplained miscarriages or preterm deliveries in the 2nd trimester with minimal symptoms.

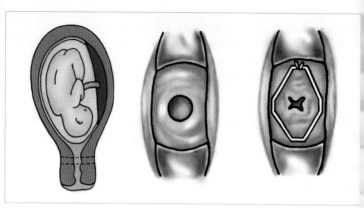

Figure 85 // Cervical insufficiency and cerclage

Hypertensive disorders during pregnancy

Gestational hypertension

(D) Gestational hypertension (SBP >140 mmHg or DBP >90 mmHg) develops after week 20 without proteinuria or other signs of organ damage. Gestational hypertension usually disappears within 12 weeks postpartum.

(E) Prevalence 6-17% in nulliparas, 2-4% in multiparas

(Ae) Idiopathic

(R) • See Pre-eclampsia
 • Risk factors for progression to pre-eclampsia: gestational age <34 wk at time of diagnosis, elevated serum uric acid, descent (Sub-Saharan African (especially West African), African-American, Afro-Caribbean)

(Hx) Asymptomatic ☺, headache ⊖, oedema ⊖

(PE) BP ↑, peripheral oedema ⊖

(Dx) • Labs: normal blood count, uric acid =, creatinine =, ASAT/ALAT = (to rule out HELLP/pre-eclampsia)
 • Urine: no proteinuria

(Tx) 💬 • Inform patient of alarm symptoms: fetal movement ↓, headache, malaise, nausea, visual disturbances, pain (upper abdomen/epigastrium between shoulder blades)
   • Frequent blood count, blood pressure and proteinuria monitoring
 🖊 Antihypertensives (methyldopa/labetalol/nifedipine)
 ✐ Consider inducing labour from wk 37

P · 10-50% risk of pre-eclampsia
· Most women become normotensive in the 1st wk postpartum, 22% recurrence risk in subsequent pregnancy, greatly increased risk of developing essential hypertension in later life

 ACE inhibitors or ARBs can lead to an increased risk of congenital malformations when used during pregnancy. Alternative antihypertensive medication should be considered.

Pre-eclampsia

D Pre-eclampsia is defined as hypertension occurring after week 20 (SBP >140 mmHg or DBP >90 mmHg), confirmed at least twice after an interval ≥4 hours, with proteinuria or signs of organ failure.

E Prevalence 2-8% of all pregnancies, 90% of cases occur after wk 34

Ae Insufficient cytotrophoblast migration to decidua with poor spiral arteries formation → placental endothelial dysfunction → hypoxia → placenta secretes inflammatory cytokines → systemic inflammation, endothelial dysfunction (see Figure 86)

R DM, pre-existent hypertension, chromosomal abnormalities, positive FHx, multiple pregnancy, chronic renal failure, molar pregnancy, nulliparity, adiposity, advanced maternal age, descent (Sub-Saharan African (esp. West African), African-American, Afro-Caribbean), PMHx: pre-eclampsia

Hx Asymptomatic ⊙, headache, nausea, vomiting, pulmonary oedema, peripheral oedema, oliguria, pain (upper abdomen/epigastrium, or between shoulder blades), retrosternal pain, visual disturbances (starry vision)

PE · BP ↑, petechiae and oedema ⊙
· Auscultation: crepitations in pulmonary oedema
· Abdominal palpation: epigastric and right upper quadrant tenderness
· Neurological exam: hyperreflexia, clonus

Dx · Labs: Hb =/↑, Ht =/↑, platelets =/↓, uric acid ↑, ASAT/ALAT =/↑, placental biomarkers for prediction of pre-eclampsia (alpha-fetoprotein (AFP) ↑, soluble fms-like tyrosine kinase-1 (sFlt-1) ↑, pregnancy-associated plasma protein-A (PAPP-A) ↓, placental growth factor (PlGF) ↓
· Urine: proteinuria (>0.3 g)
· TAU: FGR, Doppler flow (umbilical artery and MCA), oligohydramnios, placental markers (uterine artery notch)

- CTG: fetal bradycardia, variability ↓, and decelerations or preterminal CTG (see Diagnostics)

(Tx) 🗩 Hospitalisation and frequent monitoring of blood pressure (2x/d) and proteinuria (2x/wk)

    💊 • Antihypertensives (methyldopa/labetalol/nifedipine), IV in severe hypertension (>160 mmHg SBP or >110 mmHg DBP), intrapartum magnesium sulfate (eclampsia prophylaxis)
- Acetylsalicylic acid: prophylaxis during subsequent pregnancy

    ✎ Induced labour, or CS from 37 wk, or in case of clinical deterioration

(P) • Mortality: 1:100,000 pregnancies, 10-15% of maternal deaths worldwide are associated with pre-eclampsia/eclampsia
- Recurrence risk: 25-30% after severe pre-eclampsia or HELLP. A recurrence in a subsequent pregnancy usually occurs at a later gestational age.

(!) • Pre-eclampsia can occur up to 48-72h postpartum
- Vaginal delivery possible except in eclampsia
- Fetal: FGR, oligohydramnios, prematurity → perinatal mortality ↑
- Always rule out a HELLP syndrome in the lab (see HELLP syndrome for specific findings)
- Consider prescribring acetylsalicylic acid (ASA) in subsequent pregnancy in case of 1 high risk or 2 moderate risk factors (see Table 70)

INDICATION FOR ASA PRESCRIPTION	
High risk	• Pre-eclampsia in previous pregnancy • Chronic kidney disease • Autoimmune diseases (e.g. SLE, antiphospholipid syndrome) • DM type 1 or 2 • Pre-existing hypertension
Moderate risk	• Nulliparity • Maternal age ≥40 • Interval between pregnancies >10y • Pre-eclampsia in FHx (mother/sister) • Obesity (BMI >35 kg/m²) • Multiple gestation Placental insufficiency in previous pregnancy (e.g. previous child with FGR or intrauterine fetal demise (IUFD) without known cause) • Pregnancy with egg donation

Table 70 // Indications for ASA prescription

Normal

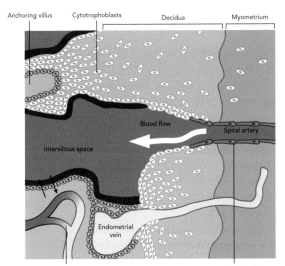

Anchoring villus   Cytotrophoblasts   Decidua   Myometrium

Blood flow

Spiral artery

Intervillous space

Endometrial
vein

Fetal blood vessels   Endothelial cell

Pre-eclampsia

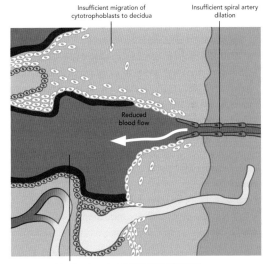

Insufficient migration of
cytotrophoblasts to decidua

Insufficient spiral artery
dilation

Reduced
blood flow

Intervillous hypoxia, prompting release of cytotoxic
substances, and systemic maternal endothelial dysfunction

Figure 86 // Placental pathophysiology of pre-eclampsia

Eclampsia

(D) Eclampsia is defined as the presence of convulsions in patients with pre-eclampsia.

(E)
- Prevalence 2-3% of patients with severe pre-eclampsia without magnesium sulfate prophylaxis, incidence 15-100:100,000 births
- Peak incidence: adolescence and age >35

(Ae) Idiopathic

(R) See Pre-eclampsia

(Hx) Loss of consciousness (possibly coma), convulsions (tonic-clonic, tongue bite, urine leakage), severe headache, epigastric/right upper quadrant pain, visual disturbances

(PE)
- Pulse =/↑, BP ↑ in 75%
- Neurological exam: cerebral nerve palsy, memory loss, hyperreflexia

(Dx)
- See Pre-eclampsia
- Cerebral MRI/CT: to rule out other causes in atypical presentations

(Tx) 🗨 • Secure and stabilise maternal health
- Secure airway to prevent aspiration (recovery position/mayo tube)

💊 • Magnesium sulfate IV (continuous until 48h postpartum), antihypertensive IV
- Oxygenation (place mother in left-lateral tilt/manual uterine displacement (MUD), and start O_2 therapy)
- Benzodiazepines: consider in case of persistent convulsion

✎ CS if persistent fetal stress after maternal stabilisation

(P)
- Mortality: 0-14%, highest mortality in low-income countries with inadequate access to prenatal care
- Fetal bradycardia improves with maternal therapy

(!)
- Eclampsia occurs intrapartum in 20% of cases and postpartum in 40% (<48h
- Maternal complications: ischaemic stroke, DIC, pulmonary oedema, acute renal failure, HELLP syndrome, risk of problems in subsequent pregnancy, death
- Fetal complications: prematurity, placental abruption, intrauterine asphyxia
- Treatment is prompt delivery. Induction or vaginal delivery can be considered if delivery is expected soon.

💡 **Right recovery position** may compress inferior vena cava and lead to maternal hypotension and shock.

Every convulsing pregnant patient is due to eclampsia until proven otherwise.

HELLP syndrome

D HELLP is short for haemolysis, elevated liver enzymes and low platelet count, and is a severe form of pre-eclampsia.

E Prevalence 0.1-0.2% of all pregnancies, prevalence 10-20% of women with pre-eclampsia or eclampsia

Ae Abnormal placental development and function with hepatic inflammation and clotting system activation

R PMHx: pre-eclampsia/HELLP

Hx Ascites, vomiting, epigastric/right upper quadrant pain, headache, jaundice, general malaise, nausea, visual disturbances (see Figure 87)

PE Pulse =/↑, BP ↑, saturation =/↓, jaundice

Dx • Labs: Hb ↓, platelets ↓, ASAT/ALAT ↑, haptoglobin ↓, indirect bilirubin ↑, creatinine ↑, LDH ↑, uric acid ↑
  • Urine: proteinuria -/+
  • TAU and CTG: fetal vitality evaluation

Tx 💊 • Magnesium sulfate IV for eclampsia prophylaxis
  • Antihypertensives, IV in severe hypertension (>160 mmHg SBP or >110 mmHg DBP): labetalol/methyldopa/nifedipine
  • Platelet transfusion: if platelets <20,000/µL before labour or <50,000/µL before CS

  🔪 Induced labour or CS

P • Gestational age is the main fetal prognostic factor
  • Maternal blood work does not affect fetal prognosis
  • HELLP recurrence risk: 1-2%
  • 25-30% chance of pre-eclampsia in next pregnancy

! • Hypertension and/or proteinuria may be absent in HELLP syndrome
  • Maternal complications: placental abruption, acute renal failure, DIC, hepatic haematoma, pulmonary oedema, eclampsia
  • Fetal complications: 7-20% mortality especially due to placental abruption, FGR, prematurity

HELLP syndrome usually occurs in primarily nocturnal episodes. The worse the episode (epigastric pain), the higher the liver parenchyma tests and the lower the platelet count.

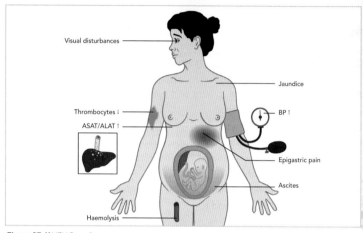

Figure 87 // HELLP syndrome

Hepatic abnormalities during pregnancy

		ACUTE FATTY LIVER IN PREGNANCY	INTRAHEPATIC CHOLESTASIS DURING PREGNANCY
	D	A sign of acute liver dysfunction or liver failure during pregnancy, typically in weeks 30-38 (see Figure 88).	Characterised by elevated maternal serum bile acids (see Figure 89). Also called gestational cholestasis.
	E	Incidence 5-15:100,000 pregnancies/year	Incidence <1-27.6%, more common in autumn and winter months, Scandinavia, Asia and South America
	Ae	Idiopathic, suspected disruption of fat metabolism during pregnancy	Idiopathic, ABCB4 mutation (10-15%), underlying liver disease, drug-induced (progestogens, oestrogens, carbamazepine, some ABx)
	R	• Maternal: BMI <20 kg/m², pre-eclampsia, HELLP, nulliparity, PMHx: acute fatty liver in pregnancy • Fetal: long-chain 3-hydroxyacyl-CoA dehydrogenase deficiency, ♂, multiple pregnancy	PMHx: gestational cholestasis, multiple gestation, chronic hepatitis C infection, positive FHx, advanced maternal age

Table 71A // Hepatic abnormalities during pregnancy

	ACUTE FATTY LIVER IN PREGNANCY	INTRAHEPATIC CHOLESTASIS DURING PREGNANCY
Hx	• Initial abdominal pain, vomiting, headache, general malaise, nausea • Long-term: ascites, jaundice	Itching (especially manual and plantar), sleep deprivation, steatorrhoea, dark urine, jaundice ⊙, nausea
PE	Long-term: jaundice, undulation	Inspection: scratch marks, no primary injuries
Dx	• Labs: leukocytes ↑, thrombocytes =/↓, aPTT/INR =/↑, fibrinogen =/↓, ALAT/ASAT ↑, total bilirubin ↑, glucose ↑, ammonia ↑, creatinine ↑, uric acid ↑ • Urine: proteinuria in accompanying HELLP syndrome or pre-eclampsia • TAU: fetal evaluation, ascites, nonspecific liver changes (fatty infiltration, hyper-echogenic) • Liver biopsy: microvesicular fatty infiltration in hepatocytes • Genetic testing in fetus: long-chain 3-hydroxyacyl-CoA dehydrogenase deficiency	• Labs: aminotransferases ↑, bile acids ↑, total and direct bilirubin ↑ • TAU: normal fetal growth, normal maternal liver
Tx	🗨 In case of abnormalities in liver function tests: delivery on short-term basis	💊 • 1st choice: ursodeoxycholic acid • 2nd choice: add cholestyramine (binds to bile salts, prevents resorption) 🔬 Induced labour at wk 36-37 (after pulmonary maturation) in case of severely elevated bile acids (>40 µmol/L) despite ursodeoxycholic acid to mitigate risk of asphyxia/IUFD
P	• Maternal mortality <5%, fetal mortality up to 30% • Liver function recovers within 7-10d postpartum • Long-term fetal liver failure in long-chain 3-hydroxyacyl-CoA dehydrogenase deficiency	• Recurrence risk: 50% • Itching disappears a few days after delivery • Serum bile acids are correlated with risk of fetal mortality
!	Complications: DIC, encephalopathy, hepatorenal syndrome, renal failure, pancreatitis	• Steatorrhoea/cholestyramine use → reduced vitamin ADEK resorption → vitamin K supplementation due to bleeding risk (maternal and fetal) • Fetal complications: asphyxia (vasoconstriction of the chorionic veins due to bile acids), fetal demise (fetal arrhythmia due to toxic effect of bile acids on cardiomyocyte), meconium-stained amniotic fluid, prematurity

able 71B // Hepatic abnormalities during pregnancy

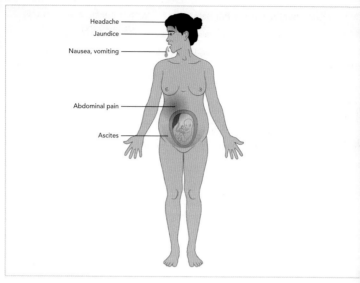

Figure 88 // Acute fatty liver in pregnancy

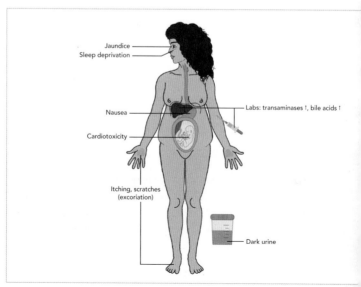

Figure 89 // Intrahepatic cholestasis in pregnancy

Maternal alloimmunisation

D Maternal alloimmunisation is caused by incompatibility with rhesus D, C, c, K, and E. Placental passage of maternal IgG erythrocyte antibodies destroys fetal erythrocytes covered with antibodies, leading to haemolytic disease of the fetus and newborn (HDFN) with impaired erythropoiesis, severe fetal anaemia, hydrops, and perinatal death.

E Prevalence of anti-D alloantibodies 1:80, prevalence of other clinically significant alloantibodies (anti-K, anti-c) 1:300

Ae Fetal maternal transfusion (FMT): ↑ gestational age → ↑ placental transfer of fetal erythrocytes to maternal circulation. Iatrogenic transfusion, non-compatible blood type in transplantation.

R Sensitising event during pregnancy (chorionic villus sampling or amniocentesis, surgical abortion >10 wk gestation, ectopic pregnancy, hydatidiform mole, immature labour, termination of pregnancy >20 wk gestation, blood loss 2nd/3rd trimester, complicated labour (CS, placental retention, multiple gestation), blunt trauma of abdomen, perinatal death

Hx Fetal movement

PE TAE: fetal growth, peak systolic velocity of middle cerebral artery (PSV-MCA), and multiples of the median (MoM)

Dx Maternal blood type, antibody status, non-invasive fetal and paternal genotyping, antibody-dependent cell-mediated cytotoxicity assay (ADCC): every 4 wk up to 28 wk gestation, and every 2 wk up to delivery

Tx 💬 Referral to fetal specialist: previous pregnancy with significant HDFN, >1.5 multiples of the median (MoM), signs of fetal anaemia

🔪 >1.5 MoM, signs of fetal anaemia: intrauterine transfusion

P Good in case of early identification and treatment, no long-term adverse effects

! Prevention with RhD prophylaxis

Placental and umbilical cord abnormalities

Placental and umbilical cord abnormalities are common but are not always diagnosed antepartum. They do not always affect fetal wellbeing. Always examine the postpartum umbilical cord and placenta for structural abnormalities. Structural placental abnormalities include:

- Ischaemic necrosis: often caused by spiral artery occlusion secondary to thrombosis, hypertension, and pre-eclampsia (20% in normal pregnancies)
- Retroplacental haematoma: placental abruption

- Calcifications: on maternal side, may initiate placental problems in early pregnancy
- Terminal villus deficiency: IUFD due to stagnation of placental development
- Chronic villitis of unknown etiology (VUE): major infiltration of immunological cells in fetal tissue. High-grade VUE can cause FGR, prematurity, IUFD, recurrent miscarriage, CNS injury, and has a relatively high risk of recurrence (25–50%)
- Circumvallate placenta: occurs when an undersized chorionic plate causes the membranes to fold around the edges of the fetal side (see Figure 90)

Structural umbilical cord abnormalities include:
- Velamentous cord insertion: umbilical vessels insert into the membranes rather than the middle of the placenta (more frequent in multiple pregnancies)
- Abnormal length: umbilical cord ↑ → risk of knots ↑ (normal ±55 cm)
- Umbilical cord cysts: no clinical significance. The presence of multiple pseudocysts may be indicative of congenital or chromosomal abnormalities
- Umbilical cord oedema: frequent in IUFD
- Single umbilical artery (SUA): associated with congenital cardiac and urogenital abnormalities

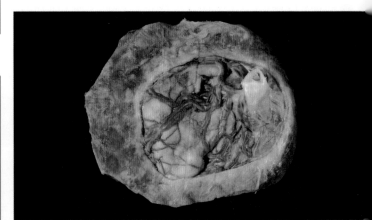

Figure 90 // Circumvallate placenta

Placental abruption

D Placental abruption is the premature partial or complete detachment of a normally implanted placenta (see Figure 91).

E Incidence 0.3-10% pregnancies/yr, highest prevalence 3rd trimester

Ae Haemorrhage caused by a ruptured blood vessel between the placenta and decidua

R Hypertensive disorders (including pre-eclampsia, eclampsia), FGR, smoking, use of cocaine, abdominal trauma, low socio-economic status, PMHx: placental abruption

Hx Acute abdominal pain, acute vaginal bleeding (66%), hypovolaemic shock (sweating, altered consciousness, dizziness), back pain (posterior placenta), fetal movements ↓

PE • Pulse =/↑, BP =/↓, capillary refill =/prolonged, saturation =, RR =/↑, oliguria/anuria
  • Abdominal palpation: hard abdomen ('uterus en bois'), fetus difficult to palpate
  • CTG: fetal distress, uterine hyperactivity

Dx • Labs: Hb ↓, blood group, PT/INR ↑, fibrinogen ↓, platelets ↓, creatinine ↑, uric acid ↑
  • TAU: normal, possible retroplacental haematoma, Doppler flow ↓

Tx 💬 Strict monitoring in case of partial abruption with stable mother and fetus before wk 34, anti-RhD in RhD-negative women
  🔪 Emergency CS in case of maternal and fetal instability

P • No correlation between vaginal blood loss and severity of fetal/maternal distress
  • Fibrinogen has the closest correlation to severity of bleeding
  • Recurrence risk: 10%

! • Complications: DIC, tubular necrosis, hypovolaemic shock
  • Heavy bleeding → extravasation of blood into the myometrium → atonic uterus → blood loss ↑

Always initiate anti-RhD immunisation if there is a risk of fetomaternal blood contact in RhD-negative pregnant women, e.g. in vaginal bleeding in pregnancy.

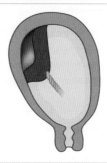

Figure 91 // Placental abruption

Placenta praevia

(D) In a placenta praevia, the placenta obstructs the internal os of the cervix. In a marginal placenta praevia, the placenta is located <2 cm from the internal os but does not obstruct it (see Figure 92).

(E) Prevalence 2-5% in the 2nd trimester, 0.4% of all live births

(Ae) Idiopathic

(R) High age, multiple pregnancy, multiparity, anatomical uterine abnormalities, smoking, cocaine, fertility treatment, PMHx: placenta praevia or CS

(Hx) Asymptomatic ☺, bright red blood loss in 2nd-3rd trimester, painless ☉

(PE) • Abdominal palpation: smooth, non-tender
  • Speculum exam: origin of bleeding

(Dx) • TAU/TVU: low-lying placenta, abnormal fetal lie/presentation
  • CTG: no fetal distress

(Tx) 💬 With limited blood loss: watchful waiting with ultrasound follow-up, bed rest, and slowly expanding activities

  🖊 • Iron supplementation or blood transfusion as needed, anti-RhD in RhD-negative pregnant patients
    • Antenatal corticosteroids in case of risk of preterm delivery

  🖊 Mode of delivery:
    • Placenta <10 mm from internal cervical os: elective CS
    • Placental tip >10 mm from internal cervical os: trial of labour

(P) • 3-5x increased risk of prematurity, neonatal death and perinatal death
  • Recurrence risk: 4-8%

(!) Elevated risk of placenta accreta (implantation near CS scar) (see Table 72), postpartum haemorrhage, and need for hysterectomy

In case of placenta praevia repeat sonographic determination of placental location at 32 weeks gestation

NUMBER OF CS	PLACENTA PRAEVIA	PLACENTA ACCRETA	PLACENTA ACCRETA WITH PRESENCE OF PLACENTA PRAEVIA
0	0.26%	0.004-0.01%	2-5%
1	0.65%	0.16-0.30%	14-24%
2	1.80%	0.26-1.6%	23-47%
3	3%	1.20-5.1%	29-40%
4	10%	2.30-9.1%	33-67%

Table 72 // Risk of abnormal placentation in subsequent pregnancy

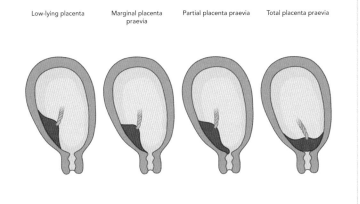

Low-lying placenta   Marginal placenta praevia   Partial placenta praevia   Total placenta praevia

Figure 92 // Types of placenta praevia

Vasa praevia

(D) In vasa praevia, the fetal vessels cross the membranes covering the interna os (see Figure 93).

(E) Prevalence 40:100,000 deliveries

(Ae) Idiopathic

(R) Low-lying placenta, placenta praevia, velamentous insertion, IVF, bilobec placenta, multiple pregnancy

(Hx) Asymptomatic, vaginal blood loss with ruptured membranes (possible vasa praevia rupture)

(PE) Avoid vaginal exam in suspected vasa praevia, as it can lead to umbilical va sospasm and fetal distress. Pulsations are rarely felt over the internal os o the cervix.

(Dx) • TAU/TVU and Doppler: vascular structures crossing the internal os of the cervix
  • CTG: variable decelerations due to compression

(Tx) 💊 • Weekly monitoring (CTG, fetal growth)
  • Individualise need for prophylactic hospitalisation 30-32 wk gestation
  💊 Antenatal corticosteroids for lung maturation (wk 28-34) due to risk o prematurity
  🔪 • CS: premature contractions, repetitive decelerations on CTG, PPROM vaginal bleeding of fetal origin, fetal tachycardia
  • Elective caesarean delivery at 34-36 wk gestation in asymptomati women

(P) Mortality 3% if diagnosed prepartum, 56% if not diagnosed prepartum

(!) Even minor vaginal blood loss can cause fetal demise due to low fetal bloo volume

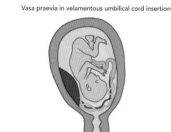
Vasa praevia in velamentous umbilical cord insertion

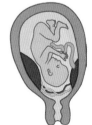
Vasa praevia in bilobed placenta

Figure 93 // Vasa praevia

Abnormalities in the third trimester

Fetal growth restriction (FGR)

FGR, previously known as intrauterine growth restriction (IUGR), or dysmaturity, is reduced fetal growth below the tenth percentile of a growth curve adjusted for genetic descent, sex, region and gestational age (see Figure 94). A distinction is made between:
- Symmetrical growth restriction: all fetal dimensions are equally undersized;
- Asymmetrical growth restriction: disproportionate fetal dimensions with relative preservation of head circumference and reduced abdominal size due to adaptive measures in response to poor environment, e.g. redistribution of energy and preferential blood supply to the brain.

Newborn prevalence 3-7%
- Symmetrical (normal growth potential): chromosomal abnormalities, congenital abnormalities/infections
- Asymmetrical (reduced growth potential): maternal disease, uteroplacental disorders

Chronic maternal disease (hypertension, kidney disease, DM, asthma, systemic lupus erythematodes), BMI <20 or >25, pre-eclampsia, smoking, infections (CMV, toxoplasmosis, rubella, varicella, parvovirus B19), PMHx: FGR

Asymptomatic 😐

Fundal height: negative discordance in 30-50%

TAU: monitor fetal growth with growth curve, looking at abdominal circumference, estimated fetal weight (EFW) and Doppler profile (uterine artery, umbilical artery, MCA)

- Regular monitoring of fetal well-being (CTG) and growth (ultrasound and Doppler) to optimise timing of delivery/induced labour
- Severe FGR at 18–20 wk: detailed fetal anatomical survey, UAPI, and MCA

Antenatal corticosteroids in preterm birth

Delivery before 40 wk (timing depends on ultrasound and Doppler findings)

Depends on gestational age at delivery and birth weight

Fetal complications: mortality, necrotising enterocolitis, respiratory distress syndrome

Fetal growth restriction is a risk factor for developing cardiovascular disease, DM type 2, metabolic syndrome, kidney disease and adiposity later in life.

 Fetal growth is monitored by tracking abdominal circumference, femoral length, biparietal diameter and head circumference.

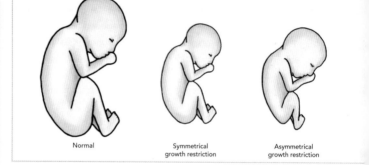

| Normal | Symmetrical growth restriction | Asymmetrical growth restriction |

Figure 94 // Types of FGR

Intrauterine fetal demise (IUFD)

Ⓓ IUFD is the death of the fetus in utero at least 16 weeks after the mother's la period and before labour has started.

Ⓔ Prevalence 0.6% of pregnancies

Ⓐₑ Fetal circulation disorder (placental abruption, placental insufficiency), infe tion (GBS, TORCHES), umbilical cord complications (prolapse, nuchal cor knots), prematurity, TTTS, rhesus antagonism, chromosomal abnormalitie hypertensive disorders of pregnancy, uterine rupture

Ⓡ Hypertensive disease (especially pre-eclampsia), age <25 or >35, smokin DM, clotting disorders, nulliparity, multiple gestation, untreated thyroid d orders, obesity, PMHx: IUFD, low socio-economic status

Ⓗₓ Asymptomatic, reduced fetal movement, vaginal bleeding

Ⓟₑ No added value

Ⓓₓ TAU: no fetal heartbeat

Ⓣₓ 💬 Psychosocial counselling for parents, induced labour

💊 Prostaglandins/oxytocin (if labour does not start spontaneously), an RhD in RhD-negative pregnant patients

· Amniocentesis/chorionic villus sampling for chromosome testing if delivery is not expected soon
· Autopsy at birth, preferably autopsy of the child and pathological testing of the placenta

P Recurrence risk depends on aetiology

! Dead fetus syndrome: prolonged retention of the dead fetus (4-6 wk) can lead to DIC. To evaluate this risk, test for fibrin degradation products and platelets weekly after 2 wk until fetal expulsion. When labor is delayed more than 48h, it is recommended to test for DIC twice a week.

 Testing after stillbirth:
· Kleihauer-Betke test
· HbA1c ↑
· Liver function and bile acid testing
· TORCHES
· Bacteriology (blood cultures, vaginal swab)
· Fetal and placental microbiology
· Maternal anti-Ro and anti-La antibodies
· Karyotypic analysis of fetal and placental tissues
· Histological examination of placenta, fetal membranes, and umbilical cord

 Registration of a stillborn child >24 weeks gestational age and legal responsibilities differ between countries.

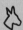 **TORCHES infections**
TORCHES is an acronym for infections that can be transmitted to the fetus in utero or during delivery. TORCHES infections have potentially serious consequences: **T**oxoplasmosis, **O**ther (enteroviruses, varicella zoster, parvovirus B19), **R**ubella, **C**ytomegalovirus, **H**erpes simplex, **S**yphilis.

Dermatoses of pregnancy

	GESTATIONAL PEMPHIGOID	**POLYMORPHIC ERUPTION IN PREGNANCY**
D	Autoimmune-mediated, bullous disease occurring in the 2nd or 3rd trimester that can persist postpartum (formerly called gestational herpes).	Consists mainly of self-limiting pruritic inflammatory dermatoses. Onset usually in 3rd trimester, after week 35 or immediately postpartum.
E	Incidence 2-5:100,000 pregnancies/year	Incidence 1:160-300 pregnancies/year
Ae	Autoimmune or as a paraneoplastic symptom of trophoblast tumours ⊖	Idiopathic: possibly due to stretching of the skin or immunological factors
R	N/A	Nulliparity
Hx	Severe itching, rash	
PE	• Umbilical papular/urticarial lesions can spread all over the body within days (bullae and vesicles) • The face and mucosa are mostly spared	• Striae and erythematous papules with white halos, may combine into urticarial plaques • Face, soles of the feet, palms of the hands and peri-umbilical region are not affected
Dx	• Labs: BP-180 antibodies • Biopsy: subepidermal vesicle with lymphocytic and eosinophilic infiltrate. Immunofluorescence: presence of C3	Biopsy (usually not needed): perivascular and interstitial lymphocytic/eosinophilic infiltrate
Tx	✏ High-dose topical/systemic corticosteroids	✏ Topic/systemic corticosteroids, non-sedative antihistamines
P	• Non-elevated risk of miscarriage • Relatively high recurrence risk, severity usually increases in subsequent pregnancies	• No effect on maternal and fetal health • Recurrence risk very low
!	• Complications: FGR, neonatal gestational pemphigoid, prematurity • Gestational pemphigoid may also present postpartum	Can be mistaken for a drug eruption, e.g. a fixed drug reaction

Table 73 // Dermatoses of pregnancy

Amniotic fluid abnormalities

	OLIGOHYDRAMNIOS	POLYHYDRAMNIOS
D	Amniotic fluid volume <5th percentile, <500 ml, amniotic fluid index (AFI) ≤5 cm or single deepest pocket (SDP) <2 cm (see Figure 95).	Amniotic fluid volume >95th percentile, >2L, AFI ≥24 cm or SDP >8 cm (see Figure 95).
E	Prevalence 11% of pregnancies at wk 40	Prevalence 1-2% of all pregnancies
Ae	• Maternal: placental dysfunction (abruption, hypertensive disorders, nephropathy, clotting disorders) • Fetal: amniotic fluid leakage, chromosomal abnormalities, congenital (urinary tract) abnormalities (dysplasia, obstruction, Potter syndrome), postterm birth	• Idiopathic ☺ • Maternal: DM, DG • Fetal: congenital abnormalities (swallowing disorder, oesophageal atresia, duodenum stenosis), chromosomal abnormalities (trisomy 18), hydrops fetalis, infection (syphilis, parvovirus B19), TTS
Hx	Asymptomatic ☺	Asymptomatic, abdominal discomfort, contractions, dyspnoea
PE	• Abdominal palpation: fetus is easy to palpate • Fundal height: negative discordance	• Abdominal palpation: fetus is difficult to palpate • Fundal height: positive discordance • Poorly audible fetal heart sounds on auscultation
	Congenital malformations: amniocentesis	
Dx	• TAU: AFI ≤5 cm, SDP <2 cm, screening for congenital abnormalities, evaluation of fetal growth, Doppler profile and fetal gastric and bladder filling • CTG: possible decelerations	• OGTT: to rule out DM/DG • Labs (abnormalities linked to aetiology): leukocytes, c-reactive protein (CRP), irregular antibodies, serology: syphilis, CMV, toxoplasmosis, rubella • TAU: >2L, AFI ≥24 cm or SDP >8 cm, evaluate hydrops fetalis
Tx	✎ Threat to fetal well-being and viable fetus: induce labour or CS	● Watchful waiting ✎ If symptomatic: amnioreduction
P	• 1st trimester: >90% end in spontaneous abortion • 2nd trimester: approx. >80% fetal mortality depending on aetiology • Anhydramnios is incompatible with life • 3rd trimester: amniotic fluid ↓ → risk of complications ↑	Depends on aetiology

Table 74A // Amniotic fluid abnormalities

OLIGOHYDRAMNIOS	POLYHYDRAMNIOS
! Complications: prematurity, umbilical cord compression	Complications: abnormal fetal lie/presentation (transverse lie or breech presentation), prematurity, umbilical cord prolapse, PPROM, postpartum uterine atony, mirror syndrome (in hydrops fetalis)

Table 74B // Amniotic fluid abnormalities

Oligohydramnios

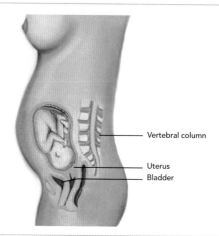

- Vertebral column
- Uterus
- Bladder

Polyhydramnios

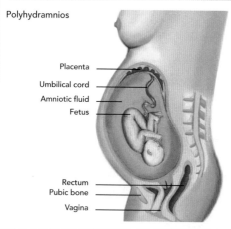

- Placenta
- Umbilical cord
- Amniotic fluid
- Fetus
- Rectum
- Pubic bone
- Vagina

Figure 95 // Amniotic fluid abnormalities

Preterm contractions

D Preterm contractions occur before week 37, with the risk of cervical dilation and/or effacement.

E 45% of preterm contractions progress to delivery, 6-8% of which end in preterm delivery

Ae No single cause, see risk factors

R Placental abruption, cervical insufficiency, congenital uterine malformation, infections, multiple pregnancy, symptomatic placenta praevia, polyhydramnios, PPROM, PMHx of preterm birth, congenital abnormalities of the fetus

Hx Contractions, vaginal pressure, menses-like cramps, vaginal bleeding (mild/spotting), vaginal discharge (mucus)

PE • T =/↑
- Speculum exam: cervical dilation >3 cm, intact membranes
- Vaginal exam: evaluate clinical impression of labour and dilation, only if membranes are intact

Dx • TVU: cervical funnelling or dilation
- Fetal fibronectin test in wk 22-34 and cervical length <30 mm (high specificity and low sensitivity for preterm birth)
- Amniotic fluid test to evaluate PPROM
- CTG: evaluate fetal condition
- Tocogram: evaluate contractions

Tx • AB ampicillin/penicillin (GBS prophylaxis), magnesium sulfate (fetal neuroprotective) in case of active contractions
- <34 wk: tocolytics (atosiban/calcium antagonists for 48h) combined with corticosteroids (fetal lung maturation)
- >34 wk: hospitalisation for delivery, discharge after 4-6h with failure to progress (FTP) and stable maternal and fetal condition

P Fetal survival at wk 24: 30-60%, fetal survival at wk 28: 90%

 If delivery is expected before week 34, administer antenatal corticosteroids to stimulate fetal lung maturation. Caffeine can be added postpartum. Planned primary CS: give corticosteroids from week 35-37 after shared-decision making. Corticosteroids are not recommended as standard from week 37 onwards.

 In the presence of preterm contractions, do not use lubricant during the speculum exam.

Braxton-Hicks contractions are false labour pains that feel like contractions and usually disappear over time. If cervical length >30 mm, chance of those contractions inducing birth <3%.

 Prevention preterm birth after previous preterm birth:
- Vaginal progesterone from 16 to 36 weeks
- Cervical length measurements: every 2 weeks between 14-16 and 24 weeks, when cervical length ≥30 mm
- Cervical length measurements: every week when cervical length <30 mm

 Indications for GBS prophylaxis to prevent vertical transmission of early-onset GBS illness:
- Previous child with GBS infection
- Maternal urinary tract infection with GBS infection

Consider GBS prophylaxis:
- Maternal GBS colonisation (positive vaginal swab)
- Preterm labour or premature rupture of membranes with unknown GBS status

Preterm prelabour rupture of membranes (PPROM)

(D) PPROM is the early (<37 weeks) rupture of membranes before labour contractions begin (see Figure 96). It is distinct from prelabour rupture of membranes (PROM).

(E) · Prevalence 3% of pregnancies
· Responsible for 30-40% of preterm births

(Ae) Urogenital infections or cervical insufficiency, idiopathic

(R) Urogenital infections, PMHx: PPROM, premature contractions, prepartum blood loss, previous cervical surgery

(Hx) Vaginal fluid loss, multiple gestation, smoking, signs of infection (fever, malodorous vaginal discharge, abdominal pain)

(PE) · Pulse =/↑, T =/↑
· Sterile speculum exam: amniotic fluid in the vaginal canal, spontaneous or after Valsalva manoeuvre

(Dx) · Labs: CRP =/↑, leukocytes =/↑ with left shift (in infection)

- TAU: fetal position, oligohydramnios (70%), fetal condition
- Vaginal culture and GBS culture: to rule out infection
- CTG: fetal tachycardia is suggestive of infection
- Amniotic fluid test: +

Tx 💬 Watchful waiting until wk 37 in the absence of signs of infection or meco-nium-containing amniotic fluid

💊 • Corticosteroids for fetal lung maturation, tocolytics in the absence of intra-amniotic infection
   • Antibiotics: reduce risk of chorioamnionitis, neonatal infection, risk of birth <48h

🔪 Induce labour from wk 37 or following signs of intra-amniotic infection (lower abdominal pain, fever, malaise, abnormal vaginal discharge, and/or reduced fetal movements)

P 50% of patients give birth prematurely

❗ Complications: intra-amniotic infection, preterm birth, oligohydramnios, umbilical cord prolapse, placental abruption

🔔 Always use a sterile speculum in PROM and avoid vaginal exam if possible to mitigate risk of intrauterine infection. Always use sterile gloves when performing a vaginal exam in PROM.

💡 Administering corticosteroids if delivery is expected <7 days and before week 34. The corticosteroids are maximally effective up to 7 days before delivery, and minimally effective after 14 days.

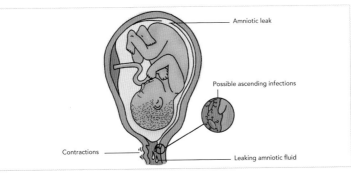

igure 96 // Complications of preterm prelabour rupture of membranes (PPROM)

Postterm pregnancy

(D) Postterm pregnancy is defined as a gestational age >42 weeks.

(E) Prevalence 0.4-4% of pregnancies

(Ae) Idiopathic ⊙, miscalculated term (relative postterm pregnancy)

(R) PMHx: postterm pregnancy, nulliparity, adiposity, advanced maternal age

(Hx) Asymptomatic

(PE) No added value

(Dx) · TAU: assess oligohydramnios, fetal Doppler profile (umbilical artery and middle cerebral artery), fetal gastric and bladder filling, and fetal movement. Consider checking gestational age by reassessing measurements of scans with crown-rump length (CRL) in wk 11-14.
· CTG: assess fetal condition

(Tx) 🔪 Induce labour from wk 41 with CTG during delivery due to fetal hypoxemia risk ↑, and risk of perinatal death

(P) · Increased risk of induced labour, assisted delivery, CS
· Perinatal mortality: 1.3-1.9:1000 births (at wk 40 0.86:1000 births)

(!) · Complications: placental insufficiency, oligohydramnios, macrosomia shoulder dystocia, meconium-containing amniotic fluid, meconium aspiration syndrome, IUFD, artificial delivery, postpartum haemorrhage
· Fetal dysmaturity syndrome: umbilical cord compression due to oligohydramnios and placental insufficiency

> 🔔 In the 3rd trimester it is difficult to assess fetal growth on ultrasound, therefore CTG is the main tool for evaluating fetal condition.

Problems during and after childbirth

Abnormal fetal presentation

Breech presentation

D In breech presentation, the presenting part is the fetal tailbone (see Figure 97).

E Prevalence at full term: 3-5%, prevalence at wk 32: 7-15%, prevalence at wk 28: 25%

R Preterm delivery, PMHx: breech presentation, intrauterine abnormality, low-lying placenta/placenta praevia, nulliparity, cervical uterus myomatosus, fetal abnormalities

Hx Kicking in lower abdomen, subcostal discomfort

PE · Leopold manoeuvres: head in uterine fundus
   · Vaginal exam: fetal tailbone or feet may be palpable in case of cervical dilation

Dx TAU: fetal head in uterine fundus, and fetal tailbone in lower segment

Tx 💬 · Possible spontaneous version (rotation) later in pregnancy
   · External version to cephalic position
   ✒ After unsuccessful version: normal delivery or consider CS

P · Recurrence risk after one pregnancy with breech presentation: 9%
  · Recurrence risk after two pregnancies with breech presentation: 25%

! · 50% of vaginal breech deliveries end in a secondary CS
  · Fetal: pressure on birthing canal ↓ → slow delivery → risk of aspiration, umbilical cord prolapse and peripartal asphyxia (difficult fetal head extraction) ↑

· **Complete breech:** flexed knee and hip joint (cross-legged).
· **Incomplete breech:** extended knee joint, flexed hip joint.
· **Complete footling breech:** extended knee and hip joint.

Requirements for breech delivery in a singleton pregnancy: no previous CS, amenorrhoea >36 weeks, spontaneous labour, skilled team, perfect or imperfect breech presentation on ultrasound (footling breech presentation is a contraindication), estimated fetal weight >2,500 and <4,000 g, no hyperextension of the head.
Guidelines and requirements for breech delivery differ between hospitals and countries.

Administer anti-RhD immunisation to an RhD-negative woman with an RhD-positive child after external version.

 Vaginal breech delivery:
- Descent of buttocks, rump and legs (spontaneous, no fetal traction).
- Delivery with Bracht's manoeuvre: grasp baby at the tailbone with both hands (like a hamburger) as soon as the scapular apices show. Once the posterior hairline becomes visible, it is used as a rotation point to turn the baby toward the mother's abdomen. At the same time, the mother pushes and pressure is applied to the fundus. Make sure the fetal back rotates to the front and correct immediately if it doesn't.
- Delivery of the arms, if not spontaneous: Løvset manoeuvre (rotating fetus back and forth, child's back facing upwards), or Van Deventer-Müllerman manoeuvre (release posterior arm followed by anterior arm).
- If fetal head is stuck, choose between: suprapubic impression, Mauriceau manoeuvre, forceps, symphysiotomy, or Zavanelli manoeuvre.
- Total breech extraction: the fetal feet are grasped and the entire fetus is extracted. Total breech extraction should only be used for a noncephalic second twin.

Transverse presentation

(D) In a transverse presentation, the fetal longitudinal axis lies perpendicular to the longitudinal axis of the uterus (see Figure 97).

(E) Prevalence 300-350:100,000 pregnancies

(Ae) Excess space in the uterus or obstruction of the lower uterine segment, preventing descent

(R) Prematurity, dysmaturity, multiparity, placenta praevia, uterine abnormalities, polyhydramnios, fetal anomaly

(Hx) Ultrasound finding, positive PMHx

(PE) Leopold manoeuvres: abnormal position in maternal abdomen with head on the side

(Dx) TAU: Abnormal fetal presentation, back facing caudally or cranially

(Tx) 💬 Eternal version to cephalic presentation if possible

✏️ If unsuccessful: CS

(P) Depending on the cause of the abnormal fetal presentation

(!) Disproportionate stretching of the lower uterine segment may occur during labour → risk of uterine rupture

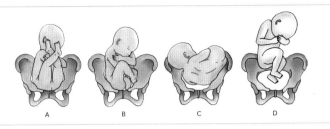

Figure 97 // Types of breech presentation and transverse presentation
A: Incomplete breech presentation **B:** Complete breech presentation **C:** Transverse presentation **D:** Complete footling breech presentation

Abnormal cephalic presentations

ABNORMALITY	DESCRIPTION OF THE PRESENTATION	POSSIBLE CONSEQUENCES
Persistent occiput posterior (sunny-side up)	Slight fetal head deflection: the occiput is the presenting part and lies posteriorly, face faced anteriorly (sunny-side up)	Vaginal delivery possible, assisted delivery often needed
Vertex presentation	Head between flexion and deflexion: occipital area around anterior fontanelle is the presenting part	Vaginal delivery possible, risk of rupture ↑
Sinciput presentation	Moderate fetal head deflection: forehead is presenting part	Vaginal delivery impossible
Face position	• Pronounced fetal head deflexion: face is presenting part (chin is presenting point, see Figure 98) • Findings in vaginal exam: facial parts palpable	• Vaginal delivery only possible if chin is in anterior orientation • Fetal complications: laryngeal oedema, stridor, respiratory difficulties
Asynclitic presentation	• Asymmetrical descent of head into the pelvic axis causing the anterior or posterior parietal bone to descend first (anterior or posterior asynclitism) • Findings in vaginal exam: ear palpable	CS in the absence of spontaneous correction
Deep transverse presentation	• Transverse head position: transverse occiput • Findings in vaginal exam: platypelloid pelvis	Promote rotation digitally (with two fingers) or manually (with the whole hand), consider proceeding to assisted delivery

Table 75 // Abnormal cephalic presentations

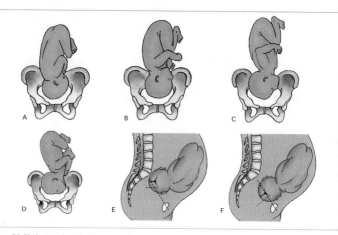

Figure 98 // Abnormal cephalic presentations
A: Occiput presentation **B:** Vertex presentation **C:** Sinciput presentation **D:** Face presentation **E:** Asynclitic presentation **F:** Deep transverse presentation

Intra-amniotic infection

(D) An intra-amniotic infection, also called chorioamnionitis, is an infection of the chorion or amniotic membrane that may also spread to the amniotic fluid, fetus, umbilical cord and/or placenta.

(E) Prevalence 1-4% of full-term deliveries, 20-25% after PPROM

(Ae) Migration of cervicovaginal flora into the cervical canal (including GBS, see Figure 99), haematogenous (especially *Listeria monocytogenes*)

(R) PROM, presence of genital pathogens, cervical insufficiency, meconium stained amniotic fluid

(Hx) Fever, abdominal/uterine pain

(PE) Pulse ↑↑, RR ↑, T ↓/↑

(Dx) • Labs: leukocytes ↑, bacteraemia, especially due to GBS or *Escherichia coli*
  • Amniotic fluid culture and gram stain exam: detect pathogen
  • CTG: fetal tachycardia

(Tx) 💊 ABx

  ✎ Augment labour or induce labour/CS

(!) • Maternal complications: dysfunctional contractions, postoperative infections, sepsis
  • Fetal/neonatal complications: asphyxia, pneumonia, brain damage, meningitis, perinatal mortality, sepsis

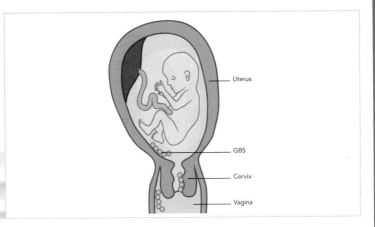

Figure 99 // Intra-amniotic infection

Placenta accreta spectrum (PAS)

(D) PAS is a pathological placental attachment to the myometrium (accreta), invasion of the myometrium (increta), or penetration through the myometrium and possibly other organs, e.g. the bladder (percreta), see Figure 100.

(E) Prevalence 4:100,000 deliveries

(Ae) Hypothesis: poor decidualisation in a scarred area

(R) Fertility procedures, adenomyosis, PMHx: uterine surgery (risk ↑ proportionate to past CS). See Table 72.

(Hx) Retained placenta, postpartum haemorrhage

(PE) Vitals (on bleeding): pulse ↑, BP ↓

(Dx) • TAU/TVU and Doppler: placental lacunae, disrupted bladder lining, hypervascularity at the placenta/bladder interface, myometrial thinning
 • MRI: heterogeneous placental signal intensity, abnormal placental vascularisation, focal myometrial interruption

(Tx) ✎ CS, possibly with prophylactic embolisation of the uterine artery and manual placental removal/resection, hysterectomy

(P) Maternal and fetal mortality and morbidity

(!) Manual placenta removal of retained placenta in case of placenta accreta/increta/percreta poses risk of life-threatening haemorrhage

> 🔔 Suspect placenta accreta spectrum in women who present with placenta praevia and previous CS.

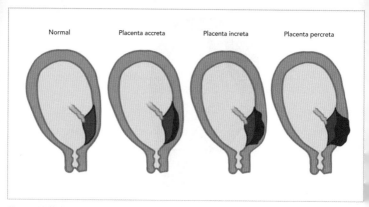

Figure 100 // Placenta accreta spectrum

Retained placenta

Ⓓ Retained placenta is diagnosed when the placenta has not been delivered in full with the Küstner and Baer's manoeuvres 60 minutes after the delivery (see Figures 44 and 101).

Ⓔ Prevalence 3% of deliveries

Ⓐₑ Placenta accreta, morbidly adherent placenta

Ⓡ PMHx: retained placenta, previous uterine surgery (e.g. curettage), premature birth, uterine abnormalities

Ⓗₓ Absence of placental delivery, vaginal bleeding

Ⓟₑ Fundal height ↑, vaginal exam/speculum exam: placenta possibly in cervix/vagina

Ⓓₓ TAU: distinction between non-detaching placenta/PAS

Ⓣₓ 🗨 Empty bladder (catheterisation), latch baby onto breast

🖋 Oxytocin injection, consider prophylactic AB, RhD prophylaxis

🖊 Manual extraction under general anaesthesia/locoregional anaesthesia

Ⓟ Recurrence risk: 25%

ⓘ Complications: postpartum endometritis, postpartum haemorrhage, uterine inversion

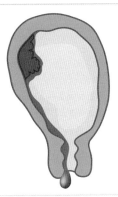

Figure 101 // Retained placenta

Failure to progress (FTP)

Ⓓ FTP is defined as active stage dilation (>3 cm dilation) that advanced by <1 cm every two hours.

Ⓔ Prevalence 10-14% of nulliparous and 3-3.5% of multiparous patients

Ⓐₑ Dysfunctional dystocia (inadequate uterine contractility) or mechanical problem (presenting part too big for birthing canal)

Ⓡ Nulliparity

Ⓟₑ Vaginal exam: evaluate progression of dilation

Ⓓₓ Partogram: monitor dilation and contractions

Ⓣₓ 💬 Fetal monitoring with CTG to evaluate fetal distress

   💊 IV oxytocin

   🔪 • Amniotomy

     • In case of cephalopelvic disproportion: CS

❗ Complications: fetal distress, postpartum infections

 Epidural anaesthesia may prolong expulsion time.

 Failure to progress in the expulsion stage is defined as an expulsion time >2 hours in nulliparas (with epidural anaesthesia: 3 hours) and ≥1 hour in multiparas (with epidural anaesthesia: 2 hours) (e.g. due to maternal exhaustion, cervical narrowing and hypotonic labour).

Fetal distress

(D) Fetal distress is caused by fetal hypoxia.

(E) Unknown

(Ae) Tachysystolia, polysystoly, oligohydramnios, maternal/fetal haemorrhage, nuchal cord, umbilical cord compression

(R) FGR, placental dysfunction, delayed expulsion, multiple pregnancy, maternal hypotension (following epidural anaesthesia)

(Hx) No added value

(PE) No added value

(Dx) CTG: reduced variability, late decelerations, complicated variable decelerations, bradycardia/tachycardia (see Diagnostics)

(Tx) 💬 Supportive therapy, e.g. IV fluids, patient in left-lateral tilt or MUD

   💊 In case of hypercontractility: stop uterine stimulants and start tocolytics (IV betamimetics or oxytocin antagonists)

   🔪 Assisted vaginal delivery, or CS as needed

(P) Depending on duration of asphyxia: ranging from no consequences to permanent brain damage

(!) Complications: meconium aspiration, metabolic acidosis, brain damage

> 💡 **Late decelerations** on a CTG occur after a contraction and are typical of fetal distress. **Complicated variable decelerations** last >60 sec.

Umbilical cord prolapse

(D) An umbilical cord prolapse occurs when the umbilical cord drops into the cervix or vagina before the presenting part of the fetus (see Figure 102).

(E) Live birth prevalence 0.2%

(Ae) Inadequate closure of the birth canal by the presenting part of the fetus

(R) Non-descended presenting part, prematurity, dysmaturity, 2nd twin, low-lying placenta, uterine abnormalities, multiparity, polyhydramnios

(PE) • Speculum exam: umbilical cord possibly visible
   • Vaginal exam: pulsations of umbilical cord possibly palpable

(Dx) • TAU and Doppler: umbilical cord location
   • CTG: bradycardia, decelerations

(Tx) 💬 Relieve pressure on umbilical cord by: manually elevating the presenting part (pushing the fetus up), placing patient in the Trendelenburg position, retrograde bladder filling through catheter (500 ml of water)

In case of fetal distress: consider tocolytics (relieve umbilical cord pressure)

Immediate delivery of the child is essential:
- Vaginal delivery, possibly assisted delivery if mother is fully dilated
- Emergency CS (after minimising pressure on the umbilical cord) if mother is not fully dilated

! Umbilical cord prolapse without full dilation rules out vaginal delivery and necessitates emergency CS

In umbilical cord prolapse, CTG changes typically start acutely after the rupture of membranes or an obstetric intervention that alters the position of the fetus.

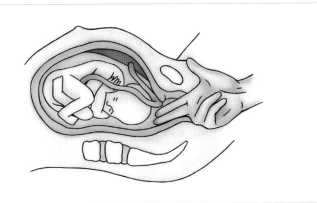

igure 102 // Umbilical cord prolapse

CONDITIONS

Uterine rupture

D A primary uterine rupture is not accompanied by scarring (rare). A secondary uterine rupture is accompanied by surgical scarring (see Figure 103).

E Prevalence of primary uterine rupture 5-17:100,000 deliveries, secondary uterine rupture 1:200 deliveries. 1% of patients with 1 previous CS, 3.9% of patients with >1 CS.

Me Uterine rupture at the level of a weak uterine segment, e.g. scar tissue

R Overstimulation of uterine contractility, macrosomia, induced labour with prostaglandins, excessive oxytocin use, advanced maternal age, PMHx: uterine rupture or uterine surgery (CS)

(Hx) Acute, abdominal pain, vaginal bleeding, macroscopic haematuria, disappearing contractions

(PE) • Pulse =/↑, BP =/↓
  • Abdominal inspection: Bandl's ring may be visible
  • Abdominal palpation: intense lower uterine tenderness, including between contractions
  • Vaginal exam: disappearance of presenting fetal part

(Dx) • TAU: haemoperitoneum, rupture of all uterine layers
  • CTG: first sign is abnormal, fetal distress

(Tx) 🔪 Emergency CS

(P) Fetal mortality: 5-25%

(!) Complications: fetal asphyxia and mortality, maternal hypovolaemic shock due to massive intra-abdominal haemorrhage, DIC

 Bandl's ring is a visible junction between the upper contralateral and lower atonic uterine segments, appearing as a ridge across the abdomen.

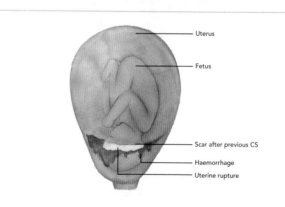

Uterus

Fetus

Scar after previous CS

Haemorrhage

Uterine rupture

Figure 103 // Secondary uterine rupture

Shoulder dystocia

(D) In shoulder dystocia, there is failure to deliver the anterior shoulder with on routine axial traction (see Figure 104).

(E) Prevalence 0.2-3% of all births

® DM/GDM, macrosomia, maternal adiposity, severe maternal weight gain during pregnancy, PMHx: shoulder dystocia

PE Turtle sign (fetal head is retracted into the vulva), downward lateral traction on the fetal head will not expedite delivery of the shoulders

Tx ✎ • Obstetric manoeuvres:
  1 External manoeuvres: McRoberts (see Figure 105) and suprapubic impression
  2 Internal manoeuvres: release posterior arm or rotate (Rubin or Woods manoeuvre)
  3 Emergency procedures: PAST manoeuvre (posterior axilla sling traction), symphysiotomy, Zavanelli manoeuvre (pushing the head back into the birth canal in preparation for CS) followed by emergency CS
  • Internal manoeuvres are often easier and more effective on all fours

P Fetal mortality: 0.35%

! • Fetal complications: brachial plexus injury, clavicle fracture, humerus fracture, hypoxic encephalopathy
  • Maternal complications: postpartum haemorrhage, tears

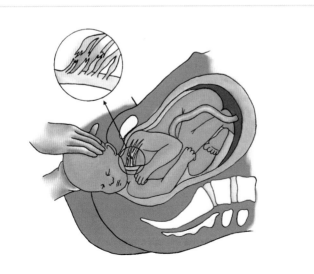

gure 104 // Shoulder dystocia with brachial plexus injury

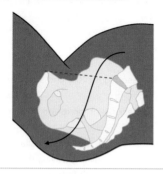
Before McRoberts manoeuvre

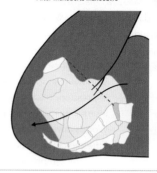
After McRoberts manoeuvre

Figure 105 // McRoberts manoeuvre

 Avoid applying fundal pressure and maternal pushing at all costs in case of shoulder dystocia: this will only worsen the impaction. Downward lateral traction on the neck can cause a brachial plexus injury.

Pubic symphysis rupture

D A pubic symphysis rupture is a traumatic tear of the symphyseal cartilage.

E Prevalence 0.005-0.8% of all deliveries

Ae Physiological weakening of pubic ligaments due to oestrogen and progesterone combined with mechanical stress during labour, traumatic assisted delivery, pelvic abnormality

R Shoulder dystocia, assisted delivery, multiparity, maternal hip dysplasia

Hx Acute pain, popping sound, pelvic instability, abnormal gait

PE Painful pubic symphysis on palpation

Dx Pelvic X-ray: >1 cm between the left and right pubic bone

Tx 🗨 Rest, consider pelvic support belt

🖊 Pubic symphysis fixation if rest is ineffective or if distance between the left and right pubic bone >4 cm

Uterine inversion

D In a uterine inversion, the uterine cavity protrudes from the cervix (see Figure 106).

E 90% complete, 10% incomplete

Ae Idiopathic

Umbilical cord traction in placental retention, uterine relaxants, macrosomia, multiparity, fast/slow delivery, short umbilical cord, placenta accreta, uterine abnormalities

ⓗ Vaginal bleeding, lower abdominal pain, urinary retention

ⓟ • Pulse ↓, BP ↓
   • Abdominal palpation: non-palpable uterine fundus
   • Vaginal exam: uterus palpable in vaginal canal

ⓓ TAU: abnormal uterine contour with inversion

ⓣ 🔖 • Discontinue uterotonic medication before intervention, restart after uterine repositioning
       • IV fluids to raise blood pressure
     🔪 • Primary interventions: repositioning with Johnson manoeuvre. If unsuccessful: new attempt after administering uterine relaxants (nitroglycerin, terbutaline, magnesium sulfate) under general anaesthesia.
       • Secondary interventions: hydrostatic repositioning (Foley-catheter or Bakri-balloon), laparotomy (Haultain procedure)

ⓟ Maternal mortality: 1.3%

⚠ Uterine inversion can cause severe haemorrhage, resulting in hypovolaemic shock

> 🔔 In case of uterine inversion, the placenta should be removed only after uterine repositioning. Removing the placenta earlier may exacerbate blood loss.

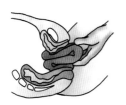 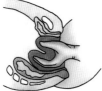 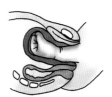

igure 106 // Uterine inversion and Johnson manoeuvre

Amniotic fluid embolism

(D) Amniotic fluid embolism can occur during labour, childbirth or immediately postpartum and is most likely caused by an anaphylactic reaction to amniotic fluid or fetal cells entering the maternal bloodstream (see Figure 107). The initial phase characterised by cardiorespiratory difficulty is followed by a second phase of DIC resulting in obstetric haemorrhage.

(E) Prevalence 1-10:100,000 deliveries

(Ae) Maternal age >35, multiparity >5, placental abnormalities, polyhydramnios, complicated labour (eclampsia, placental abruption, forceps delivery, CS), blunt abdominal trauma, invasive procedures (abortion, amniocentesis)

(Hx) · Aura (33%), convulsions (33%), ischaemic stroke, agitation, vomiting, nausea, chills
· Cardiorespiratory failure: dyspnoea, risk of cardiac arrest

(PE) · Pulse ↓/↑, BP ↓, saturation ↓, RR ↑
· Cyanosis, pulmonary auscultation: crackles, wheezing
· Neurological exam to evaluate cerebral embolisms

(Dx) · Labs: Hb ↓, D-dimers (DIC) ↑, fibrinogen (DIC) ↓, leukocytes ↑, platelets (DIC) ↓
· Arterial blood gas: hypoxaemia without hypercapnia, if persistent cardiac failure → metabolic acidosis
· Chest X-ray: pulmonary oedema or haemorrhage
· CTG: decelerations, variability ↓, bradycardia
· ECG: normal, ventricular fibrillation, pulseless electrical activity (PEA), asystole

(Tx) 🖊 Supporting therapy: O_2, NaCl, clotting factors for clotting disorder
🖊 Intrapartum embolism → assisted delivery/CS as soon as possible

(P) Maternal mortality 25-66%

(!) DIC is characterised by bleeding time ↑ and obstetric haemorrhage ↑

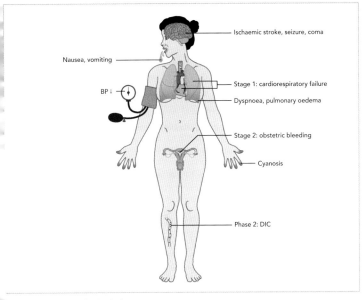

Figure 107 // Amniotic fluid embolism

Postpartum haemorrhage

D Postpartum haemorrhage is defined as blood loss ≥1000 ml within 24 hours of delivery (see Figure 108).

E Prevalence 1-5% of deliveries

Ae The 4 Ts (in order of frequency): tone ↓, tissue (retained placental remnant), trauma, thrombus (coagulopathy)

Hx Vaginal blood loss (≥1000 ml <24h)

R Retained placental remnants, macrosomia, slow progress in labour, induced labour, instrumental delivery, multiple pregnancy, full bladder

PE · Pulse ↓, BP =/↓
 · Bimanual exam: evaluate uterine tone

Dx · Labs: Hb ↓, platelets =/↓, evaluate clotting parameters, cross-match testing
 · TAU/TVU: evaluate retained placental remnant

Tx Keep the patient warm (blankets, warmed infusion of fluids)
 · Uterotonics IV (oxytocin, prostaglandins, methylergometrine, or carbo-prost)
 · Tranexamic acid IV

- Correct coagulation disorders (e.g. platelet transfusion, whole blood, fresh frozen plasma, specific factor concentrate)

- Catheter for urine drainage
- Local pressure: continuous bimanual uterine compression and massage, uterine balloon catheter (Bakri® balloon)
- Surgical correction of soft-tissue injury
- If blood loss persists: manual exam under anaesthesia (with removal of placental remnant if applicable), embolisation, B-Lynch procedure, hysterectomy

Ⓟ Recurrence risk: 15-20%

ⓘ Watch out for hypovolaemic shock (see Table 3) and Sheehan syndrome (secondary to hypovolaemic shock)

Postpartum bleeding: 4 Ts: **T**rauma, **T**one ↓, **T**issue (placental remnants), **T**hrombus (clotting disorder).

Sheehan syndrome: damage to the anterior pituitary gland due to excessive drop in blood pressure caused by heavy blood loss during or after childbirth → reduced perfusion of the pituitary gland following pituitary growth in preparation for hormone production, e.g. for breastfeeding. Released hormone production may initiate decreased milk production (prolactin ↓), absence of menstruation (FSH/LH ↓), hypothyroidism (TSH ↓) and adrenal function disorders (ACTH ↓).

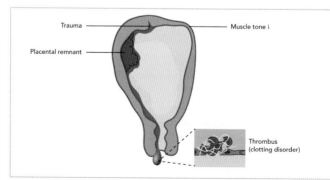

Trauma — Muscle tone ↓

Placental remnant

Thrombus (clotting disorder)

Figure 108 // Postpartum haemorrhage: causes

Puerperal pathology

 The puerperium is a period of six weeks after childbirth marked by a large number of physiological changes.

Fever

Some women come down with a fever during the puerperium. Fever may occur on the first day, especially after vaginal delivery. The timing of the fever may be indicative of the aetiology (see Table 76).

TIME AFTER DELIVERY	CONSIDER
<24u	Idiopathic (80%), maternal fever (group A streptococcus (GAS)), post-CS wound infection
Day 1	UTI
Day 2-3	Wound infection (episiotomy, CS scar)
Day 3-4	Endometritis
Day 4-5	Salpingitis, PID
Day 6-7	Parametritis
Week 2	Thrombo-embolic processes
Week 2 and later	Puerperal mastitis

Table 76 // Overview of the most common infections after childbirth and time of presentation

 STIs rarely cause postpartum endometritis, but are a common cause of endometritis outside pregnancy.

 The most common foci of postpartum infections are the chest, breasts, bladder, pelvis, abdomen, legs and womb.

SYSTEMIC INFLAMMATORY RESPONSE SYNDROME (SIRS) (≥2 of the following 4 criteria)	
Temperature	<36°C or >38°C, <96.8°F or >100.4°F
Heart rate	>90/min
Respiratory rate	>20/min, or PaCO$_2$ <32 mm Hg
White blood cell count	>12,000/mm, <4,000/mm, and/or >10% band cells
SEPSIS (≥2 SIRS criteria with suspected or confirmed underlying infection)	
SEVERE SEPSIS (sepsis with dysfunction of at least one organ or system)	

Table 77 // Severity of sepsis based on SIRS criteria

Sepsis protocol (start when ≥2 SIRS criteria)
- Measure blood lactate level, remeasure if initial lactate >2 mmol/L;
- Obtain blood cultures prior to administering antibiotics;
- Administer broad-spectrum antibiotic;
- Rapid administration of 30 ml/kg crystalloid for hypotension or lactate >2 mmol/L;
- Administer vasopressors if patient is hypotensive during or after fluid resuscitation to maintain MAP >65 mmHg.

Puerperal sepsis

(D) Puerperal sepsis is a decidual infection that can consist of endometritis alon
or of myometritis or parametritis (see Figure 109).

(E) • Prevalence endomyometritis 1-8% of deliveries, puerperal sepsis 1(
60:100,000
- Typically occurs around 3-4d postpartum (watch out for Group A strep
tococcus (GAS) → typical, highly dramatic onset at 1-2d postpartum)

(Ae) Polymicrobial infection (e.g. streptococcus (especially GAS), staphylococcu.
Escherichia coli)

(R) Intra-amniotic infection, placental remnant, manual placental removal, pro
longed expulsion, frequent vaginal exam, meconium-stained amniotic fluic
DM

(Hx) Lower abdominal pain, malodorous lochia, chills, headache, general malaise
anorexia, fever

• T ↓/↑, pulse ↑, RR ↑

  • Abdominal palpation: uterine discomfort

  • Vaginal exam: cervical motion tenderness, open cervix

  • Bimanual exam: uterine subinvolution, uterine tenderness

Dx • Labs: leukocytes ↑ with left shift, CRP ↑, lactate ↑, blood cultures

  • Urine output ↓

Tx 🔊 Measurement urine-output

  🖉 AB, thrombosis prophylaxis with LMWH

P Good with timely treatment, mortality as high as 11% in Asia and Africa

❗ • Possible local, haematogenous and lymphogenous spread of infection to
    lesser pelvis with possible abscess formation

  • Treatment based on systemic inflammatory respons syndrome (SIRS), and
    sepsis protocol (see Table 77)

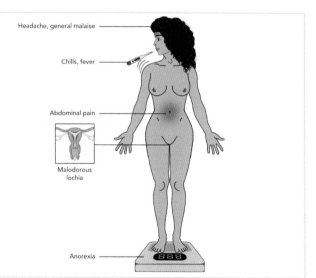

Headache, general malaise

Chills, fever

Abdominal pain

Malodorous
lochia

Anorexia

gure 109 // Puerperal sepsis

Moderate vaginal blood loss >24h postpartum

  • Uterine blood loss: can be caused by retained placental remnant, open ex-
    ternal os and subinvolution of the uterus.

  • Vaginal or perineal blood loss: may be caused by a poorly sutured tear, clotting disorder, or cervical or vaginal abnormalities.

 · Prophylactic ABx and surgical curettage in cases of placental remnants
 · Vaginal/perineal: re-suture, leave drain, adequate clotting management and embolisation as needed

> Normal vaginal bleeding may persist for up to 6 weeks after childbirth.

Urinary tract infection (UTI)
(D) Puerperal UTI is usually caused by delayed urine discharge during pregnancy.

(Ae) 75% of UTIs are caused by *Escherichia coli*

(Dx) Urine culture (mid-stream urine sample is best, as urine may otherwise be contaminated with postpartum vaginal fluid loss)

(Tx) ABx

Urinary retention
(D) Caused by increased residual urine as a result of increased capacity and mild hypotonia secondary to temporal neural function impairment.

(E) Prevalence 3-5%

(R) Epidural anaesthesia, assisted delivery, nulliparity, episiotomy, CS

(Dx) · Labs: urinalysis and culture (UTI, haematuria, glycosuria, crystals, electrolytes), renal function (BUN, creatinine, electrolytes), glucose
 · Abdominal US: hydronephrosis, distension of ureter, kidney stones, bladder distension

(Tx) Pelvic floor physiotherapy
 If residue >500 ml: bladder catheter

Urinary incontinence
(D) Postpartum stress incontinence is especially common after vaginal deliveries and may be accompanied by urge incontinence.

(E) Prevalence 33% in the first 3 mo postpartum

(R) Multiparity, assisted delivery, sphincter tears

(Tx) Watchful waiting
 Pelvic floor physiotherapy if persistent

Clotting

Clotting factors peak around childbirth, causing hypercoagulability in the early puerperium (thrombotic tendency is five times higher than normal). Two other contributing factors are venous stasis in the lower extremities due to mechanical obstruction (uterus compressing inferior vena cava) and vascular damage due to e.g. pre-eclampsia or surgical procedures. These three factors are known collectively as Virchow's triad and increase the risk of thromboembolic events.

 Virchow's triad: hypercoagulability, stasis and endothelial dysfunction due to vascular damage.

Digestive system

Women often experience constipation in the first days of the puerperium. This may be caused by temporary intestinal hypotonia or a lack of exercise. The pelvic floor muscles and nerves are compressed during childbirth. When this pressure disappears after childbirth, the body may fail to properly recognise the signs that the intestines are full, resulting in constipation. Constipation can also be caused by perineal tenderness, causing women to hold their bowel movements. Constipation can also be caused by iron supplements prescribed in anticipation of blood loss during labour. In addition to constipation, women may also develop haemorrhoids postpartum resulting from venous congestion during labour.

Psychological problems

Pregnancy and delivery are profound events and have great psychological impact. After childbirth, women undergo major hormonal changes that can be accompanied by an unstable emotional state.

Crying spells ('baby blues')

- Up to 80% of childbirths
- Acute, possibly severe complications during delivery
- Irritation, forgetfulness, headaches, crying spells, insomnia, lethargy
- Usually disappears after 10-14d

Posttraumatic stress disorder (PTSD)
- R Acute (serious) complications during delivery
- Hx Flashbacks, nightmares, active avoidance of pregnancy-related issues, irritability, concentration ↓, skittishness

Postpartum depression
- E Incidence 13% of childbirths
- Hx Classical symptoms of depression (<4 wk of delivery), dissatisfaction with child care, dissatisfaction with motherhood
- Tx Social support, psychological therapy, and pharmacological therapy (SSRI as first-line treatment)

Postpartum psychosis
- E Prevalence 200:100,000
- R FHx +, PMHx: psychosis, bipolar disorder, primigravity
- Hx Anxiety, restlessness, mania, paranoia, delusion (<2-4 wk of delivery)
- Tx 🖊 Antipsychotics, lithium, electroconvulsive therapy (ECT)
- P 50% recurrence rate, lower recurrence rate if time between pregnancies >2

Benign tumours

Fibroids
- D Fibroids, also called uterine myomas, are benign myometrial tumours composed of smooth muscle and connective tissue (see Figure 110).
- E Prevalence: ±25% age >30, rare age <20
- Ae Oestrogen-dependent growth → regression after menopause
- R FHx +, oestrogen exposure ↑ (early menarche, prolonged postmenopause oestrogen replacement), person with dark skin with an uterus, nullipari, obesity
- Hx Asymptomatic (66%), menorrhagia, lower abdominal pain, compression surrounding organs in advanced stages (haemorrhoids, hydronephrosis, po lakisuria, tenesmus)
- PE Bimanual exam: possibly palpable uterine enlargement
- Dx • TAU/TVU/hysterosonography: myometrial tumours
  • Hysteroscopy: to rule out fibroid in uterine cavity

- Pelvic MRI: determine location and size for preoperative planning

 Asymptomatic: watchful waiting, ultrasound monitoring for large fibroids

Symptomatic: NSAIDs, tranexamic acid, cycle suppression (OC, progestogens, levonorgestrel, hormone-containing IUD, GnRH analogue), progesterone receptor modulators (ulipristal acetate, prescribed in exceptional cases)

Symptomatic: myomectomy (hysteroscopic/laparoscopic), embolisation, or hysterectomy

0.1% risk of myosarcoma

Rapid growth after menopause → consider myosarcoma (cramping lower abdominal pain; watch out for nascent fibroid (expulsion fibroid); 'mottled' appearance during surgery → pay attention to the presence of adenomyosis)

 OC use and smoking reduce fibroid risk.

Uterine fibroid symptoms may worsen in combination with a copper IUD.

ESHGE CLASSIFICATION		
S M - Submucosal	0	Pedunculated intracavitary
	1	<50% intramural
	2	≥50% intramural
) - Other	3	Endometrial contacts; 100% intramural
	4	Intramural
	5	Subserosal ≥50% intramural
	6	Subserosal <50% intramural
	7	Subserosal pedunculated
	8	Other (e.g. cervical, parasitic)

le 78 // ESHGE classification of uterus myomatosus

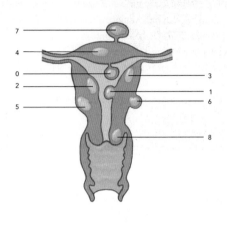

Figure 110 // Different types of fibroids according to the ESHGE classification
0: Pedunculated submucosal fibroid **1:** <50% intramural fibroid **2:** ≥50% intramural fibroid **3:** Submuco
fibroid **4:** Intramural fibroid **5:** Subserosal fibroid **6:** Subserosal fibroid **7:** Pedunculated subserosal fibro
8: Cervical fibroid

Dermoid cyst

(D) A dermoid cyst, also called a mature teratoma, is an ovarian cyst compose
of mature tissue from one or several mature germ layers (see Figure 111).

(E) 10-20% of all ovarian neoplasms, peak age 10-30

(Ae) Excessive growth of one or more ovarian germ layers

(Hx) Asymptomatic ⊙, abdominal bloating, abdominal pain, abnormal vagir
bleeding

(PE) Possibly palpable abdominal mass

(Dx) • TAU/TVU: cyst site, size, appearance
• Labs: tumour markers β-hCG =/↑, AFP =/↑, LDH ↑, CA125 =/↑
• MRI: for site, size and appearance as needed, if TAU/TVU is not sufficier

(Tx) 🗨 Watchful waiting preferred if <5 cm

✎ Laparoscopic/laparotomic ovariectomy or cystectomy (1st choice wh
>10 cm or symptomatic)

(P) 0.2-2% malignancy

(!) In case of acute onset of pain, consider ovarian torsion; may contain hair ar
or teeth; 10-15% develop a dermoidcyst on the contralateral side

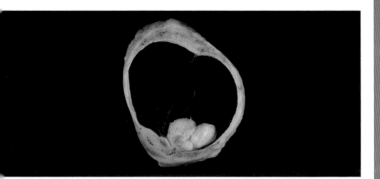

Figure 111 // Dermoid cyst

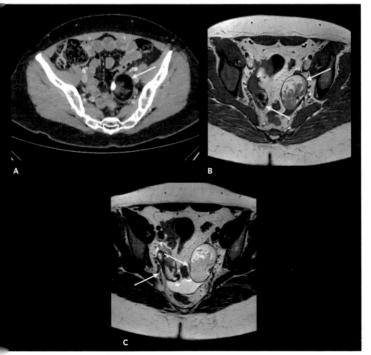

Figure 112 // Additional imaging of a dermoid cyst.

CT-scan of a left ovarial mass containing fat, soft-tissue, and calcification. **B** and **C:** The subsequent T1 and T2 weighted MRI sequence confirm the findings of an inclusion cyst with fatty and soft-tissue components, and a normal right ovary.

Borderline ovarian tumour

(D) A borderline ovarian tumour has low malignant potential. Borderline ovarian tumours do not always undergo malignant degeneration and are not necessarily a precursor of ovarian carcinoma.

(E) Prevalence 150-200, incidence 1.8-5.5:100,000/year, 15% of epithelial ovarian tumours are borderline tumours, serous borderline ovarium tumours: 60%, mucinous borderline ovarium tumours: 30%

(Hx) Asymptomatic ☺

(PE) Bimanual exam: enlarged ovary or ovaries

(Dx) • TAU/TVU/MRI: detect ovarian tumour
   • Labs: tumour markers (CA125 =/↑ in serous carcinomas, CEA =/↑ in mucinous carcinomas)
   • Biopsy: histology to distinguish benign/malignant tumours, watch out for risk of tissue spill, is still done but very rarely

(Tx) 🔪 In fertile life stage: unilateral salpingo-oophorectomy, postmenopausal bilateral salpingo-oophorectomy (BSO), hysterectomy, omentectomy, peritoneal biopsies, and appendix (risk of intestinal type in mucinous tumours) via laparoscopy or laparotomy

(P) 5-year survival >95%

(!) Serous type occurs in 25-40% bilaterally, mucinous type occurs in 5-10% bilaterally

  33% of women with a borderline ovarian tumour are aged <40. Preservation of fertility is therefore an important consideration when choosing treatment.

Cervical polyp

(D) A cervical polyp is generally a benign tumour that grows from the cervix (see Figure 113).

(E) During the reproductive phase, mainly at age >40

(R) Chronic inflammation of the cervix

(Ae) Exact aetiology unknown

(Hx) Asymptomatic ☺, contact bleeding, menorrhagia, abnormal discharge, intermenstrual blood loss

(PE) • Speculum exam: visible polyp, haemorrhage
   • Vaginal exam: cervical abnormalities, blood on glove

Ⓓ No added value

Ⓣ🖊️ • For benign, small polyps: outpatient resection with polyp forceps
   • For larger polyps: surgical resection

Ⓟ Unknown

❗ Pay attention to risk of malignancy: send polyps for pathology

Endometrial polyp

Ⓓ An endometrial polyp is a benign tumour arising from the endometrium (see Figure 113).

Ⓔ Just before menopause, sometimes during menopause

Ⓐₑ Endometrial hyperplasia

Ⓡ Oestrogen ↑, tamoxifen use, adiposity

Ⓗₓ Asymptomatic ⊙, menorrhagia, bloody discharge, dysmenorrhoea

ⓅE Speculum exam: may reveal polyp

Ⓓₓ • TVU, hysterosonography and possible hysteroscopy: polyp and endometrial thickening
   • Pipelle biopsy: to rule out malignancy

Ⓣ🖊️ Hysteroscopic polyp resection

Ⓟ Malignant transformation: 1.7% premenopausal, 5% postmenopausal

❗ Pay attention to risk of endometrial carcinoma or malignant degeneration

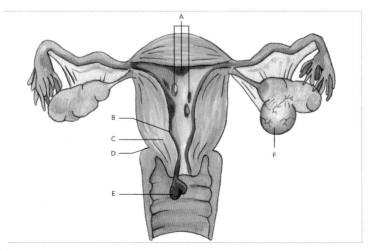

Figure 113 // Benign tumours
A: Endometrial polyps **B:** Endometrium **C:** Myometrium **D:** Perimetrium **E:** Cervical polyp **F:** Ovarian cyst

Endometrial cyst

(D) An endometrial cyst, also called a chocolate cyst or endometrioma, consists of endometrial tissue and is often filled with old blood (see Figure 114).

(E) Prevalence 1.2-1.5%

(Ae) Presence of endometrial tissue outside the uterus due to endometriosis

(R) Endometriotic foci, endogenous oestrogen exposure ↑ (early menarche/ late menopause)

(Hx) Dysmenorrhoea, acute abdominal pain associated with rupture/leakage, abnormal vaginal bleeding, low back pain

(PE) Vaginal exam: cervical/adnexal motion tenderness

(Dx) • TAU/TVU: blood-filled cyst
   • Pelvic MRI: presence of deep infiltrating endometriosis

(Tx) ✎ Laparoscopic cystectomy: fast growth, changing sonographic characteristics, insufficient pain relief with medication, infertility, or cyst >10 cm

(P) Recurrence in 25%

(!) Pay attention to risk of developing of ovarian carcinoma in women with endometriosis, endometrial cysts are benign

> 💡 Bilateral endometriomas and trying to conceive: be careful with surgical intervention because of risk of iatrogenic damage and permanent effects on ovarian reserve.

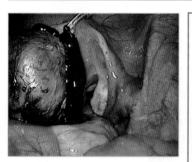

Figure 114 // Perforated chocolate cyst

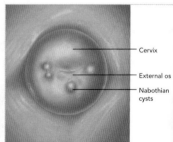

Cervix

External os

Nabothian cysts

Figure 115 // Nabothian cysts

Nabothian cysts

(D) Nabothian cysts are benign cervical cysts filled with mucus (see Figure 115). They can measure several millimetres to several centimetres across.

(E) Unknown

- (Ae) Blocked cervical gland
- (R) Cervicitis, after childbirth
- (Hx) Asymptomatic ☉, full feeling in vagina
- (PE) Speculum exam: multiple fluid-filled cysts visible on cervix
- (Dx) For borderline benign/malignant cases: biopsy
- (Tx) 💬 Asymptomatic: watchful waiting
- (P) Not a precursor to cervical carcinoma

Malignant tumours

BRCA mutations

(D) *BRCA* mutations cause hereditary breast and ovarian cancer (HBOC) syndrome associated with a high risk of developing breast and ovarian carcinoma. The *BRCA1* and *BRCA2* genes help in repair of DNA defects (especially double-strand breaks) through homologous recombination.

(E) 5-10% of breast carcinomas and 25% of ovarian carcinomas occur in patients with a *BRCA* mutation

(Ae) Mutation in *BRCA1* gene (chromosome 17) or *BRCA2* gene (chromosome 13)

(R) Positive family history, genetically autosomal-dominant, Jewish-Ashkenazi ancestry (5-10x increased risk)

(Hx) FHx +

(PE) • Breast carcinoma (see Breast carcinoma)
- • Ovarian carcinoma: often asymptomatic for a long time ☉, abdominal pain, 'full' feeling, constipation

(Dx) • DNA diagnostics
- • Periodic exam
  - Age 25-29: annual breast MRI and clinical appointment every 6-12 mo
  - Age 30-75: annual breast MRI, and mammography, and clinical appointment
  - Age >75: individualised screening, consider mammography every 2y

(Tx) 📏 Risk-reducing surgeries: bilateral mastectomy (breast carcinoma), bilateral salpingo-oophorectomy (ovarian carcinoma): age 35-45

(P) See Table 79

💡 Timing of *BRCA1/2* mutations screening differ between countries.

Positive family history:
- ≥1 1st/2nd degree relatives with:
  - Breast carcinoma diagnosed age <50
  - Triple negative breast cancer age <60
  - Primary carcinoma both breasts
  - Ovarian and breast carcinoma in same person
  - Male with breast carcinoma
  - Ovarian cancer
- ≥2 1st/2nd degree relatives same side of family with:
  - ≥1 breast carcinoma age <50
  - ≥1 breast carcinoma and 1 relative with high grade pancreatic or prostate carcinoma any age
- ≥3 1st/2nd degree relatives with:
  - ≥1 breast carcinoma and 2 relatives with breast carcinoma
  - Prostate carcinoma at any age.

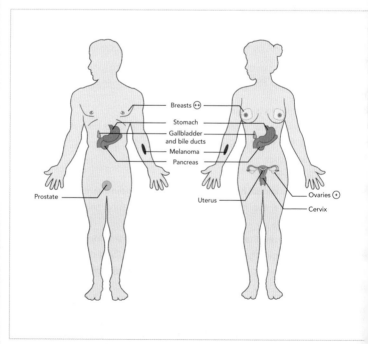

Figure 116 // Sites of *BRCA* mutation tumours

TUMOUR TYPE	*BRCA1* GENE DEFECT	*BRCA2* GENE DEFECT
Breast carcinoma	60-85% (♂ 1%)	60-85% (♂ 7%)
Ovarian carcinoma	30-60%	5-20%
Miscellaneous	Pancreatic, uterine, cervical carcinoma	Prostate, pancreatic, gallbladder, bile duct, gastric carcinoma, melanoma

Table 79 // Lifetime risk of carcinoma

- **BRCA: br**east **ca**ncer
- Pay attention to: also increases risk of ovarian carcinoma and other tumours (see Figure 116), depending on type of *BRCA* mutation (see Table 79).

Cervical carcinoma

D Cervical carcinoma is a common gynaecological malignancy that is most common in developing countries.

E Incidence 7:100,000/year, squamous cell carcinoma (74%), adenocarcinoma (18%) or other carcinomas (8%) arising from the cervix

Ae HPV infection

R HPV 16/18/31/33 infection, cervical intraepithelial neoplasia (CIN), age 30-45, immunosuppression, smoking, multiple sexual partners

Ix Abnormal vaginal bleeding, contact bleeding, discharge symptoms (purulent, malodorous), abdominal pain, back pain, micturition and defaecation disorders ⊖

°E · Lymph nodes: inguinal and supraclavicular
   · Speculum exam: tumour appearance and size
   · Vaginal exam: irregular cervix, decreased mobility, tumour consistency
   · Rectovaginal exam: invasion of surrounding structures, parametrial invasion

Ix · Smear test: >PAP3b/HSIL and HPV status
   · Colposcopy: localisation of abnormal CIN and possible biopsy
   · Labs: tumour markers (SCC ↑)
   · MRI: assessment of local tumour extension (size, parametrial, and vaginal involvement)
   · CT/PET-CT: rule out distant metastases, PET-CT also for planning of primary chemoradiation

- Cervical biopsy: staging, histology

(Tx) 💬 Prevention: population screening, HPV vaccination

🔍 Radiotherapy and/or chemotherapy

🔬 Conisation, simple hysterectomy, radical hysterectomy, radical trachelectomy (preserving fertility), sentinel node dissection, or pelvic lymphadenectomy

(P) 5-year survival stage Ia-IIb >80%, IIb-IIIb 56-68%, IVa-IVb 10-22%, avg. 65%,
in early stage 98%

(!) • Surgical complications (after conisation/trachelectomy): gestational problems → cervical insufficiency, difficult dilation
- Complications after radiotherapy: bladder dysfunction, bowel problems
pelvic fibrotic abnormalities, sexual dysfunction, infertility
- Mortality rate 2.2:100.000 patients/y

Consultation about fertility preservation is recommended in young
patients prior to treatment of cervical carcinoma.

Metastatic spread of cervical carcinoma:
- Infiltrative: vagina, rectum, bladder
- Lymphogenic: pelvic, para-aortic lymph nodes
- Haematogenic: rare

- Cervical dysplasia is traditionally classified based on cytology (PAP
smear or Bethesda system) and histology (biopsy), see section on
Diagnostics.
- CIN 1 does not require treatment. Treatment options for CIN 2 and
3 include medication (imiquimod), ablation or LLETZ.
- LLETZ removal of the entire transformation zone: recurrence risk
of CIN 2-3 ↓.

Before pregnancy, perform a laparoscopic abdominal cerclage if cervix <1 cm.

Cervical screening for cervical dysplasia: see Diagnostics // Smear
test

Sedlis criteria (at least 2 out of 3) to indicate the need for adjuvant radiotherapy:
- Positive lymphovascular space involvement (LVSI)
- Invasion depth >1/3 (of ≥15 mm)
- Tumour diameter ≥4 cm

Endometrial carcinoma

D Endometrial carcinoma is the most common gynaecological malignancy and can be classified into endometrioid, serous, clear cell and mucinous adenocarcinoma (see Figure 117).

E Incidence 20-28:100,000/year, 75% postmenopausal

Ae Long-term oestrogen stimulation and genetic predisposition

R Oestrogen stimulation (advanced age, adiposity, no/few pregnancies, late menopause, oestrogen supplementation), genetic (Lynch syndrome)

Hx Postmenopausal blood loss, premenopausal menometrorrhagia, abnormal discharge

PE Bimanual palpation: possible uterine enlargement and/or fixation, evaluate pelvic masses

Dx • TVU/MRI: suspicious endometrium >4 mm
   • Chest and abdominal CT with venous contrast: to rule out metastases
   • Cervical cytology: 50% positive
   • Pipelle biopsy/hysteroscopy: staging, histology

Tx ✂ Curative: hysterectomy/adnexectomy, lymphadenectomy (sentinel node or pelvic), tumour debulking surgery (all sites), omentectomy in selected cases

   💊 • Curative: adjuvant radiotherapy (external or brachytherapy), chemotherapy
      • Palliative: radiotherapy, chemotherapy or hormone therapy

P 5-year survival stage I: 87-96%, stage II: 72-86%, stage III: 42-53%, stage IV: 15-19%

! Atypical hyperplasia is a premalignant endometrial abnormality

Metastatic spread of endometrial carcinoma:
- Infiltrative: myometrial, cervical, intra-abdominal
- Lymphoid: pelvic, left clavicular
- Haematogenous: pulmonary, hepatic

Lynch syndrome: increased risk of malignancies of the ovaries, intestines, stomach, pancreas, gall bladder, ureter, kidneys, and brain.

 Referral for genetic analysis in case of:
- Endometrial carcinoma age <50
- Microsatellite instability (MSI), or abnormal mismatch repair (MMR) in immunohistochemistry
- Personal history of endometrial carcinoma AND ≥1 1st or 2nd degree relatives with endometrial or colorectal cancer (age <50)
- ≥3 1st or 2nd degree relatives with Lynch syndrome associated cancer

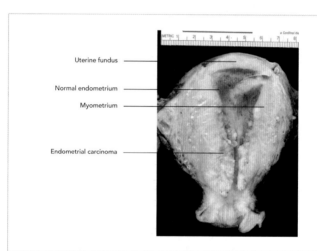

Uterine fundus

Normal endometrium

Myometrium

Endometrial carcinoma

Figure 117 // Endometrial carcinoma

Breast carcinoma

D Breast carcinoma, also called breast cancer, is a malignant abnormality of the breast. Breast carcinoma develops in breast tissue and is associated with early haematogenous metastasis and lymph node metastasis. Breast carcinomas are classified according to the site from which they originate: ductal (in a milk duct) or lobular (in a mammary gland). A distinction is also made between carcinoma in situ (confined to the glandular ducts, does not penetrate the basal lamina) and invasive breast cancer (invades the basement membrane and spreads to fatty and supporting tissue).

E · Incidence 2,100,000/year
  · ♀: most common malignancy in the Western world
  · Breast carcinoma is rarely diagnosed in patients aged <30, 80% are aged ≥50

Ae Genetic predisposition 5-15%: *BRCA/CHEK2/PALB2*-mutation, Li-Fraumeni syndrome, Cowden syndrome, Klinefelter syndrome

R Age 50-75, genetic predisposition, hormonal replacement/supplementation, menstruation age <12 and/or menopause age >55, low parity, dense glandular tissue, adiposity, PMHx: breast carcinoma, radiotherapy, atypical hyperplasia

Hx · See Figure 118
  · Lump or thickening in the breast attached to the skin, skin dimpling or pitting, nipple changes (nipple discharge, retraction, redness, scaling, spot resembling eczema (Paget's disease, see Figure 119))
  · Mastitis persisting after 1 wk of ABx
  · Suspected lymph node swelling in the axilla, supraclavicular or infraclavicular

PE · See Figure 118
  · Breast: abnormal shape, asymmetry, swelling
  · Skin: colour, retractions, orange peel, ulcerations, eczema, elevations, unilateral enhanced vein definition
  · Nipples: colour, shape, swelling, bleeding, skin pathology
  · Lymph nodes: axillary, parasternal, and supraclavicular

Dx · Mammography: irregular mass with indistinct or spiculated margins, architectural distortion, microcalcifications (see Figure 120)
  · Ultrasound: after inconclusive mammography or positive mammography (1st choice in patients aged <30 due to dense glandular tissue), target ultrasound of the axilla to rule out lymph node metastases
  · MRI: in mutation carriers aged >25, to evaluate response to neo-adjuvant chemotherapy, to diagnose and follow up lobular carcinomas
  · Histology: biopsy

Tx ✐ Breast-conserving surgery or modified radical mastectomy (with sentinel node procedure or axillary lymph node dissection). Breast reconstruction can either be performed during surgery or after the recovery period.

  ℘ · Chemotherapy: adjuvant or neo-adjuvant, before or after radiotherapy, various regimens available
  · Radiotherapy: irradiation of the breast and/or axilla, parasternal or me-

dial subclavicular irradiation according to various regimens

- Targeted therapy: in HER2neu positive breast cancer (10-15%), consisting of monoclonal antibodies that target proteins on the tumour cell wall, e.g. trastuzumab
- Antihormonal therapy: in oestrogen and/or progesterone receptor-positive breast cancer (65-80%), drugs inhibiting hormone action or production, e.g. tamoxifen (blocks hormone receptor), and aromatase inhibitors (block conversion of androgen to oestrogen). Menopausal status is a factor in therapy selection (aromatase inhibitors: only for postmenopausal women), as is the patient's history of e.g. thrombo-embolic events (contraindication to tamoxifen).

P · Lifetime risk ♀ 11-13%
- The 5-year survival rate ranges from 99% in stage I to 28% in stage IV (see Table 80)
- Depends on factors including lymph node metastases, tumour size, degree of differentiation, presence or absence of oestrogen, and/or progesterone receptors, overexpression of HER2neu, metastases, skin oedema (orange skin)
- Remote metastases: incurable
- The 5-year survival rate has increased to 90% in recent years, partly thanks to population screening

STAGE	EXPLANATION
I	Tumour <2 cm, no metastases
II	Tumour 2-5 cm, possible lymph node metastases
III	Tumour >5 cm, possible lymph node metastases
IV	Remote metastases

Table 80 // Breast carcinoma staging

A triple-negative breast carcinoma (TNBC) is characterised by negative HER2neu, progesterone and oestrogen receptor tests. TNBC often has a worse prognosis because it offers fewer options for targeted therapy and hormone therapy. TNBC occurs in 15-20% of all patients and is more common in younger women (with a *BRCA* mutation).

Screening: it is recommended women aged 50-70 have a mammography biannually for breast cancer screening. In the USA, breast cancer screening continues until the age of 74. Screening between ages 40-49 can be considered, where patient preferences and potential harms and benefits should be discussed. The mortality rate has decreased by 20% over recent years (see Table 81).

 Mammography test results are scored with BI-RADS. Radiologists use this score to estimate the chance of malignancy and decide on follow-up treatment (see Table 82).

INDICATION FOR ANNUAL MRI AND/OR MAMMOGRAPHY

- Increased risk based on FHx
- (50% chance of) carrying a *BRCA1* or *BRCA2* mutation or mutation in other risk genes *(PTEN, TP53, STK11, CDH1, CHEK2, ATM, NF1, PALB2)*
- PMHx: invasive breast carcinoma
- PMHx: ductal carcinoma in situ (DCIS)
- Thoracic/axillary radiotherapy age <40

Table 81 // Indication for additional screening

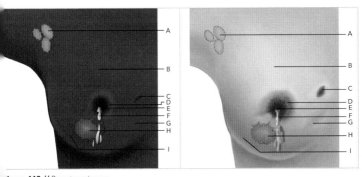

Figure 118 // Breast carcinoma

A: Swollen axillary lymph nodes **B:** Chest pain **C:** Non-healing wound **D:** Redness, scaling (Paget's disease) **E:** Nipple retraction **F:** Nipple discharge **G:** Skin dimpling **H:** Firm lump that does not change in size with patient's menstrual cycle **I:** Mastitis

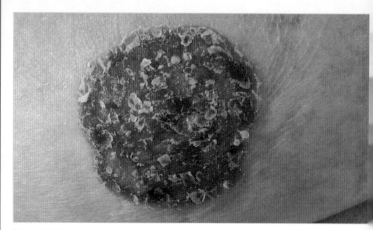

Figure 119 // Paget nipple

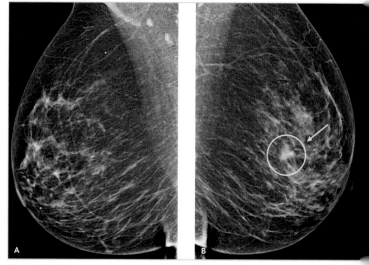

Figure 120 // A screening mammogram (craniocaudal view, **A:** right breast, **B:** left breast) in a post-menopausal woman reveals a new mass in the left breast, suspected for breast carcinoma and classified as BI-RADS 5

BI-RADS	ESTIMATED PROBABILITY OF MALIGNANCY
0	Incomplete assessment, mainly reserved for primary screening mammography
1	No abnormalities
2	Benign findings
3	Probable benign finding (probability of malignancy <2%)
4	Suspicious finding (probability of malignancy 2-95%)
5	Highly suggestive of malignancy (probability of malignancy >95%)
6	Biopsy-proven malignancy

Table 82 // BI-RADS classification

Ovarian carcinoma

D Ovarian carcinoma is a predominantly epithelial tumour arising from the ovarian surface epithelium (80%). Ovarian carcinoma is classified into serous cysteadenocarcinoma (60%), mucinous/endometrial/transitional/clear cell, and Brenner tumours (20%). The remainder consists of non-epithelial ovarian malignancies (20%) originating from ovarian germ cells, the sex cord, stroma cells, or ovarian metastases.

E Incidence 14:100,000/year, prevalence 1,200 women/year, life-time risk 2%

Ae 20% hereditary

R <2 pregnancies, no ovulation inhibitors, genetic (*BRCA1/2* gene mutation, HBOC family)

Hx Asymptomatic ⊙, nonspecific abdominal symptoms, abdominal distention due to tumour (ball feeling in abdomen) or ascites, abnormal blood loss, abnormal defaecation or micturition

PE • Palpable abdominal mass, shifting dullness (in ascites)
   • Vaginal exam: relationship to surrounding structures, tumour mobility

Dx • TAU/TVU: primary tumour, use risk prediction models to assess risk of malignancy (IOTA simple rules or adnex model, see Tables 83 and 84)
   • Chest and abdominal CT with venous contrast: metastases and relationship to surrounding structures
   • Labs: tumour markers (CA125 ↑ and CEA ↑ in epithelial tumours, β-hCG ↑, LDH ↑ and AFP ↑ in non-epithelial tumours, inhibine ↑ in granulosa cell tumours)
   • Biopsy: in case of diagnostic uncertainty (see Figure 121)

Tx 🖋 Adjuvant and neo-adjuvant chemotherapy, hyperthermic intraperitoneal chemotherapy (HIPEC) in stage IIIC ovarium carcinoma

🖋 Laparotomic staging surgery in early stage, laparotomic debulking surgery in advanced stage

P • 5-year survival stage I-II 78-100%, stage III-IV 25%
  • Mortality 2.7-9.9:100,000/y worldwide

! 'Silent lady killer' due to early peritoneal metastasis and late symptoms. 60-75% of ovarian carcinomas have reached stage III or IV by the time of diagnosis.

💡 Metastatic spread of ovarian carcinoma:
  • Infiltrative: peritoneum of the abdominal wall, paracolic gutter, visceral peritoneum of the colon, diaphragm, small intestine
  • Lymphogenic: para-aortic, paracaval, pelvic, axillary
  • Haematogenous: liver, spleen (less common)

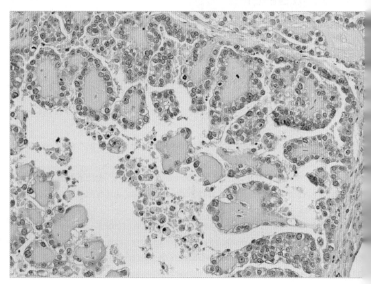

Figure 121 // Biopsy of ovarian carcinoma

 💡 The ovarian-adnexal imaging-reporting-data system (O-RADS) is a radiology reporting tool for ultrasound and MRI to assess the risk of malignancy based on the characteristics of ovarian lesions.

RULES FOR PREDICTING A MALIGNANT TUMOUR (M-RULES)		RULES FOR PREDICTING A BENIGN TUMOUR (B-RULES)	
M1 Irregular solid tumour	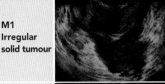	**B1** Unilocular	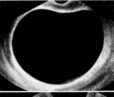
M2 Presence of ascites	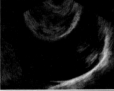	**B2** Presence of solid components with largest diameter <7 mm	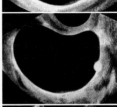
M3 At least 4 papillary structures	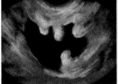	**B3** Presence of acoustic shadows	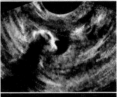
M4 Irregular multilocular-solid tumour with largest diameter ≥100 mm	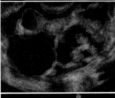	**B4** Smooth multilocular tumour with largest diameter <100 mm	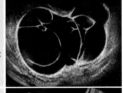
M5 Very strong blood flow (color score 4)	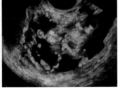	**B5** No blood flow (color score 1)	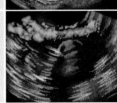

Table 83 // IOTA simple rules

A RISK PREDICTION MODEL THAT CAN RELIABLY DISTINGUISH BETWEEN BENIGN, BORDERLINE, STAGE I INVASIVE, STAGE II-IV INVASIVE, AND SECONDARY METASTATIC ADNEXAL OVARIAN TUMOURS

1. Age of patient at examination (years)
2. Oncology centre (referral centre for GYN oncology)
3. Maximal diameter of lesion (mm)
4. Maximal diameter of largest solid part (mm)
5. More than 10 locules?
6. Number of papillary projections
7. Acoustic shadows present?
8. Ascites (fluid outside pelvis) present?
9. Serum CA125 (U/ml)

Table 84 // IOTA adnex model

- OC, bilateral tubectomy, breastfeeding, and pregnancy lower the risk of developing ovarian carcinoma.
- For women with a stage I tumour who want to have children, a unilateral adnexectomy with staging may be performed first until they no longer intend to have children.
- Unilateral ovarian masses are suspect for metastases.
- Ovarium tumours can develop from the fallopian tube from serous tubal intraepithelial carcinoma (STIC).

Vaginal carcinoma

Ⓓ More than 90% of vaginal carcinomas are squamous cell carcinomas, 5% adenocarcinomas originating from the vagina. Melanomas and sarcomas are very rare.

Ⓔ Incidence 0.6:100,000 women/year, 2% of all female tract malignancies

Ⓐⓔ HPV infection, in utero exposure to synthetic hormone DES

Ⓡ Vaginal intraepithelial neoplasia (VAIN), malignant or premalignant cervical abnormality, DES exposure in utero, multiple sexual partners, young age at first intercourse, smoking, endometriosis

Ⓗⓧ Abnormal bleeding, contact bleeding, discharge symptoms, micturition disorders, defaecation disorders, vaginal pain

Ⓟⓔ • Vaginal inspections: visible malignant lesion, premalignant lesions may manifest as red discolouration

- Inguinal lymph node palpation
- (Dx) Colposcopy: vaginal mapping preinvasive and invasive disease
- Chest and abdominal CT with venous contrast: assess primary tumour and relationship to surrounding structures, and rule out metastases
- Labs: tumour markers (SCC 1)
- Biopsy: tumour size, location, lymph node metastases, histological tumour type, and presence of lymphovascular space invasion (LVSI)

(Tx) 🦠 Radiotherapy, possibly in conjunction with chemotherapy

🔪 Surgical resection is possible in exceptional cases

(P) 5-year survival stage I 83-92%, stage II 68-78%, stage III-IV 44-58%

> 💡 Vaginal carcinomas may go unnoticed during a speculum exam because the blades of the speculum obstruct the anterior and posterior vaginal walls. These walls can be inspected by rotating the speculum 90° or by using a transparent speculum.

Vulvar carcinoma

(D) Vulvar carcinoma arises from the vulva and are usually squamous cell carcinomas, but can also be melanomas and adenocarcinomas.

(E) Incidence 2:100,000/year

(Ae) HPV infection or chronic inflammation and/or dystrophy (at older age)

(R) Vulvar intra-epithelial neoplasia (VIN), dystrophy, HPV infection, age >65, lichen sclerosus et atrophicus, smoking

(Hx) Itching, vulvar mass, burning sensation on micturition, bloody discharge, vulvar pain

(PE) • Tumour labia minora/majora: size and localisation of the lesion (unifocal/multifocal, distance to midline, urethra, anus, and clitoris)
- Lymph nodes: inguinal

(Dx) • Ultrasound, PET/CT, MRI: unifocal, <4 cm, and no suspicious inguinal lymph nodes
- Chest and abdominal CT with venous contrast: >4 cm or multifocal, or suspicious inguinal lymph nodes
- PET-CT: in locally advanced disease, or treatment planning
- Biopsy: nodal status, histological tumour type, and LVSI

(Tx) 🦠 Depending on stage: chemotherapy/radiotherapy

🔪 • For squamous cell carcinoma: wide local excision, depending on stage

(→ sentinel node procedure, lymph node dissection)

- For larger abnormalities: radical vulvectomy

(P) 5-year survival: stage I: 79%, stage II: 59%, stage III: 43%, stage IV: 13%

(!) Premalignant form: VIN (see Table 85)

VIN CLASSIFICATION		
Class	Old terminology	New terminology
VIN 1 VIN 2 and VIN 3	Flat condylomata or HPV effect VIN, usual type: (a) VIN, warty type (b) VIN, basaloid type (c) VIN, mixed	LSIL HSIL
Differentiated VIN	VIN, differentiated type	Differentiated VIN (dVIN)

Table 85 // Classification of vulvar intraepithelial neoplasia (VIN)

Gestational trophoblastic neoplasia (GTN)

(D) GTN, or malignant gestational trophoblastic disease (GTD), is a collective of pregnancy-related diseases: choriocarcinoma, invasive mola, epithelioid trophoblastic tumour (ETT), and placental site trophoblastic tumour (PSTT).

(E) Choriocarcinoma incidence 0.072:1,000; invasive mole (complete mole 15-20%, partial mole 1-5%), ETT, and PSTT are very rare

(Ae) 95% preceded by hydatidiform mole, abortion, termination of pregnancy, tubal pregnancy

(R) Extreme reproductive age, previous hydatidiform molar pregnancy, history of spontaneous abortions, oral contraceptives, paternal and environmental factors, vitamin A deficiency, serum hCG levels >100,000 mIU/ml

(Hx) Vaginal bleeding, uterus larger than gestational age, pelvic pain or pressure, severe nausea or vomiting, hypertensive signs (headache, oedema), fatigue, dyspnoea, dizziness, irregular palpitations

(PE) · In case of vaginal bleeding: BP =/↓, HR ↑
· Abdomen (palpation): enlarged uterus, pain at palpation

(Dx) · Labs: crossmatch, Hb, hCG levels
· TVU: intrauterine typical grape-like structures
· Thoracoabdominal CT: presence of pulmonary and/or liver metastases
· Brain MRI: screening for brain metastases if CT shows pulmonary metastases

(Tx) 💬 Follow-up hCG every 1-2 wk

• FIGO stage I-II: chemotherapy
  • FIGO stage III-IV: multiagent chemotherapy, brain metastasis → radio-therapy
  • FIGO III-IV: adjuvant radiotherapy, cytoreductive surgery

Hysterectomy if chemotherapy is ineffective, treatment of extreme haem-orrhage, women not trying to conceive, and age >40

Risk of metastasis (lungs, ovaries, vagina). Cure rate approx. 90%, prognosis depends on histologic type, extent of spread, hCG level, duration of disease, site, and number of metastases, nature of preceding pregnancy, extent of prior treatment

Chemotherapy-related fertility problems, recurrence risk 0.6%-2%

Follow-up hCG after treatment:
  • Partial hydatidiform molar: single normal hCG level 1 month after first hCG normalisation.
  • Complete hydatidiform molar: monthly hCG levels for 6 months after hCG normalisation.

Clinical reasoning

 This section lists several examples of diagnoses to consider for specific complaints.

Primary amenorrhoea

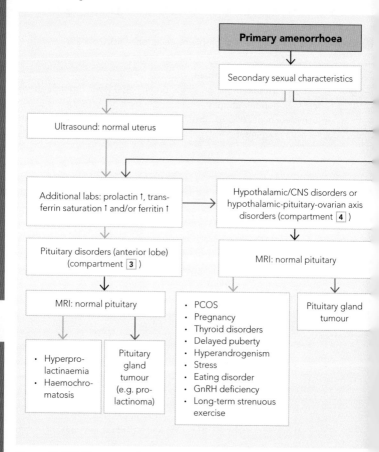

Diagram 12 // DD Primary amenorrhoea

In **primary amenorrhoea** several causal compartments can be distinguished:

1. Anatomic abnormalities of the hymen, vagina, and/or Müllerian ducts (uterus, upper 1/3 of the vagina)
2. Ovarian/gonadal disorders (ovarian failure)
3. Anterior pituitary disorders
4. Disorders causing abnormal hypothalamic and upper CNS function

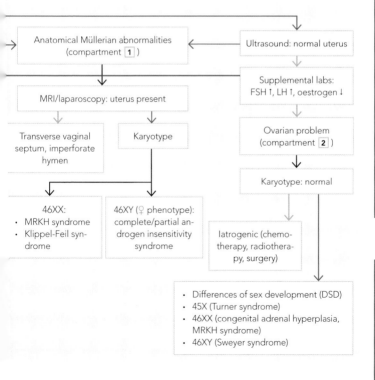

Secondary amenorrhoea

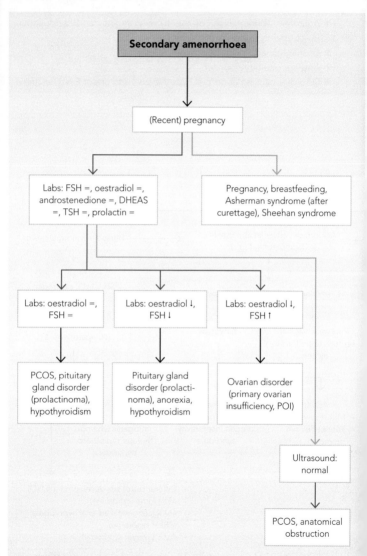

Secondary amenorrhoea

(Recent) pregnancy

Labs: FSH =, oestradiol =, androstenedione =, DHEAS =, TSH =, prolactin =

Pregnancy, breastfeeding, Asherman syndrome (after curettage), Sheehan syndrome

Labs: oestradiol =, FSH =

Labs: oestradiol ↓, FSH ↓

Labs: oestradiol ↓, FSH ↑

PCOS, pituitary gland disorder (prolactinoma), hypothyroidism

Pituitary gland disorder (prolactinoma), anorexia, hypothyroidism

Ovarian disorder (primary ovarian insufficiency, POI)

Ultrasound: normal

PCOS, anatomical obstruction

Diagram 13 // DDx Secondary amenorrhoea

Hypertension during pregnancy

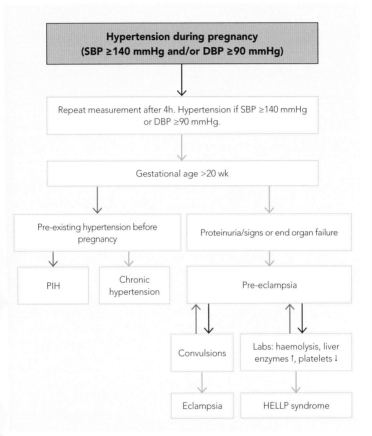

**Hypertension during pregnancy
(SBP ≥140 mmHg and/or DBP ≥90 mmHg)**

Repeat measurement after 4h. Hypertension if SBP ≥140 mmHg or DBP ≥90 mmHg.

Gestational age >20 wk

Pre-existing hypertension before pregnancy

Proteinuria/signs or end organ failure

PIH

Chronic hypertension

Pre-eclampsia

Convulsions

Labs: haemolysis, liver enzymes ↑, platelets ↓

Eclampsia

HELLP syndrome

Diagram 14 // DDx Hypertension during pregnancy

 BP ≥140/90 mmHg is defined as hypertension. In cases of severe hypertension (SBP≥160 mmHg or DBP ≥110 mmHg), drug therapy is advised.

 Pre-eclampsia can also occur without proteinuria and hypertension.

Vaginal bleeding outside pregnancy

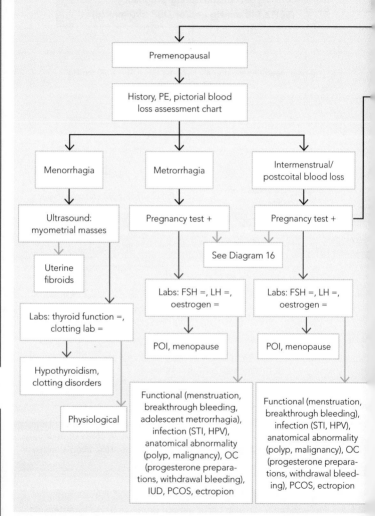

Diagram 15 // DDx Vaginal bleeding outside pregnancy

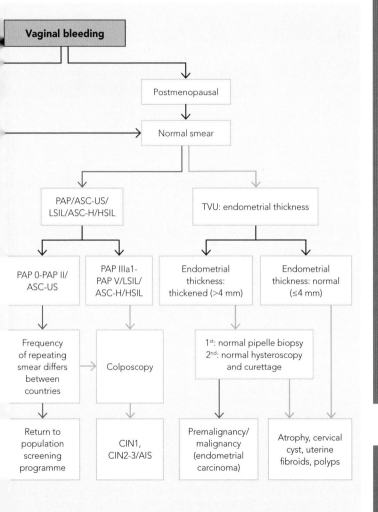

CLINICAL REASONING

Vaginal bleeding during pregnancy

 In pregnant patients with vaginal blood loss, consider a smear (see Diagram 10).

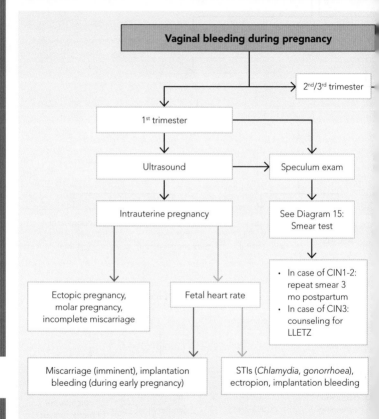

Diagram 16 // DDx Vaginal bleeding during pregnancy

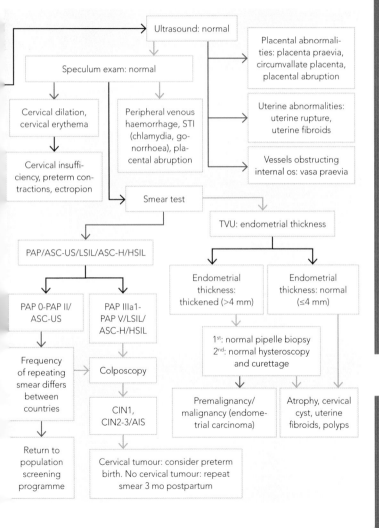

Ultrasound: normal

Speculum exam: normal

Cervical dilation, cervical erythema

Cervical insufficiency, preterm contractions, ectropion

Peripheral venous haemorrhage, STI (chlamydia, gonorrhoea), placental abruption

Placental abnormalities: placenta praevia, circumvallate placenta, placental abruption

Uterine abnormalities: uterine rupture, uterine fibroids

Vessels obstructing internal os: vasa praevia

Smear test

TVU: endometrial thickness

PAP/ASC-US/LSIL/ASC-H/HSIL

PAP 0-PAP II/ ASC-US

PAP IIIa1-PAP V/LSIL/ ASC-H/HSIL

Frequency of repeating smear differs between countries

Colposcopy

CIN1, CIN2-3/AIS

Return to population screening programme

Cervical tumour: consider preterm birth. No cervical tumour: repeat smear 3 mo postpartum

Endometrial thickness: thickened (>4 mm)

Endometrial thickness: normal (≤4 mm)

1st: normal pipelle biopsy
2nd: normal hysteroscopy and curettage

Premalignancy/ malignancy (endometrial carcinoma)

Atrophy, cervical cyst, uterine fibroids, polyps

Appendices

Appendix 1: FIGO classification

 In gynaecological oncology, the FIGO classification is used instead of the TNM classification. In addition to staging I to IV, additional information is provided by the subclassification (A to C) to describe invasive characteristics and metastases.

FIGO STAGE	ENDOMETRIUM	OVARY, FALLOPIAN TUBES AND PERITONEUM	CERVIX
I	Confined to uterine corpus and ovary	Confined to ovaries or fallopian tubes	Confined to cervix (disregard extension to uterine corpus)
II	Invasion of cervical stroma without extrauterine extension or with substantial LVSI, or aggressive histological types with myometrial invasion	Involvement of one or both ovaries or fallopian tubes with pelvic extension	Invasion beyond uterus, but not extended onto lower third of vagina or to pelvic wall
III	Local and/or regional spread of tumour of any histological subtype	Involvement of one or both ovaries or fallopian tubes or peritoneal cancer, with cytologically or histologically confirmed spread to peritoneum outside the pelvis and/or metastasis to retroperitoneal lymph nodes	Involvement of lower third of the vagina and/or extension to pelvic wall and/or causing hydronephrosis or non-functioning kidney and/or involvement of pelvic and/or para-aortic lymph nodes
IV	Spread to bladder mucosa and/or intestinal mucosa and/or distant metastasis	Distant metastasis excl. peritoneal metastases	Extension beyond true pelvis or involvement (i.e. biopsy-proven) of bladder/rectal mucosa

Table 86 // FIGO classification per gynaecological malignancy

VULVA	VAGINA	GESTATIONAL TROPHO-BLASTIC NEOPLASIA
Confined to vulva	Confined to vaginal wall	Confined to uterine corpus
Extension to adjacent perineal structures ($1/3$ lower urethra, $1/3$ lower vagina, anus) without lymph node metastases	Invasion of subvaginal tissue, but not extended to pelvic wall	Extension to adnexa or vagina, but limited to the genital structures
Tumour of any size with extension to upper part of adjacent perineal structures, or with any number of nonfixed, nonulcerated lymph node	Extension to pelvic wall	Extension to lungs, with or without genital tract involvement
Tumour of any size fixed to bone; fixed, ulcerated lymph node metastases; or distant metastases	Extended beyond true pelvis or involvement of bladder/rectal mucosa	All other metastatic sites

Appendix 2: Caesarean section

Pre-OR checklist

Prior to surgery, the following should be discussed/completed:
- OR: type of procedure, purpose of surgery, risks and complications
- MRSA checklist completed?
- SURPASS completed?
- Allergies documented?
- Do not resuscitate (DNR) discussed/advance decision to refuse treatment agreed
- Preoperative labs: Hb, Ht, blood crossmatching, coagulation status
- Premedication prescribed (e.g., paracetamol as needed)
- Pre- and post-operative orders prepared? Anticoagulants discontinued?
- Time-out completed?

 An advance decision to refuse all treatment can be abbreviated as DNR (fo not resuscitate) or DNACPR (do not apply cardiopulmonary resuscitation).

 This CS report serves as an example only. Different hospitals/countries may have different requirements.

 Layers to be passed during CS: cutis, subcutis, fascia of Camper, fascia of Scarpa, abdominal linea alba and rectus abdominis muscle, transverse fascia, preperitoneal fat, peritoneum, perimetrium, myometrium, endometrium and membranes.

Example C-section OR report

- Indication: [primary/secondary due to breech presentation/fetal distress]
- Anaesthesia [general/spinal]
- Position in left-lateral tilt
- The surgical area is disinfected and covered
- Incision [Pfannenstiel/Joel-Cohen/Maylard, or lower midline incision in case of prior laparotomy or extreme urgency]
- The subcutis and fascia are first opened by [blunt/sharp] expansion. The bladder peritoneum is opened by sharp expansion and dissected by hand, after which a large bladder retractor is placed behind the bladder.
- A transverse incision is made in the lower uterine segment.
- The uterus is expanded medially along the marking incision and digitally
- After rupture of the membranes, the large bladder retractor is removed and the presenting part of the child is pulled from the lesser pelvis
- Appearance of amniotic fluid [clear/meconium]
- A child was born at [time] in [cephalic/breech presentation] in [good/moderate/bad] condition, Apgar score [...]
- After childbirth, [IV kefzol/flagyl/augmentin] is administered
- Atraumatic spring clips are used to clamp the uterine wound edges
- Oxytocin [5 IE] is administered to the mother. The placenta is delivered through controlled cord traction.
- The large bladder retractor is reinserted and the cavum uteri is checked for placental remnants which are [present/absent] [and are removed]. The internal os of the cervix is localised.
- When the corner sutures are in place, the uterus is closed in [one/two layers] with [dissolvable multifilament suture], haemostasis is checked. The uterus and adnexa are checked. After a second haemostasis check and mesh check, the abdominal wall is closed [with suture material]. The skin is closed with [staples/intracutaneous sutures].
- CS had [complications/no complications]. [Explanation if applicable]
- Total blood loss: [... ml]

Elements in italics should be specified on a case-by-case basis

PROCEDURE	TECHNIQUE	ADVANTAGE	DISADVANTAGE
Pfannenstiel incision	Horizontal incision just above the pubic symphysis	Small, inconspicuous scar under the bikini line, heals fast	Poor uterine access
Joel-Cohen incision	Horizontal suprapubic incision	Deep layers are opened by blunt expansion, shortening the procedure and reducing tissue damage	More proximal scar than Pfannenstiel
Maylard incision	Horizontal interiliac incision	High exposure, gives best access in patients with adiposity	Penetrates all abdominal wall layers, more postoperative pain
Lower midline incision	Vertical incision from navel to pubic symphysis	Quick and easy access	Large scar with risk of incisional hernia

Table 87 // CS surgical techniques

 The patient is positioned in left-lateral tilt to prevent inferior vena cava syndrome.

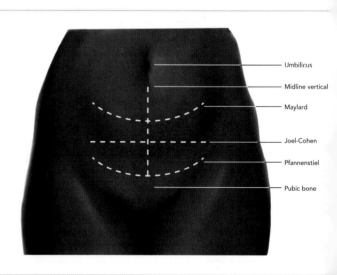

- Umbilicus
- Midline vertical
- Maylard
- Joel-Cohen
- Pfannenstiel
- Pubic bone

Figure 122 // Incisions CS

References

1. Abdelshafi S, Okasha A, Elsirgany S, Khalil A, El-Dessouky S, AbdelHakim N, Elanwary S, Elsheikhah A. Peak systolic velocity of fetal middle cerebral artery to predict anemia in Red Cell Alloimmunization in un-transfused and transfused fetuses. Eur J Obstet Gynecol Reprod Biol. 2021 Mar;258:437-442. doi 10.1016/j.ejogrb.2021.01.046. Epub 2021 Jan 29. PMID: 33571914.

2. Adams TS, Rogers LJ, Cuello MA. Cancer of the vagina: 2021 update. Int J Gynaecol Obstet. 202° Oct;155 Suppl 1(Suppl.1):19-27. doi: 10.1002/ijgo.13867. PMID: 34669198; PMCID: PMC9298013.

3. Alexander EK, Marqusee E, Lawrence J, Jarolim P, Fischer GA, Larsen PR. Timing and magnitude of in creases in levothyroxine requirements during pregnancy in women with hypothyroidism. N Engl J Mec 2004 Jul 15;351(3):241-9. doi: 10.1056/NEJMoa040079. PMID: 15254282.

4. AlJulaih GH, Muzio MR. Gestational Trophoblastic Neoplasia. In: StatPearls [Internet]. Treasure Island (FL, United States): StatPearls Publishing; 2023 Jan [Updated 2023 Nov 12] [cited 2023 nov 29]. Availabl from: https://www.ncbi.nlm.nih.gov/books/NBK562225/

5. American Academy of Pediatrics, American College of Obstetricians and Gynecologists. Guidelines fc Perinatal Care (8th ed.). [Internet]. Elk Grove Village, IL and Washington DC, United States; 2017. Availa ble from: https://www.acog.org/clinical-information/physician-faqs/-/media/3a22e153b67446a6b31fb0 1e469187c.ashx

6. American College of Obstetrics and Gynecologists' Committee on Practice Bulletins—Obstetrics. ACOG Practice Bulletin No. 49: Dystocia and augmentation of labor. Obstet Gynecol. 2003 Dec;102(6):1445-54 doi: 10.1016/j.obstetgynecol.2003.10.011. PMID: 14662243.

7. American College of Obstetrics and Gynecologists' Committee on Practice Bulletins. ACOG Practic Bulletin No. 122: Breast cancer screening. Obstet Gynecol. 2011 Aug;118(2 Pt 1):372-382. doi: 10.1097 AOG.0b013e31822c98e5. PMID: 21775869.

8. American College of Obstetricians and Gynecologists' Committee on Practice Bulletins—Gynecolog ACOG Practice Bulletin No. 190: Gestational Diabetes Mellitus. Obstet Gynecol. 2018 Feb;131(2):e4¹ e64. doi: 10.1097/AOG.0000000000002501. PMID: 29370047.

9. American College of Obstetricians and Gynecologists' Committee on Practice Bulletins—Gynecolog ACOG Practice Bulletin No. 200: Early Pregnancy Loss. Obstet Gynecol. 2018 Nov;132(5):e197-e207. do 10.1097/AOG.0000000000002899. PMID: 30157093.

10. American College of Obstetrics and Gynecologists' Committee opinion No 797: Prevention of Group Streptococcal Early-Onset Disease in Newborns. Obstet Gynecol. 2020 Feb;135(2):e51-e72. doi: 10.109 AOG.0000000000003668. Erratum in: Obstet Gynecol. 2020 Apr;135(4):978-979. PMID: 31977795.

11. American Psychiatric Association. Diagnostic and Statistical Manual of Mental Disorders. Ame can Psychiatric Association, Washington DC, USA; 2013. Available from: https://doi.org/10.1176/app books.9780890425787.

12. Ananth CV, Kinzler WL. Acute placental abruption: Pathophysiology, clinical features, diagnosis, and co sequences [Internet]. UpToDate. 2022 Jul 12 [cited 2022 nov 23]. Available from: https://medilib.ir/upt date/show/6826

13. Anderson M, Kutzner S, Kaufman RH. Treatment of vulvovaginal lichen planus with vaginal hydrocortis ne suppositories. Obstet Gynecol. 2002 Aug;100(2):359-62. doi: 10.1016/s0029-7844(02)02117-8. PMI 12151163.

14. Anum EA, Brown HL, Strauss JF 3rd. Health disparities in risk for cervical insufficiency. Hum Repro 2010 Nov;25(11):2894-900. doi: 10.1093/humrep/deq177. Epub 2010 Jul 19. PMID: 20643692; PMC. PMC2955555.

15. Aronson SL, Lopez-Yurda M, Koole SN, Schagen van Leeuwen JH, Schreuder HWR, Hermans RHM, « Hingh IHJT, van Gent MDJM, Arts HJG, van Ham MAPC, van Dam PA, Vuylsteke P, Aalbers AGJ, Verwa VJ, Van de Vijver KK, Aaronson NK, Sonke GS, van Driel WJ. Cytoreductive surgery with or without h perthermic intraperitoneal chemotherapy in patients with advanced ovarian cancer (OVHIPEC-1): fir survival analysis of a randomised, controlled, phase 3 trial. Lancet Oncol. 2023 Oct;24(10):1109-1118. d 10.1016/S1470-2045(23)00396-0. Epub 2023 Sep 11. PMID: 37708912.

16. Ayres-de-Campos, D., Spong, C.Y., Chandraharan, E. and (2015), FIGO consensus guidelines on int

partum fetal monitoring: Cardiotocography. International Journal of Gynecology & Obstetrics, 131: 13-24. https://doi.org/10.1016/j.ijgo.2015.06.020

17. Ball E, Waters N, Cooper N, Talati C, Mallick R, Rabas S, Mukherjee A, Sri Ranjan Y, Thaha M, Doodia R, Keedwell R, Madhra M, Kuruba N, Malhas R, Gaughan E, Tompsett K, Gibson H, Wright H, Gnanachandran C, Hookaway T, Baker C, Murali K, Jurkovic D, Amso N, Clark J, Thangaratinam S, Chalhoub T, Kaloo P, Saridogan E. Evidence-Based Guideline on Laparoscopy in Pregnancy: Commissioned by the British Society for Gynaecological Endoscopy (BSGE) Endorsed by the Royal College of Obstetricians & Gynaecologists (RCOG). Facts Views Vis Obgyn. 2019 Mar;11(1):5-25. Erratum in: Facts Views Vis Obgyn. 2020 Jan 24;11(3):261. PMID: 31695854; PMCID: PMC6822954.

18. Becker CM, Bokor A, Heikinheimo O, Horne A, Jansen F, Kiesel L, King K, Kvaskoff M, Nap A, Petersen K, Saridogan E, Tomassetti C, van Hanegem N, Vulliemoz N, Vermeulen N; ESHRE Endometriosis Guideline Group. ESHRE guideline: endometriosis. Hum Reprod Open. 2022 Feb 26;2022(2):hoac009. doi: 10.1093/hropen/hoac009. PMID: 35350465; PMCID: PMC8951218.

19. Beckmann CRB, Ling FW, Barzansky BM, Herbert WNP, Laube DW, Smith RP. Obstetrics and Gynaecology (6th ed.). Lippincott Williams & Wilkins, Philadelphia, PA, United States; 2010.

20. Berek JS, Renz M, Kehoe S, Kumar L, Friedlander M. Cancer of the ovary, fallopian tube, and peritoneum: 2021 update. Int J Gynaecol Obstet. 2021 Oct;155 Suppl 1(Suppl 1):61-85. doi: 10.1002/ijgo.13878. PMID: 34669199; PMCID: PMC9298325.

21. Bhatla N, Aoki D, Sharma DN, Sankaranarayanan R. Cancer of the cervix uteri: 2021 update. Int J Gynaecol Obstet. 2021 Oct;155 Suppl 1(Suppl 1):28-44. doi: 10.1002/ijgo.13865. PMID: 34669203; PMCID: PMC9298213.

22. Birge O, Bakır MS, Karadag C, Dinc C, Doğan S, Tuncer HA, Simsek T. Risk factors that increase recurrence in borderline ovarian cancers. Am J Transl Res. 2021 Jul 15;13(7):8438-8449. PMID: 34377341; PMCID: PMC8340170.

23. Broekhuijsen K, van Baaren GJ, van Pampus MG, Ganzevoort W, Sikkema JM, Woiski MD, Oudijk MA, Bloemenkamp KW, Scheepers HC, Bremer HA, Rijnders RJ, van Loon AJ, Perquin DA, Sporken JM, Papatsonis DN, van Huizen ME, Vredevoogd CB, Brons JT, Kaplan M, van Kaam AH, Groen H, Porath MM, van den Berg PP, Mol BW, Franssen MT, Langenveld J; HYPITAT-II study group. Immediate delivery versus expectant monitoring for hypertensive disorders of pregnancy between 34 and 37 weeks of gestation (HYPITAT-II): an open-label, randomised controlled trial. Lancet. 2015 Jun 20;385(9986):2492-501. doi: 10.1016/S0140-6736(14)61998-X. Epub 2015 Mar 25. Erratum in: Lancet. 2016 Feb 27;387(10021):848. PMID: 25817374.

24. Broeze KA, Opmeer BC, Coppus SF, Van Geloven N, Alves MF, Anestad G, Bhattacharya S, Allan J, Guerra-Infante MF, Den Hartog JE, Land JA, Idahl A, Van der Linden PJ, Mouton JW, Ng EH, Van der Steeg JW, Steures P, Svensrup HF, Tiitinen A, Toye B, Van der Veen F, Mol BW. Chlamydia antibody testing and diagnosing tubal pathology in subfertile women: an individual patient data meta-analysis. Hum Reprod Update. 2011 May-Jun;17(3):301-10. doi: 10.1093/humupd/dmq060. Epub 2011 Jan 12. PMID: 21227996.

25. Capobianco G, Tinacci E, Saderi L, Dessole F, Petrillo M, Madonia M, Virdis G, Olivari A, Santeufemia DA, Cossu A, Dessole S, Sotgiu G, Cherchi PL. High Incidence of Gestational Trophoblastic Disease in a Third-Level University-Hospital, Italy: A Retrospective Cohort Study. Front Oncol. 2021 May 5;11:684700. doi: 10.3389/fonc.2021.684700. PMID: 34026657; PMCID: PMC8135795.

26. Carr RR, Ensom MH. Fluoxetine in the treatment of premenstrual dysphoric disorder. Ann Pharmacother. 2002 Apr;36(4):713-7. doi: 10.1345/aph.1A265. PMID: 11918525.

27. Cleveland AA, Harrison LH, Farley MM, Hollick R, Stein B, Chiller TM, Lockhart SR, Park BJ. Declining incidence of candidemia and the shifting epidemiology of Candida resistance in two US metropolitan areas, 2008-2013: results from population-based surveillance. PLoS One. 2015 Mar 30;10(3):e0120452. doi: 10.1371/journal.pone.0120452. PMID: 25822249; PMCID: PMC4378850.

28. Cohlen B, Bijkerk A, Van der Poel S, Ombelet W. IUI: review and systematic assessment of the evidence that supports global recommendations. Hum Reprod Update. 2018 May 1;24(3):300-319. doi: 10.1093/humupd/dmx041. PMID: 29452361.

29. Colombo N, Sessa C, Bois AD, Ledermann J, McCluggage WG, McNeish I, Morice P, Pignata S, Ray-Coquard I, Vergote I, Baert T, Belaroussi I, Dashora A, Olbrecht S, Planchamp F, Querleu D; ESMO–ESGO Ovarian Cancer Consensus Conference Working Group. ESMO-ESGO consensus conference recommendations on ovarian cancer: pathology and molecular biology, early and advanced stages, borderline tumours and recurrent disease. Int J Gynecol Cancer. 2019 May 2:ijgc-2019-000308. doi: 10.1136/ijgc-2019-000308. Epub ahead of print. PMID: 31048403.

30. Darragh TM, Colgan TJ, Cox JT, Heller DS, Henry MR, Luff RD, McCalmont T, Nayar R, Palefsky JM, Stoler MH, Wilkinson EJ, Zaino RJ, Wilbur DC; Members of LAST Project Work Groups. The Lower Anogenital Squamous Terminology Standardization Project for HPV-Associated Lesions: background and consensus recommendations from the College of American Pathologists and the American Society for Colposcopy and Cervical Pathology. Arch Pathol Lab Med. 2012 Oct;136(10):1266-97. doi: 10.5858/arpa.LGT200570. Epub 2012 Jun 28. Erratum in: Arch Pathol Lab Med. 2013 Jun;137(6):738. PMID: 22742517.

31. Davis E, Sparzak PB. Abnormal Uterine Bleeding. In: StatPearls [Internet]. Treasure Island (FL, United States): StatPearls Publishing; 2023 Jan [Updated 2023 Sep 4] [cited 2023 nov 18]. Available from: https://www.ncbi.nlm.nih.gov/books/NBK532913/

32. Derbala Y, Grochal F, Jeanty P. Vasa previa. J Prenat Med. 2007 Jan;1(1):2-13. PMID: 22470817; PMCID PMC3309346.

33. Dodd JM, Flenady VJ, Cincotta R, Crowther CA. Progesterone for the prevention of preterm birth: a systematic review. Obstet Gynecol. 2008 Jul;112(1):127-34. doi: 10.1097/AOG.0b013e31817d0262. PMID 18591318.

34. Earls MF, Yogman MW, Mattson G, Rafferty J; COMMITTEE ON PSYCHOSOCIAL ASPECTS OF CHILD AND FAMILY HEALTH. Incorporating Recognition and Management of Perinatal Depression Into Pediatric Practice. Pediatrics. 2019 Jan;143(1):e20183259. doi: 10.1542/peds.2018-3259. PMID: 30559120.

35. Einarson TR, Piwko C, Koren G. Prevalence of nausea and vomiting of pregnancy in the USA: a meta analysis. J Popul Ther Clin Pharmacol. 2013;20(2):e163-70. Epub 2013 Jul 14. PMID: 23863545.

36. ElSayed NA, Aleppo G, Aroda VR, Bannuru RR, Brown FM, Bruemmer D, Collins BS, Hilliard ME, Isaacs D, Johnson EL, Kahan S, Khunti K, Leon J, Lyons SK, Perry ML, Prahalad P, Pratley RE, Seley JJ, Stanton RC, Gabbay RA, on behalf of the American Diabetes Association. 2. Classification and Diagnosis of Diabetes: Standards of Care in Diabetes-2023. Diabetes Care. 2023 Jan 1;46(Suppl 1):S19-S40. doi: 10.2337/dc23-S002. Erratum in: Diabetes Care. 2023 Feb 01;: Erratum in: Diabetes Care. 2023 Sep 1;46(9):1715. PMID: 36507649; PMCID: PMC9810477.

37. Elson CJ, Salim R, Potdar N, Chetty M, Ross JA, Kirk EJ on behalf of the Royal College of Obstetricians and Gynaecologists. Diagnosis and management of ectopic pregnancy. BJOG 2016;. 123: e15–e55.

38. Fertility problems: assessment and treatment. London, United Kingdom: National Institute for Health and Care Excellence (NICE); 2017 Sep. PMID: 32134604.

39. Giblin J, Coad B, Lamb C, Berlin C, Rea G, Hanson H, Snape K, Berner K & Consensus Meeting attendees. UK recommendations for the management of transgender and gender-diverse patients with inherited cancer risks. BJC Rep 1, 1 (2023). https://doi.org/10.1038/s44276-023-00002-0

40. Gilroy AM, MacPherson BR, Ross LM. Prometheus: Anatomische atlas [Atlas of Anatomy]. Dutch. Houten, Netherlands: Bohn Stafleu van Loghum; 2014.

41. Groves MJ. Genital Herpes: A Review. Am Fam Physician. 2016 Jun 1;93(11):928-34. PMID: 27281837

42. Guideline Group on Unexplained Infertility; Romualdi D, Ata B, Bhattacharya S, Bosch E, Costello M, Gersak K, Homburg R, Mincheva M, Norman RJ, Piltonen T, Dos Santos-Ribeiro S, Scicluna D, Somers S, Sunkara SK, Verhoeve HR, Le Clef N. Evidence-based guideline: unexplained infertility†. Hum Reprod 2023 Oct 3;38(10):1881-1890. doi: 10.1093/humrep/dead150. PMID: 37599566; PMCID: PMC10546081.

43. Gundersen TD, Krebs L, Loekkegaard ECL, Rasmussen SC, Glavind J, Clausen TD. Postpartum urinary tract infection by mode of delivery: a Danish nationwide cohort study. BMJ Open. 2018 Mar 14;8(3):e018479. doi: 10.1136/bmjopen-2017-018479. PMID: 29540408; PMCID: PMC5857667.

44. Harlow SD, Gass M, Hall JE, Lobo R, Maki P, Rebar RW, Sherman S, Sluss PM, de Villiers TJ; STRAW 10 Collaborative Group. Executive summary of the Stages of Reproductive Aging Workshop + 10: addressing the unfinished agenda of staging reproductive aging. Menopause. 2012 Apr;19(4):387-95. doi: 10.1097/gme.0b013e31824d8f40. PMID: 22343510; PMCID: PMC3340903.

45. Harlow BL, Kunitz CG, Nguyen RH, Rydell SA, Turner RM, MacLehose RF. Prevalence of symptoms consistent with a diagnosis of vulvodynia: population-based estimates from 2 geographic regions. Am J Obstet Gynecol. 2014 Jan;210(1):40.e1-8. doi: 10.1016/j.ajog.2013.09.033. Epub 2013 Sep 28. PMID 24080300; PMCID: PMC3885163.

46. Hembree WC, Cohen-Kettenis PT, Gooren L, Hannema SE, Meyer WJ, Murad MH, Rosenthal SM, Safer JD, Tangpricha V, T'Sjoen GG. ENDOCRINE TREATMENT OF GENDER-DYSPHORIC/GENDER-INCONGRUENT PERSONS: AN ENDOCRINE SOCIETY CLINICAL PRACTICE GUIDELINE. Endocr Pract. 2017 Dec;23(12):1437. doi: 10.4158/1934-2403-23.12.1437. PMID: 29320642.

47. Hickok DE, Gordon DC, Milberg JA, Williams MA, Daling JR. The frequency of breech presentation by gestational age at birth: a large population-based study. Am J Obstet Gynecol. 1992 Mar;166(3):851-

doi: 10.1016/0002-9378(92)91347-d. PMID: 1550152.

48. Hill DA, Taylor CA. Dyspareunia in Women. Am Fam Physician. 2021 May 15;103(10):597-604. PMID: 33983001.

49. Hofmeister S, Bodden S. Premenstrual Syndrome and Premenstrual Dysphoric Disorder. Am Fam Physician. 2016 Aug 1;94(3):236-40. PMID: 27479626.

50. Honein MA, Kirby RS, Meyer RE, Xing J, Skerrette NI, Yuskiv N, Marengo L, Petrini JR, Davidoff MJ, Mai CT, Druschel CM, Viner-Brown S, Sever LE; National Birth Defects Prevention Network. The association between major birth defects and preterm birth. Matern Child Health J. 2009 Mar;13(2):164-75. doi: 10.1007/s10995-008-0348-y. Epub 2008 May 17. PMID: 18484173.

51. Hypertension in pregnancy: diagnosis and management. London: National Institute for Health and Care Excellence (NICE); 2019 Jun 25. PMID: 31498578.

52. Jamieson DJ, Steege JF. The prevalence of dysmenorrhea, dyspareunia, pelvic pain, and irritable bowel syndrome in primary care practices. Obstet Gynecol. 1996 Jan;87(1):55-8. doi: 10.1016/0029-7844(95)00360-6. PMID: 8532266.

53. Jarvis CI, Lynch AM, Morin AK. Management strategies for premenstrual syndrome/premenstrual dysphoric disorder. Ann Pharmacother. 2008 Jul;42(7):967-78. doi: 10.1345/aph.1K673. Epub 2008 Jun 17. PMID: 18559957.

54. Jauniaux E, Alfirevic Z, Bhide AG, Belfort MA, Burton GJ, Collins SL, Dornan S, Jurkovic D, Kayem G, Kingdom J, Silver R, Sentilhes L; Royal College of Obstetricians and Gynaecologists. Placenta Praevia and Placenta Accreta: Diagnosis and Management: Green-top Guideline No. 27a. BJOG. 2019 Jan;126(1):e1-e48. doi: 10.1111/1471-0528.15306. Epub 2018 Sep 27. PMID: 30260097.

55. Keulen JK, Bruinsma A, Kortekaas JC, van Dillen J, Bossuyt PM, Oudijk MA, Duijnhoven RG, van Kaam AH, Vandenbussche FP, van der Post JA, Mol BW, de Miranda E. Induction of labour at 41 weeks versus expectant management until 42 weeks (INDEX): multicentre, randomised non-inferiority trial. BMJ. 2019 Feb 20;364:l344. doi: 10.1136/bmj.l344. PMID: 30786997; PMCID: PMC6598648.

56. Key Statistics for Cervical Cancer [Internet]. Updated: 2023 Jan 12 [cited 2023 Dec 1]. Available from: https://www.cancer.org/cancer/cervical-cancer/about/key-statistics.html.

57. Khieu M, Butler SL. High Grade Squamous Intraepithelial Lesion. In: StatPearls [Internet]. Treasure Island (FL, United States): StatPearls Publishing; 2023 Jan [Updated 2022 Jan 5] Available from: https://www.ncbi.nlm.nih.gov/books/NBK430728/

58. Kilby, MD, Bricker, L on behalf of the Royal College of Obstetricians and Gynaecologists. Management of monochorionic twin pregnancy. BJOG 2016; 124: e1–e45. doi: 10.1111/1471-0528.14188. Epub 2016 Nov 16. PMID: 27862859.

59. Kim M, Ishioka S, Endo T, Baba T, Akashi Y, Morishita M, Adachi H, Saito T. Importance of uterine cervical cerclage to maintain a successful pregnancy for patients who undergo vaginal radical trachelectomy. Int J Clin Oncol. 2014 Oct;19(5):906-11. doi: 10.1007/s10147-013-0631-9. Epub 2013 Oct 31. PMID: 24170246.

60. Koopmans CM, Bijlenga D, Groen H, Vijgen SM, Aarnoudse JG, Bekedam DJ, van den Berg PP, de Boer K, Burggraaff JM, Bloemenkamp KW, Drogtrop AP, Franx A, de Groot CJ, Huisjes AJ, Kwee A, van Loon AJ, Lub A, Papatsonis DN, van der Post JA, Roumen FJ, Scheepers HC, Willekes C, Mol BW, van Pampus MG; HYPITAT study group. Induction of labour versus expectant monitoring for gestational hypertension or mild pre-eclampsia after 36 weeks' gestation (HYPITAT): a multicentre, open-label randomised controlled trial. Lancet. 2009 Sep 19;374(9694):979-988. doi: 10.1016/S0140-6736(09)60736-4. Epub 2009 Aug 3. PMID: 19656508.

61. Koskas M, Amant F, Mirza MR, Creutzberg CL. Cancer of the corpus uteri: 2021 update. Int J Gynaecol Obstet. 2021 Oct;155 Suppl 1(Suppl 1):45-60. doi: 10.1002/ijgo.13866. PMID: 34669196; PMCID: PMC9297903.

62. Kreisel K, Torrone E, Bernstein K, Hong J, Gorwitz R. Prevalence of Pelvic Inflammatory Disease in Sexually Experienced Women of Reproductive Age - United States, 2013-2014. MMWR Morb Mortal Wkly Rep. 2017 Jan 27;66(3):80-83. doi: 10.15585/mmwr.mm6603a3. PMID: 28125569; PMCID: PMC5573882.

63. Kudela G, Wiernik A, Drosdzol-Cop A, Machnikowska-Sokolowska M, Gawlik A, Hyla-Klekot L, et al. Multiple variants of obstructed hemivagina and ipsilateral renal anomaly (OHVIRA) syndrome—one clinical center case series and the systematic review of 734 cases. J Pediatr Urol. (2021) 17(5):653 e651–e659. doi: 10.1016/j.jpurol.2021.06.023

64. Kwee A, Bots ML, Visser GH, Bruinse HW. Emergency peripartum hysterectomy: A prospective study in The Netherlands. Eur J Obstet Gynecol Reprod Biol. 2006 Feb 1;124(2):187-92. doi: 10.1016/j.ejogrb.2005.06.012. Epub 2005 Jul 18. PMID: 16026917.

65. Lee KH, Hong JS, Jung HJ, Jeong HK, Moon SJ, Park WH, Jeong YM, Song SW, Suk Y, Son MJ, Lim JJ,

Shin JI. Imperforate Hymen: A Comprehensive Systematic Review. J Clin Med. 2019 Jan 7;8(1):56. doi: 10.3390/jcm8010056. PMID: 30621064; PMCID: PMC6352236.

66. Levy MM, Evans LE, Rhodes A. The Surviving Sepsis Campaign Bundle: 2018 update. Intensive Care Med. 2018 Jun;44(6):925-928. doi: 10.1007/s00134-018-5085-0. Epub 2018 Apr 19. PMID: 29675566.

67. Lindor, KD, Lee, RH. Intrahepatic cholestasis of pregnancy. Uptodate. 2023 Oct 9 [cited 2023 nov 28]. Available from: https://www.uptodate.com/contents/intrahepatic-cholestasis-of-pregnancy

68. Lindsay TJ, Vitrikas KR. Evaluation and treatment of infertility. Am Fam Physician. 2015 Mar 1;91(5):308-14. Erratum in: Am Fam Physician. 2015 Sep 15;92 (6):437. PMID: 25822387.

69. Lorber B. Listeriosis. Clin Infect Dis. 1997 Jan;24(1):1-9; quiz 10-1. doi: 10.1093/clinids/24.1.1. PMID: 8994747.

70. Lu MC. Recommendations for preconception care. Am Fam Physician. 2007 Aug 1;76(3):397-400. PMID: 17708141.

71. Luger RK, Kight BP. Hypertension In Pregnancy. In: StatPearls [Internet]. Treasure Island (FL, United States): StatPearls Publishing; 2023 Jan [Updated 2022 Oct 3] [cited 2023 nov 28]–. Available from: https://pubmed.ncbi.nlm.nih.gov/28613589/.

72. Man JK, Parker AE, Broughton S, Ikhlaq H, Das M. Should IUI replace IVF as first-line treatment for unexplained infertility? A literature review. BMC Womens Health. 2023 Oct 27;23(1):557. doi: 10.1186/s12905-023-02717-1. PMID: 37891606; PMCID: PMC10612289.

73. Mastrolia SA, Baumfeld Y, Hershkovitz R, Yohay D, Trojano G, Weintraub AY. Independent association between uterine malformations and cervical insufficiency: a retrospective population-based cohort study. Arch Gynecol Obstet. 2018 Apr;297(4):919-926. doi: 10.1007/s00404-018-4663-2. Epub 2018 Feb 1 PMID: 29392437.

74. Mavrides, E, Allard, S, Chandraharan, E, Collins, P, Green, L, Hunt, BJ, Riris, S, Thomson, AJ on behalf of the Royal College of Obstetricians and Gynaecologists. Prevention and management of postpartum haemorrhage. BJOG 2016; 124: e106–e149.

75. Med-Info. Illustratieve anatomie en chirurgische anatomie [Illustrative anatomy and surgical anatomy]. Dutch; 2014 Dec 3. Available from: http://www.med-info.nl/anatomie_0_Overzicht.

76. Mekinian A, Kolanska K, Cheloufi M, Coulomb A, Cohen J, Abisror N, Bornes M, Kayem G, Alijotas-Reig J, Fain O. Chronic Villitis of unknown etiology (VUE): Obstetrical features, outcome and treatment. J Reprod Immunol. 2021 Nov;148:103438. doi: 10.1016/j.jri.2021.103438. Epub 2021 Oct 23. PMID: 34710823

77. Muller DRP, Stenvers DJ, Malekzadeh A, Holleman F, Painter RC, Siegelaar SE. Effects of GLP-1 agonists and SGLT2 inhibitors during pregnancy and lactation on offspring outcomes: a systematic review of the evidence. Front Endocrinol (Lausanne). 2023 Oct 10;14:1215356. doi: 10.3389/fendo.2023.1215356 PMID: 37881498; PMCID: PMC10597691.

78. Mustonen S, Ala-Houhala IO, Vehkalahti P, Laippala P, Tammela TL. Kidney ultrasound and Doppler ultrasound findings during and after acute urinary retention. Eur J Ultrasound. 2001 Mar;12(3):189-96. doi: 10.1016/s0929-8266(00)00115-4. PMID: 11423242.

79. Muzii L, Di Tucci C, Di Feliciantonio M, Galati G, Verrelli L, Donato VD, Marchetti C, Panici PB. Management of Endometriomas. Semin Reprod Med. 2017 Jan;35(1):25-30. doi: 10.1055/s-0036-1597126. Epub 2016 Dec 7. Erratum in: Semin Reprod Med. 2017 Jul;35(4):390-392. PMID: 27926971.

80. National Collaborating Centre for Women's and Children's Health (UK). Antibiotics for Early-Onset Neonatal Infection: Antibiotics for the Prevention and Treatment of Early-Onset Neonatal Infection. London RCOG Press; 2012 Aug. PMID: 23346609.

81. National Collaborating Centre for Women's and Children's Health (UK). Fertility: Assessment and Treatment for People with Fertility Problems. London: Royal College of Obstetricians & Gynaecologists; 2013 Feb. PMID: 25340218.

82. Nelson-Piercy C, Fayers P, de Swiet M. Randomised, double-blind, placebo-controlled trial of corticosteroids for the treatment of hyperemesis gravidarum. BJOG. 2001 Jan;108(1):9-15. doi: 10.1111/j.1471-0528.2001.00017.x. PMID: 11213010.

83. Newman L, Rowley J, Vander Hoorn S, Wijesooriya NS, Unemo M, Low N, Stevens G, Gottlieb S, Kiarie J, Temmerman M. Global Estimates of the Prevalence and Incidence of Four Curable Sexually Transmitted Infections in 2012 Based on Systematic Review and Global Reporting. PLoS One. 2015 Dec 8;10(12):e0143304. doi: 10.1371/journal.pone.0143304. PMID: 26646541; PMCID: PMC4672879.

84. Nikolajsen S, Løkkegaard EC, Bergholt T. Reoccurrence of retained placenta at vaginal delivery: an observational study. Acta Obstet Gynecol Scand. 2013 Apr;92(4):421-5. doi: 10.1111/j.1600-0412.2012.01520.x. Epub 2012 Sep 18. PMID: 22882191.

35. Nout RA, Calaminus G, Planchamp F, Chargari C, Lax S, Martelli H, McCluggage WG, Morice P, Pakiz M, Schmid MP, Stunt J, Timmermann B, Vokuhl C, Orbach D, Fotopoulou C. ESTRO/ESGO/SIOPe Guidelines for the management of patients with vaginal cancer. Int J Gynecol Cancer. 2023 Aug 7;33(8):1185-1202. doi: 10.1136/ijgc-2023-004695. PMID: 37336757.

36. Oeffinger KC, Fontham ET, Etzioni R, Herzig A, Michaelson JS, Shih YC, Walter LC, Church TR, Flowers CR, LaMonte SJ, Wolf AM, DeSantis C, Lortet-Tieulent J, Andrews K, Manassaram-Baptiste D, Saslow D, Smith RA, Brawley OW, Wender R; American Cancer Society. Breast Cancer Screening for Women at Average Risk: 2015 Guideline Update From the American Cancer Society. JAMA. 2015 Oct 20;314(15):1599-614. doi: 10.1001/jama.2015.12783. Erratum in: JAMA. 2016 Apr 5;315(13):1406. PMID: 26501536; PMCID: PMC4831582.

37. Olawaiye AB, Cuello MA, Rogers LJ. Cancer of the vulva: 2021 update. Int J Gynaecol Obstet. 2021 Oct;155 Suppl 1(Suppl 1):7-18. doi: 10.1002/ijgo.13881. PMID: 34669204; PMCID: PMC9298362.

38. Ovarian Cancer: The Recognition and Initial Management of Ovarian Cancer. Cardiff (UK): National Collaborating Centre for Cancer (UK); 2011 Apr. PMID: 22479719.

39. Ovarian Stimulation TEGGO, Bosch E, Broer S, Griesinger G, Grynberg M, Humaidan P, Kolibianakis E, Kunicki M, La Marca A, Lainas G, Le Clef N, Massin N, Mastenbroek S, Polyzos N, Sunkara SK, Timeva T, Töyli M, Urbancsek J, Vermeulen N, Broekmans F. ESHRE guideline: ovarian stimulation for IVF/ICSI†. Hum Reprod Open. 2020 Apr 1;2020(2):hoaa009. doi: 10.1093/hropen/hoaa009. Erratum in: Hum Reprod Open. 2020 Dec 29;2020(4):hoaa067. PMID: 32395637; PMCID: PMC7203749.

40. Pados G, Gordts S, Sorrentino F, Nisolle M, Nappi L, Daniilidis A. Adenomyosis and Infertility: A Literature Review. Medicina (Kaunas). 2023 Aug 26;59(9):1551. doi: 10.3390/medicina59091551. PMID: 37763670; PMCID: PMC10534714.

41. Park KJ, Soslow RA. Neoplastic lesions of the cervix. Elsevier, 2020. P.227-293

42. Peebles K, Velloza J, Balkus JE, McClelland RS, Barnabas RV. High Global Burden and Costs of Bacterial Vaginosis: A Systematic Review and Meta-Analysis. Sex Transm Dis. 2019 May;46(5):304-311. doi: 10.1097/OLQ.0000000000000972. PMID: 30624309.

43. Pelisse M, Leibowitch M, Sedel D, Hewitt J. Un nouveau syndrome vulvo-vagino-gingival. Lichen plan érosif plurimuqueux [A new vulvovaginogingival syndrome. Plurimucous erosive lichen planus]. Ann Dermatol Venereol. 1982;109(9):797-8. French. PMID: 7158935.

44. Perlman NC, Carusi DA. Retained placenta after vaginal delivery: risk factors and management. Int J Womens Health. 2019 Oct 7;11:527-534. doi: 10.2147/IJWH.S218933. PMID: 31632517; PMCID: PMC6789409.

45. Pillay J, Donovan L, Guitard S, Zakher B, Gates M, Gates A, Vandermeer B, Bougatsos C, Chou R, Hartling L. Screening for Gestational Diabetes: Updated Evidence Report and Systematic Review for the US Preventive Services Task Force. JAMA. 2021 Aug 10;326(6):539-562. doi: 10.1001/jama.2021.10404. PMID: 34374717.

46. Price S, McManus J, Barrett J. The transgender population: improving awareness for gynaecologists and their role in the provision of care. Obstet Gynaecol. 2019;21:11–20. https://doi.org/10.1111/tog.12521

47. Romani L, Steer AC, Whitfeld MJ, Kaldor JM. Prevalence of scabies and impetigo worldwide: a systematic review. Lancet Infect Dis. 2015 Aug;15(8):960-7. doi: 10.1016/S1473-3099(15)00132-2. Epub 2015 Jun 15. PMID: 26088526.

48. Rowley J, Vander Hoorn S, Korenromp E, Low N, Unemo M, Abu-Raddad LJ, Chico RM, Smolak A, Newman L, Gottlieb S, Thwin SS, Broutet N, Taylor MM. Chlamydia, gonorrhoea, trichomoniasis and syphilis: global prevalence and incidence estimates, 2016. Bull World Health Organ. 2019 Aug 1;97(8):548-562P. doi: 10.2471/BLT.18.228486. Epub 2019 Jun 6. PMID: 31384073; PMCID: PMC6653813.

49. Royal College of Obstetricians and Gynaecologists. Best Practice in Abortion Care. Londen: RCOG; 2022.

50. Royal College of Obstetricians and Gynaecologists. Non-invasive prenatal testing for chromosomal abnormality using maternal plasma DNA. RCOG Scientific Impact Paper No 15. Londen: RCOG; 2014.

51. Royal College of Obstetricians and Gynaecologists. The Management of Nausea and Vomiting of Pregnancy and Hyperemesis Gravidarum. Green-top Guideline No. 69. London: RCOG; 2016.

52. Royal College of Obstetricians and Gynaecologists. Green-top guideline 31: the investigation and management of the small-for-gestational-age Fetus. Londen: RCOG; 2014.

53. Royal College of Obstetricians and Gynaecologists. The Management of Ovarian Hyperstimulation Syndrome. Green-top Guideline No. 5. London: RCOG; 2016

54. Royal College of Obstetricians and Gynaecologists. The Management of Women with Red Cell Antibodies during Pregnancy. Green-top Guideline No. 65. London: RCOG; 2014.

105. Sato N, Tanaka KA, Szlam F, Tsuda A, Arias ME, Levy JH. The vasodilatory effects of hydralazine, nicardipine, nitroglycerin, and fenoldopam in the human umbilical artery. Anesth Analg. 2003 Feb;96(2):539-44, table of contents. doi: 10.1097/00000539-200302000-00044. PMID: 12538209.

106. Schünke M, Schulte E, Schumacher U. Prometheus: Anatomische atlas. Inwendige organen [Atlas of Anatomy. Internal organs]. Dutch. Houten, Netherlands: Bohn Stafleu van Loghum; 2020.

107. Sedlis A, Bundy BN, Rotman MZ, Lentz SS, Muderspach LI, Zaino RJ. A randomized trial of pelvic radiation therapy versus no further therapy in selected patients with stage IB carcinoma of the cervix after radical hysterectomy and pelvic lymphadenectomy: A Gynecologic Oncology Group Study. Gynecol Oncol. 1999 May;73(2):177-83. doi: 10.1006/gyno.1999.5387. PMID: 10329031.

108. Selius BA, Subedi R. Urinary retention in adults: diagnosis and initial management. Am Fam Physician. 2008 Mar 1;77(5):643-50. PMID: 18350762.

109. Shrestha D, La X, Feng HL. Comparison of different stimulation protocols used in in vitro fertilization: a review. Ann Transl Med. 2015 Jun;3(10):137. doi: 10.3978/j.issn.2305-5839.2015.04.09. PMID: 26207230; PMCID: PMC4486909.

110. Singh N, Ghatage P. Etiology, Clinical Features, and Diagnosis of Vulvar Lichen Sclerosus: A Scoping Review. Obstet Gynecol Int. 2020 Apr 21;2020:7480754. doi: 10.1155/2020/7480754. PMID: 32373174; PMCID: PMC7191405.

111. Sit D, Rothschild AJ, Wisner KL. A review of postpartum psychosis. J Womens Health (Larchmt). 2006 May;15(4):352-68. doi: 10.1089/jwh.2006.15.352. PMID: 16724884; PMCID: PMC3109493.

112. Sleiman Z, Zreik T, Bitar R, Sheaib R, Al Bederi A, Tanos V. Uncommon presentations of an uncommon entity: oHVIRA syndrome with hematosalpinx and pyocolpos. Facts Views Vis Obgyn. (2017) 9(3):167–76. PMCID: PMC5819326; PMID: 29479403

113. Sloane PD, Slatt LM, Ebell MH, Jacques LB, Smith MA. Essentials of family medicine. Lippincott William & Wilkins; 2008.

114. Spector IP, Carey MP. Incidence and prevalence of the sexual dysfunctions: a critical review of the empirical literature. Arch Sex Behav. 1990 Aug;19(4):389-408. doi: 10.1007/BF01541933. PMID: 2205172.

115. Stewart DE, Vigod S. Postpartum Depression. N Engl J Med. 2016 Dec 1;375(22):2177-2186. doi: 10.1056/NEJMcp1607649. PMID: 27959754.

116. Tahseen S, Griffiths M. Vaginal birth after two caesarean sections (VBAC-2)-a systematic review with meta-analysis of success rate and adverse outcomes of VBAC-2 versus VBAC-1 and repeat (third) caesarean sections. BJOG. 2010 Jan;117(1):5-19. doi: 10.1111/j.1471-0528.2009.02351.x. PMID: 19781046.

117. Takakura S, Tanaka H, Enomoto N, Maki S, Ikeda T. The Successful Use of Nitroglycerin for Uterine Hyperstimulation with Fetal Heart Rate Abnormality Caused by a Controlled-Release Dinoprostone Vaginal Delivery System (PROPESS): A Case Report. Medicina (Kaunas). 2021 May 12;57(5):478. doi: 10.3390/medicina57050478. PMID: 34065827; PMCID: PMC8151635.

118. Teal S, Edelman A. Contraception Selection, Effectiveness, and Adverse Effects: A Review. JAMA. 2021 Dec 28;326(24):2507-2518. doi: 10.1001/jama.2021.21392. PMID: 34962522.

119. Teede HJ, Tay CT, Laven J, Dokras A, Moran LJ, Piltonen TT, Costello MF, Boivin J, Redman LM, Boyle JA, Norman RJ, Mousa A, Joham AE; International PCOS Network. Recommendations from the 2023 International Evidence-based Guideline for the Assessment and Management of Polycystic Ovary Syndrome†. Hum Reprod. 2023 Sep 5;38(9):1655-1679. doi: 10.1093/humrep/dead156. PMID: 37580037; PMCID: PMC10477934.

120. Thom DH, Rortveit G. Prevalence of postpartum urinary incontinence: a systematic review. Acta Obstet Gynecol Scand. 2010 Dec;89(12):1511-22. doi: 10.3109/00016349.2010.526188. Epub 2010 Nov 5. PMID: 21050146.

121. Tonguc EA, Var T, Yilmaz N, Batioglu S: Intrauterine device or estrogen treatment after hysteroscopic uterine septum resection. Int J Gynaecol Obstet. 2010, 109: 226-229. 10.1016/j.ijgo.2009.12.015.

122. Torre LA, Trabert B, DeSantis CE, Miller KD, Samimi G, Runowicz CD, Gaudet MM, Jemal A, Siegel RL. Ovarian cancer statistics, 2018. CA Cancer J Clin. 2018 Jul;68(4):284-296. doi: 10.3322/caac.21456. Epub 2018 May 29. PMID: 29809280; PMCID: PMC6621554.

123. Tsakiridis I, Giouleka S, Mamopoulos A, Athanasiadis A, Dagklis T. Investigation and management of stillbirth: a descriptive review of major guidelines. J Perinat Med. 2022 Feb 21;50(6):796-813. doi: 10.1515/jpm-2021-0403. PMID: 35213798.

124. Vaginitis in Nonpregnant Patients: ACOG Practice Bulletin, Number 215. Obstet Gynecol. 2020 Jan;135(1):e1-e17. doi: 10.1097/AOG.0000000000003604. PMID: 31856123.

125. Valle RF, Sciarra JJ. Intrauterine adhesions: hysteroscopic diagnosis, classification, treatment, and repr

ductive outcome. Am J Obstet Gynecol. 1988 Jun;158(6 Pt 1):1459-70. doi: 10.1016/0002-9378(88)90382-1. PMID: 3381869.

126. Van den Broeck J, Willie D, Younger N. The World Health Organization child growth standards: expected implications for clinical and epidemiological research. Eur J Pediatr. 2009 Feb;168(2):247-51. doi: 10.1007/s00431-008-0796-9. Epub 2008 Aug 1. PMID: 18670787.

127. Van Lankveld JJ, Granot M, Weijmar Schultz WC, Binik YM, Wesselmann U, Pukall CF, Bohm-Starke N, Achtrari C. Women's sexual pain disorders. J Sex Med. 2010 Jan;7(1 Pt 2):615-31. doi: 10.1111/j.1743-6109.2009.01631.x. PMID: 20092455.

128. Van Wagoner N, Qushair F, Johnston C. Genital Herpes Infection: Progress and Problems. Infect Dis Clin North Am. 2023 Jun;37(2):351-367. doi: 10.1016/j.idc.2023.02.011. PMID: 37105647.

129. Venetis CA, Papadopoulos SP, Campo R, Gordts S, Tarlatzis BC, Grimbizis GF. Clinical implications of congenital uterine anomalies: a meta-analysis of comparative studies. Reprod Biomed Online. 2014 Dec;29(6):665-83. doi: 10.1016/j.rbmo.2014.09.006. Epub 2014 Sep 21. PMID: 25444500.

130. Vergani P, Ornaghi S, Pozzi I, Beretta P, Russo FM, Follesa I, Ghidini A. Placenta previa: distance to internal os and mode of delivery. Am J Obstet Gynecol. 2009 Sep;201(3):266.e1-5. doi: 10.1016/j.ajog.2009.06.009. Epub 2009 Jul 24. PMID: 19631924.

131. Vieira-Baptista P, Pérez-López FR, López-Baena MT, Stockdale CK, Preti M, Bornstein J. Risk of Development of Vulvar Cancer in Women With Lichen Sclerosus or Lichen Planus: A Systematic Review. J Low Genit Tract Dis. 2022 Jul 1;26(3):250-257. doi: 10.1097/LGT.0000000000000673. Epub 2022 Mar 11. PMID: 35285455.

132. Wang X, Chen C, Wang L, Chen D, Guang W, French J. Conception, early pregnancy loss, and time to clinical pregnancy: a population-based prospective study. Fertil Steril. 2003 Mar;79(3):577-84. PubMed PMID: 12620443.

133. Wennerholm UB, Saltvedt S, Wessberg A, Alkmark M, Bergh C, Wendel SB, Fadl H, Jonsson M, Ladfors L, Sengpiel V, Wesström J, Wennergren G, Wikström AK, Elden H, Stephansson O, Hagberg H. Induction of labour at 41 weeks versus expectant management and induction of labour at 42 weeks (SWEdish Post-term Induction Study, SWEPIS): multicentre, open label, randomised, superiority trial. BMJ. 2019 Nov 20;367:l6131. doi: 10.1136/bmj.l6131. Erratum in: BMJ. 2021 Dec 15;375:n3072. PMID: 31748223; PMCID: PMC6939660.

134. WHO guideline for screening and treatment of cervical pre-cancer lesions for cervical cancer prevention [Internet]. 2nd ed. Geneva: World Health Organization; 2021. PMID: 34314129.

135. World Health Organization. Haemoglobin concentrations for the diagnosis of anaemia and assessment of severity [Internet]. 2011 [cited 2017 Aug 4]. Available from: http://www.who.int/vmnis/indicators/haemoglobin.pdf.

136. Yoshimi K, Inoue F, Odai T, Shirato N, Watanabe Z, Otsubo T, Terauchi M, Takeda T. Current status and problems in the diagnosis and treatment of premenstrual syndrome and premenstrual dysphoric disorder from the perspective of obstetricians and gynecologists in Japan. J Obstet Gynaecol Res. 2023 May;49(5):1375-1382. doi: 10.1111/jog.15618. Epub 2023 Feb 23. PMID: 36822597.

137. Youssef MA, Abou-Setta AM, Lam WS. Recombinant versus urinary human chorionic gonadotrophin for final oocyte maturation triggering in IVF and ICSI cycles. Cochrane Database Syst Rev. 2016 Apr 23;4(4):CD003719. doi: 10.1002/14651858.CD003719.pub4. PMID: 27106604; PMCID: PMC7133782.

138. Younis JS, Shapso N, Fleming R, Ben-Shlomo I, Izhaki I. Impact of unilateral versus bilateral ovarian endometriotic cystectomy on ovarian reserve: a systematic review and meta-analysis. Hum Reprod Update. 2019 May 1;25(3):375-391. doi: 10.1093/humupd/dmy049. PMID: 30715359.

Are you missing a resource or topic? Or is there a new guideline that isn't yet listed here? Let us know! Together we can keep Compendium Medicine up to date.

Illustrations & figures

Illustrators

Yente S. Beentjes: *figure 80, modification figures 33, 39, and 40*
Hebe T.A. Boerhout: *figures 10,11, modification figures 89, 92, 93 and 118*
Cas van Cruchten: *figure 57*
Susan Deelstra: *figures 9, 12, 37 and 58*
Jasmijn van Es: *figure 103, modification figures 21, 22, 31, 82, 88, 104 and 105*
Astrid A.H. Feikema: *figures 68 and 82*
Dite L.C. de Jong: *figures 29, 86, and 116*
Didi D.J. Juin: *modification figures 7, 8, 19, 20, 23, 32, 41, 48, 100 and table 83*
Jasmin Kaur: *figures 42, 43, 95, modification figures 72, 73, 103 and 122*
Koen L.C. Ketelaars: *figures 1, 2, 3, 4, 6, 7, 8, 14, 15, 16, 17, 19, 21, 22, 25, 27, 28, 31, 32, 33, 34, 35, 46, 47, 51, 52, 59, 60, 69, 71, 79, 88, 89, 91, 92, 93, 96, 99, 100, 101, 105, 107, 108, and 110*
Rosalie C. Krijl: *figures 23, 49, 83, 85, 94, 98, 102 and 104, modification figures 42, 43, 68, 71, 75, 79, 97, 102, and 106*
Sibylle Lange: *figures 61, 73, 87, and 109*
Juliëtte M.E. Linskens: *figure 56*
Kim van den Nobelen: *modification figure 50*
Belle van Rosmalen: *figures 74 and 75*
Laura Sanchez: *modification figures 74, 96 and 99*
Esther Simons: *figures 13, 24, 38, 39, 40, 41 and 44*
Flori W. Sintenie: *figure 5*
Carlijn Sturm: *figures 45, 48, 50, 55, 72, 77, 81, 84, 115, and 118*
Isabel Versmissen: *figures 36, 37, 76, and 113*
Linda Xie: *figure 1, modification figures 59 and 109*

Sources

01. Figure 18: This is a picture of a cervix of a lactating woman with no STDs and who has given birth vaginally twice. / Ep11904 / https://commons.wikimedia.org/wiki/File:Cervix. jpg/ Public domain

02. Figure 26: Hysteroscopic view of a submucous fibroid of the posterior uterine wall / Hic et nunc / https://commons.wikimedia.org/wiki/File:Myoma.jpg / Public domain

03. Figure 30: Vaginal wet mount of candidal vulvovaginitis / Mikael Häggström / https:// nl.m.wikipedia.org/wiki/Bestand:Vaginal_wet_mount_of_candidal_vulvovaginitis.jpg / CC0 1.0 Universal Public Domain Dedication (https://creativecommons.org/publicdomain/zero/1.0/)

04. Figure 53: University of New Mexico (z.j.). Photo Gallery of Skin Conditions. From https://hsc.unm.edu/medicine/departments/dermatology/inclusive-dermatology/gallery.html

05. Figures 54, 64, 65, 67 en 119: Huidziekten.nl

06. Figure 62: Infectious Cervicitis / Dr Paul Wiesner, Center for Disease Control, Publicm-Health Information Library / https://commons.wikimedia.org/wiki/File:Infectious_CervicitisCDC_PHIL6495.jpg / Public domain

07. Figure 63: Perihepatic adhesions following a chlamydia infection / Hic et nunc / https://commons.wikimedia.org/wiki/File:Perihepatic_adhesions_2.jpg / Public domain

08. Figure 66: This is an enlargement of a Phthirus pubis, or more commonly known as the pubic or crab louse. / W.H.O., (World Health Organization) / http://www.publicdomainfiles.com/show_file.php?id=13519422618930 / Public domain

09. Figure 69: Picture tongue: Primary stage syphilis sore (chancre) on the surface of a tongue. / CDC/ https://commons.wikimedia.org/wiki/File: Primary_stage_syphilis_sore_(chancre)_on_the_surface_of_a_tongue-CDC.jpg / Public domain. Picture exanthema: Secondary syphilitic rash / CDC / https://cs.wikipedia.org/wiki/Soubor: Secondary_syphilitic_rash_Treponema_pallidum_6756_lores.jpg / Public domain. Picture hand and foot: www.huidziekten.nl.

Picture gumma: Gumma of nose due to a long standing tertiary syphilitic Treponema pallidum infection / CDC, J. Pledger / https://commons.wikimedia.org/wiki/File:Gumma_of_nose_due_to_a_long_standing_tertiary_syphilitic_Treponema_pallidum_infection_5330_lores.jpg / Public domain

10. Figure 70: trichomonas pics / isis325 / https://ccsearch.creativecommons.org/photos/ed87697a-3b8a-4253-8df1-754fe454d103 / CC BY 2.0 (https://creativecommons.org/licenses/by/2.0/)

11. Figure 78: Polycystic ovary / Schomynv / https://en.m.wikipedia.org/wiki/File:Polycystic_ovary.jpg / CC0 1.0 Universal Public Domain Dedication (https://creativecommons.org/publicdomain/zero/1.0/)

12. Figure 90: Circumvallate placenta / Ed Uthman / https://www.flickr.com/photos/euthman/533599728 / CC BY 2.0 (https://creativecommons.org/licenses/by/2.0/)

13. Figure 111: Mature cystic teratoma of ovary 2 / Ed Uthman / https://commons.wikimedia.org/wiki/File:Mature_cystic_teratoma_of_ovary_2.jpg / Public domain

14. Figures 112 and 120: Gwendolyn Vuurberg

15. Figure 114: Perforierte Endometriosezyste / Hic et nunc / https://en.wikipedia.org/wiki/File:Perforierte_Endometriosezyste.jpg / Public domain

16. Figure 117: Endometrial Carcinoma / Ed Uthman / https://www.flickr.com/photos/euthman/414637011/in/photostream/ / CC BY 2.0 (https://creativecommons.org/licenses/by/2.0/) / Aanwijslijnen en verklarende tekst toegevoegd

17. Figure 121: Ovarian clear cell carcinoma / cnicholsonpath / https://www.flickr.com/photos/76113756@N07/7070710927/in/photostream/ / CC BY 2.0 (https://creativecommons.org/licenses/by/2.0/)

18. Photos cover and About us, page 344: https://www.ivarpel.nl

19. Figure cover and first pages: Traité complet de l'anatomie de l'homme: comprenant la médecine opératoire 1831-1844 / Bourgery, Jean Baptiste Marc; Jacob, Nicolas

Epilogue

Through the collaborative effort of an incredible team consisting of students, illustrators, graphic designers, and medical specialists, with this pocket we have successfully translated our vision into reality. Our goal was to ensure that you, as students and doctors, have access to essential information – literally at your fingertips, regardless of your location.

A heartfelt thank you, Maaike, for spearheading the publication of our fourth English pocket! We extend our gratitude to Gwen, for her comprehensive involvement in the *Obstetrics and Gynaecology* project. To Nathasja and Sherdina – what an incredible journey we have embarked upon together! Your contributions and enthusiasm have been instrumental every step of the way. This has been an intense yet uniquely rewarding process, for which we also want to thank the authors of the previous edition: Carlijn, Paul, Floortje, Guusje, Kelly, Hagma, and Lizzy-Sara.

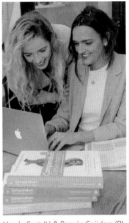

Veerle Smit (L) & Romée Snijders (R)

We are enormously grateful to all the medical professionals who provided valuable feedback and content support, elevating the quality of the text. Your contributions were integral to achieving this result.

This pocket could not have turned out so visually successful without all the illustrators – also often medical students – who collaborated on this pocket. Thanks to our team for their exceptional ability to comprehensibly cover the specialty in their graphic work.

We gratefully acknowledge our graphic heroes, Maria and Ivana, whose efforts gave this pocket its recognisable *Compendium Medicine* look. Special thanks also go to Vera, Melanie, Pauline, Delano, and Jasmijn for ensuring the smooth functioning of the entire process.

Last, a sincere thank you to all our colleagues who have *Compendium Medicine* on their bookshelves. Your support has been indispensable in realising our dreams.

We are incredibly proud of this team and hope to see you again soon, in or outside the hospital!

Amsterdam, August 2024

Veerle Smit, MD & Romée Snijders, MD
Doctors and founders of *Compendium Medicine*

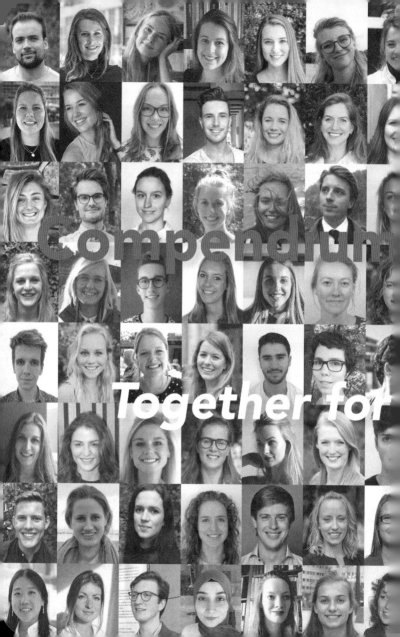

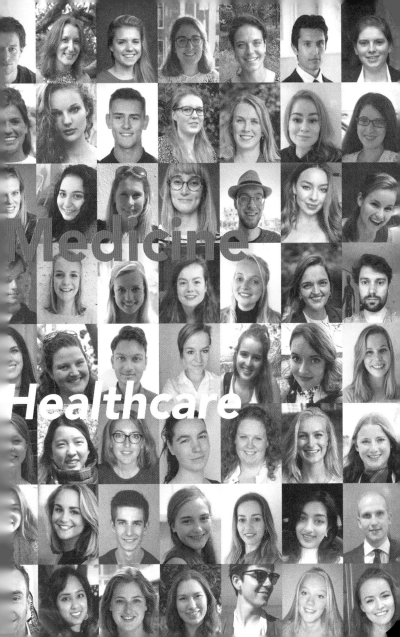

Medicine

Healthcare

About us

As medical students, we felt overwhelmed by the amount of medical knowledge available. An overview was lacking. Fueled by this need for change, we embarked on a journey that has now brought together over 500 students and doctors to create the entire *Compendium Medicine* book series. Our mission is to help and connect healthcare professionals globally by providing accessible knowledge.

The bigger picture

In 2015, at VU University in Amsterdam, the Netherlands, our paths crossed as we were both pursuing our medical educations. The vast sea of medical knowledge overwhelmed us, highlighting the need for a comprehensive overview. We were surprised by the isolated efforts of every hospital and university, each working on its own 'island', publishing individual books and reference works instead of fostering collaboration.

Motivated to make a difference, we envisioned a solution: a comprehensive guide encompassing all 35 subspecialties, enriched with figures, icons, charts, and mnemonics. Our vision was clear – our books had to be visual, concise, and to the point. With a dedicated team of students and doctors, we started writing an encyclopedia using our unique method. *Compendium Medicine* was born!

Book series

Following almost two years of dedicated effort, the first edition achieved sold-out status even before its official launch: a remarkable start to the ongoing rollercoaster journey. The most rewarding aspect of this experience has been – and still is – the overwhelmingly positive feedback from medical students and specialists. Our narrative caught the attention of prominent Dutch and Belgian newspapers and journals, leading to invitations to feature on popular talk shows on national television.

Compendium Medicine book series

Our white-coat pockets

One year later, both of us had started our clinical rotations. We recognized a common challenge faced by many peers: the need for quick and easy access to practical information. In response, we started creating our first series of pockets – concise yet comprehensive pocket-sized booklets designed to provide essential and practical information during a shift.

A period of many milestones followed. Our team expanded every month: from authors to medical specialists, from ambassadors to illustrators. With a growing number of followers on social media, a real community was born. With this team, we worked incredibly hard on new pockets as well as new additions like flashcards and pocket cards. As of now, we have launched a total of 18 different pockets!

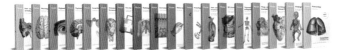

Compendium Medicine pockets

Expanding our mission globally

With the experience gained over the past years, we are committed to making a positive impact on medical students and healthcare professionals worldwide. This new phase kicked off with the distribution of our *Radiology* pocket to all continents. We were amazed to have reached readers from over 80 countries! Their positive feedback was instrumental in propelling us forward, and we are excited to present our fourth pocket in English: *Obstetrics and Gynaecology*. And this is just the beginning: we are actively working on bringing more pockets to you!

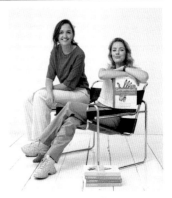

Romée Snijders & *Veerle Smit*

Doctors and founders of *Compendium Medicine*

Compendium Compass

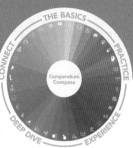

We believe that on your journey from medical student to retirement you continuously navigate these five steps. The Compendium Compass assists you along the way.

1 THE BASICS

Start at the foundation. Explore all 35 medical specialisms through our comprehensive series, featuring clear diagrams, tables, and illustrations. Visit our website for additional details.

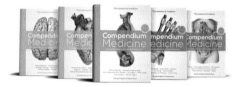

2 PRACTICE

Reinforce your foundational knowledge with our 'Compendium Medicine' app and through our social media platforms! The app, which can be downloaded from the Apple and Android app stores, enables you to practice questions on a daily basis and participate in the monthly challenge.

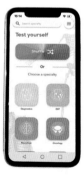

Scan this QR code for more information.

3 EXPERIENCE

Learn on-the-go by carrying our pockets and pocket cards with you on the ward, during your shifts and rounds, anytime. Our first pockets are already available worldwide, with many more to come. See below for details!

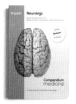
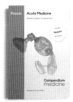
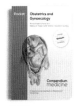
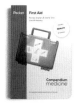

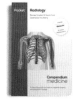
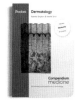

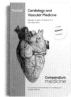

4 DEEP DIVE

Explore medical knowledge through extensive reading, immersing yourself in a variety of literature, guidelines, and the latest scientific articles.

5 CONNECT

Interested in connecting with individuals in your field? Become a member of our community through our social media platform – a network of students, physicians, specialists, and other healthcare professionals.

Abbreviations

(e)FAST	(extended) focused assessment sonography for trauma	BSO	bilateral salpingo-oophorectomy
°C	degrees Celsius	BTC	basal temperature chart
AB	antibiotics	CA125	cancer antigen 125
ABx	AB therapy	CA19-9	cancer antigen 19-9
AC	abdominal circumference	CAH	congenital adrenal hyperplasia
ACE	angiotensin converting enzyme	cAMP	cyclic adenosine monophosphate
aCGH	array comparative genomic hybridization	CAT	chlamydia antibody test
		CBT	cognitive behavioural therapy
ACTH	adrenocorticotropic hormone	cc	cubic centimeter
ADCC	antibody-dependent cell-mediated cytotoxicity	CF	cystic fibrosis
		CI	contraindication
ADL	activities of daily living	CIN	cervical intraepithelial neoplasia
Ae	aetiology	CIS	carcinoma in situ
AFC	antral follicle count	cm	centimetre
AFI	amniotic fluid index	CMV	cytomegalovirus
AFP	alpha fetoprotein	CNS	central nervous system
AGS	adrenogenital syndrome	CO_2	carbon dioxide
AIS	adenocarcinoma in situ	COH	controlled ovarian hyperstimulation
AIS	androgen insensitivity syndrome		
ALAT	alanine aminotransferase	COPD	chronic obstructive pulmonary disease
AMH	anti-Müllerian hormone		
approx.	approximately	CPR	cardiopulmonary resuscitation
AP	angina pectoris	CRL	crown-rump length
aPTT	activated partial thromboplastin time	CRP	c-reactive protein
		CS	caesarean section
ARB	angiotensin II receptor blockers	CT	chlamydia trachomatis
ARDS	acute respiratory distress syndrome	CT	computed tomography
		CTG	cardiotocography
ASA	antisperm antibodies	CVA	cerebrovascular accident
ASAT	aspartate aminotransferase	CVP	central venous pressure
ASC-H	atypical squamous cells for which a high-grade lesion cannot be excluded	D	definition
		d	day/days
		DBP	diastolic blood pressure
ASC-US	atypical squamous cells of undetermined significance	DCDA	dichorionic diamniotic
		DCIS	ductal carcinoma in situ
ATLS	advanced trauma life support	DDx	differential diagnosis
AUS	advanced ultrasound scanning	DES	diethylstilbestrol
AV	atrioventricular	DEXA	dual x-ray absorptiometry
AVF	anteversion-flexion	DFA	direct fluorescent antibody
avg.	average	DHEA-S	dehydroepiandrosterone sulfate
AVPU	alert, verbal, pain, unresponsive	DHT	dihydrotestosterone
AVRF	anteversion-retroflexion	DIC	disseminated intravascular coagulation
BCG	blood glucose curve		
BHR	basal heart rate	dl	deciliter
BMI	body mass index	DM	diabetes mellitus
BP	blood pressure	DNA	deoxyribonucleic acid
BPD	biparietal diameter	DNACRP	do not attempt cardiopulmonary resuscitation
bpm	beats per minute		
BRCA	breast cancer	DNR	do not resuscitate
		DRE	dynamic rectovaginal examination

DSD	differences in sex development
DVT	deep vein thrombosis
Dx	diagnostics
D&E	dilation and evacuation
E	epidemiology
e.g.	exempli gratia (for example)
ECG	electrocardiogram
ECT	electroconvulsive therapy
EFW	estimated fetal weight
ELISA	enzyme-linked immunosorbent assay
esp.	especially
etc.	et cetera
EPO	erythropoietin
ETT	epithelioid trophoblastic tumor
FAS	fetal alcohol syndrome
FAST	focus assessment with sonography in trauma
FD	full dilation
FGM	female genital mutilation
FGR	fetal growth restriction
FHx	family history
FIGO	International Federation of Gynaecology and Obstetrics
FISH	fluorescence in situ hybridization
FL	femoral length
FMT	fetal maternal transfusion
FSH	follicle-stimulating hormone
FTP	failure to progress
FTT	failure to thrive
g	gram(s)
GAS	group A Streptococcus
GBS	group B Streptococcus
GCS	Glasgow Coma Scale
GD	gender dysphoria
GDC	glucose day curve
GDM	gestational diabetes mellitus
GH	genital hiatus
GIS	gel infusion sonography
gluc	glucose
GnRH	gonadotropin-releasing hormone
GP	general practice
GTD	gestational trophoblastic disease
GTN	gestational trophoblastic neoplasia
Hb	haemoglobin
HBOC	hereditary breast and ovarian cancer syndrome
HBsAg	hepatitis B surface antigen
HC	head circumference
hCG	human chorionic gonadotropin
Hct	haematocrit test
HDFN	haemolytic disease of the fetus and newborn
HELLP	haemolysis, elevated liver enzymes and low platelet count
HER2	human epidermal growth factor receptor 2
HIV	human immunodeficiency virus
HPV	human papilloma virus
hr	hour/hours
HSG	hysterosalpingography
HSIL	high-grade squamous intraepithelial lesion
HSV	herpes simplex virus
Ht	haematocrit
Hx	patient history
i.e.	id est (that is)
ICSI	intra-cytoplasmic sperm injection
IE/IU	international units
IEA	irregular erythrocyte antibodies
IgG	immunoglobulin G
IGF	insulin-like growth factor
IGT	impaired glucose tolerance
IM	intramuscular
INR	international normalised ratio
IRAB	irregular antibodies
IU	international unit
IUD	intrauterine device
IUFD	intrauterine fetal demise
IUI	intrauterine insemination
IV	intravenous
IVF	in vitro fertilisation
kg	kilogram
L	litres
LAM	lactational amenorrhea method
LDH	lactate dehydrogenase
LH	luteinizing hormone
LLETZ	large loop excision of the transformation zone
LMWH	low-molecular-weight heparin
LOA	left occiput anterior
LOP	left occiput posterior
LOT	left occiput transverse
LP	lichen planus
LP	lumbar puncture
LSEA	lichen sclerosus et atrophicus
LSIL	low-grade squamous intraepithelial lesion
LVSI	lymphovascular space involvement
m^2	square meter
MAP	mean arterial pressure
MAR	mixed antiglobulin reaction
max.	maximum
MCA	middel cerebral artery
MCDA	monochorionic diamniotic
MCMA	monochorionic monoamniotic
MCV	mean corpuscular volume

MDMA	3,4-methylenedioxy methamphetamine		PI	pulsatility index
MEOWS	Modified Early Obstetric Warning Score		PlGF	placental growth factor
			PID	pelvic inflammatory disease
mg	miligram(s)		PIH	pregnancy-induced hypertension
MI	myocardial infarction		PKA	protein kinase A
min	minute/minutes		PMDD	premenstrual dysphoric disorder
min.	minimum		PMHx	patient medical history
ml	mililitres		PMS	premenstrual syndrome
mm	millimeter		POI	premature ovarian insufficiency
mmHg	millimetres of mercury		POH	potassium hydroxide
mmol	millimole		PPROM	preterm prelabour rupture of membranes
MMR	mismatch repair		PROM	prelabour rupture of membranes
mo	month/months		PSTT	placental site trophoblastic tumor
MoM	multiples of the median		PSV	peak systolic velocity
MRI	magnetic resonance imaging		PTNS	posterior tibial nerve stimulation
MRKH	Mayer-Rokitansky-Küster-Hauser syndrome		PTSD	posttraumatic stress disorder
MRSA	methicillin-resistant Staphylococcus aureus		PUL	pregnancy of unknown location
			PVD	provoked vulvodynia
MSI	microsatellite instability		R	risk factors
MUD	manual uterine displacement		RE	rectal exam
N/A	not applicable		Rhc	rhesus C
NaCl	sodium chloride		RhD	rhesus D
ng	nanogram		ROA	right occiput anterior
NIPT	noninvasive prenatal test		ROP	right occiput posterior
nl	nanolitre		ROT	right occiput transverse
NO	nitrous oxide		RPR	rapid plasma reagin
NSAID	non-steroidal anti-inflammatory drug		RR	respiratory rate
			RVF	retroversion-flexion
O₂	oxygen		S	symptoms
OA	occiput anterior		SBP	systolic blood pressure
OAT	oligoasthenoteratozoospermia		SCC	squamous cell carcinoma
OC	oral contraceptives		SDP	single deepest pocket
OGTT	oral glucose tolerance test		SE	speculum exam
OHSS	ovarian hyperstimulation syndrome		sec	second/seconds
			SES	socio-economic status
OHVIRA	obstructed hemivagina and ipsilateral renal anomaly		sFlt-1	soluble fms-like tyrosine kinase-1
			SHx	social history
OP	occiput posterior		SIL	squamous intraepithelial lesion
OR	operating room		SIRS	systemic inflammatory response syndrome
ORT	ovarian reserve test			
OS	ovarian stimulation		SIS	saline infusion sonography
P	prognosis		SLE	systemic lupus erythematodes
PA	pathology		SNRI	serotonin and norepinephrine reuptake inhibitor
PAPP-A	pregnancy-associated plasma protein-A			
			SRY	sex-determining region Y gene
PAST	posterior axilla sling traction		ssp.	subspecies
PBAC	pictorial blood assessment chart		SSRI	selective serotonin reuptake inhibitor
PCOS	polycystic ovarian syndrome			
PCR	polymerase chain reaction		STI	sexually transmitted infection
PCR NAAT	polymerase chain reaction nucleic acid amplification test		SUA	single umbilical cord artery
			SURPASS	surgical patient safety system
PE	physical examination		T	temperature
PEA	pulseless electrical activity		TAPS	twin anaemia polycythaemia sequence

TAU	transabdominal ultrasound
TENS	transcutaneous electrical neurostimulation
TESE	testicular sperm extraction
TNBC	triple-negative breast carcinoma
TOA	tubo-ovarian abscess
TORCHES	toxoplasmosis, other, rubella, cytomegalovirus, herpes simplex, syphilis
TOT	trans obturator tape
TPHA	Treponema pallidum haemagglutination assay
TSH	thyroid stimulating hormone
TTPA	Treponema pallidum particle agglutination
TTTS	twin-to-twin transfusion syndrome
TVT	tension-free vaginal tape
TVU	transvaginal ultrasound
Tx	treatment
U	units
UAPI	umbilical artery pulsatility index
UDT	urodynamic test
UTI	urinary tract infection
VA	vaccuum aspiration
VAIN	vaginal intraepithelial neoplasia
VE	vaginal exam
VEGF	vascular endothelial growth factor
VIN	vulvar intra-epithelial neoplasia
VUE	chronic villitis of unknown etiology
VVS	vulvar vestibulitis syndrome
wk	week/weeks
µg	micrograms

Index